New Frontiers in Otolaryngology

New Frontiers in Otolaryngology

Edited by **Chad Downs**

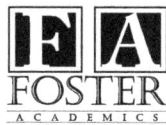

FA
FOSTER
ACADEMICS

New Jersey

Published by Foster Academics,
61 Van Reypen Street,
Jersey City, NJ 07306, USA
www.fosteracademics.com

New Frontiers in Otolaryngology
Edited by Chad Downs

© 2016 Foster Academics

International Standard Book Number: 978-1-63242-430-3(Hardback)

Contents

Preface

The world is advancing at a fast pace like never before. Therefore, the need is to keep up with the latest developments. This book was an idea that came to fruition when the specialists in the area realized the need to coordinate together and document essential themes in the subject. That's when I was requested to be the editor. Editing this book has been an honour as it brings together diverse authors researching on different streams of the field. The book collates essential materials contributed by veterans in the area which can be utilized by students and researchers alike.

Otolaryngology is the branch of medical science that deals with the diagnosis and treatment of diseases related to ear, nose and throat. It is generally concerned with rhinology, reconstructive and plastic surgeries, neurotology, cancerous and non-cancerous tumors in head and neck, laryngology, and allergies. This book has been compiled in such a manner that it will provide in-depth knowledge about the theory and practice of otolaryngology. It strives to provide a fair idea about this discipline and to help develop a better understanding of the latest advances within this field. The topics included in this book are of utmost significance and bound to provide incredible insights to the readers.

Each chapter is a sole-standing publication that reflects each author's interpretation. Thus, the book displays a multi-facetted picture of our current understanding of applications and diverse aspects of the field. I would like to thank the contributors of this book and my family for their endless support.

Editor

Hearing Preservation after Cochlear Implantation: UNICAMP Outcomes

Guilherme Machado de Carvalho, Alexandre C. Guimaraes, Alexandre S. M. Duarte, Eder B. Muranaka, Marcelo N. Soki, Renata S. Zanotello Martins, Walter A. Bianchini, Jorge R. Paschoal, and Arthur M. Castilho

Otology, Audiology and Implantable Ear Prostheses, Ear, Nose, Throat and Head & Neck Surgery Department, P.O. Box 6111, Campinas University, UNICAMP, 13081-970 São Paulo, SP, Brazil

Correspondence should be addressed to Guilherme Machado de Carvalho; guimachadocarvalho@gmail.com

Academic Editor: Peter S. Roland

Background. Electric-acoustic stimulation (EAS) is an excellent choice for people with residual hearing in low frequencies but not high frequencies and who derive insufficient benefit from hearing aids. For EAS to be effective, subjects' residual hearing must be preserved during cochlear implant (CI) surgery. *Methods*. We implanted 6 subjects with a CI. We used a special surgical technique and an electrode designed to be atraumatic. Subjects' rates of residual hearing preservation were measured 3 times postoperatively, lastly after at least a year of implant experience. Subjects' aided speech perception was tested pre- and postoperatively with a sentence test in quiet. Subjects' subjective responses assessed after a year of EAS or CI experience. *Results*. 4 subjects had total or partial residual hearing preservation; 2 subjects had total residual hearing loss. All subjects' hearing and speech perception benefited from cochlear implantation. CI diminished or eliminated tinnitus in all 4 subjects who had it preoperatively. 5 subjects reported great satisfaction with their new device. *Conclusions*. When we have more experience with our surgical technique we are confident we will be able to report increased rates of residual hearing preservation. Hopefully, our study will raise the profile of EAS in Brazil and Latin/South America.

1. Introduction

Just over a decade ago people with sensorineural hearing loss had 2 main hearing (re)habilitation options: (1) a hearing aid (HA) if they had mild to moderate hearing loss and (2) a cochlear implant (CI) if they had severe to profound hearing loss. These 2 device options improved most users' hearing. However, people who could hear in the low frequencies (up to 1000 Hz) but not the medium and high frequencies—the downward or "ski slope" audiogram—had too much high frequency hearing loss to benefit from their hearing aid(s) but were not CI candidates because surgeons feared the surgery would destroy their residual hearing.

A solution for such people is electric-acoustic stimulation (EAS), a concept developed by von Ilberg and colleagues in 1999 [1]. EAS provides synergistic unilateral acoustic (via the HA) and electrical (via the CI) stimulation and provides its users with better hearing than they had had with their HA or

HAs [2–4] and better hearing than enjoyed by unilateral CI-only users [1–5], especially in noisy environments [2–4, 6–9]. EAS also provides better sound quality and more natural hearing than unilateral CIs or HAs [4, 10]. These benefits are, however, only possible if surgeons do not damage the cochlea (and thus the person's residual hearing) during CI surgery. To this end, technology and "soft surgical" techniques have been—and are continuing to be—developed.

"Soft" surgery was first described by Lehnhardt and Laszig in 1994 [11] and multiple surgeons and their teams have since refined it [12–16]. Electrode insertion is of utmost importance in atraumicity: the round window approach [15] has shown to cause minimal cochlear damage and is thus better for residual hearing preservation [4, 10].

Electrode design (shape, length, and bundle flexibility) is also critical to reducing cochlear trauma [17–21]; both MED-EL (Innsbruck, Austria) and Cochlear Limited (Sydney,

TABLE 1: Subject demographics.

Subject number	Age at implantation (years)	Sex	Duration of hearing loss (years)	Insertion
1	63	M	5	Round window
2	62	M	10	Cochleostomy
3	40	F	10	Round window
4	29	M	8	Round window
5	42	M	20	Round window
6	46	M	15	Round window

Australia) have designed electrodes to meet this specific need. Focusing on MED-EL's FLEX[24] (formerly known as the FLEX[EAS]), as it is the electrode we used in our study, recently surgeons have used it to achieve partial or complete hearing preservation in 100% of their study subjects [10, 16]. Although such perfection is not always possible, regardless of the surgeon's skill or the implanted device's technical wizardry [22], it was our aim to preserve the residual hearing in each of the 6 subjects we implanted between March 2010 and October 2011.

2. Materials and Methods

2.1. Subjects. 6 subjects (mean age 47 years) were implanted with MED-EL cochlear implants with FLEX[24] electrodes. Study inclusion criteria were as follows: all subjects had to (1) be older than 18 years, (2) have sensorineural bilateral hearing loss with little or no benefit from HA (less than 40% of auditory discrimination in monosyllables), (3) have pure-tone thresholds of ≤60 dB hearing loss in at least 1 frequency between 250 and 500 Hz and of ≥80 dB in frequencies above 1000 Hz, (4) have had stable hearing loss for at least the past two years, and lastly (5) pass a psychological examination ensuring they had realistic expectations about the potential benefits of receiving a cochlear implant and/or using EAS (Table 1). All subjects underwent pure tone audiometry (PTA) and speech tests, pre- and postoperatively.

2.2. Surgical Technique. We used the same surgical technique on all subjects. The technique, which we have named the UNICAMP approach, is a mastoidectomy approach. It is based on techniques developed in various otology centers.

2.3. Description of Surgical Technique. Patients were under general anesthesia, tracheal intubation, and placed in a supine position with their head turned to the contralateral side. The operative field was prepared through extensive shaving, cleaned with chlorhexidine 2%, and the attachment of the electrodes to monitor CN VII.

We used a micropore to isolate the operative field from the rest of the scalp and gave prophylaxis with cefazolin (50 mg/kg) intravenously during induction of anesthesia.

(1) The main landmarks are marked: tip of the mastoid, temporal line, retroauricular incision line, area of the internal component, and area of the microphone with the help of an implant template;

(2) antisepsis with 0.2% aqueous chlorhexidine, placement of sterile drapes and steri-drape 2;

(3) rectilinear retroauricular incision and dissection along anatomical planes; preparation of a "cross" Palva flap (periosteal muscle) raising the four segments of the flap over the subperiosteal plane;

(4) removal of small fragments of fascia and temporal muscle to occlude the cochleostomy;

(5) simple mastoidectomy, identifying the lateral semicircular canal, the short ramus of the anvil, the posterior wall of the outer ear canal, the tegmen timpani, and the lateral sinus; gathering a small amount of bone dust;

(6) thinning of the posterior wall of the outer ear canal, posterior tympanotomy, preservation of the incus buttress;

(7) preparation of the receiver bed for the implant on the squamous portion of the temporal bone (well) using a specific implant template;

(8) irrigation of the cavity with povidone-iodine (10% povidone-iodine/1% active iodine) for two minutes followed by abundant irrigation with lactated Ringer's solution;

(9) irrigation of the cavity with ciprofloxacin (4 mg/mL) for two minutes followed by irrigation with lactated Ringer's solution;

(10) intravenous administration of dexamethasone (8 mg) before approaching the inner ear via a cochleostomy or through the round window;

(11) application of topical triamcinolone (40 mg/mL) over the round window;

(12) opening the membrane of the round window; if this approach is impossible, the endosteum is opened by means of a cochleostomy;

(13) positioning of the implant into the prior drilled bed;

(14) Preparation of the fascia graft; making a pinhole central orifice to allow the electrode to pass snugly to be placed in the cochleostomy/round window site;

(15) insertion of the electrode slowly and continuously during three minutes;

(16) positioning the muscle graft around the electrode to seal the cochleostomy; placing bone dust to close the posterior tympanotomy;

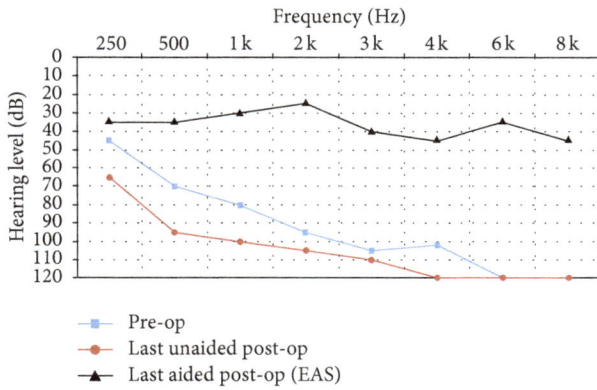

FIGURE 1: Audiometric results for Subject 1.

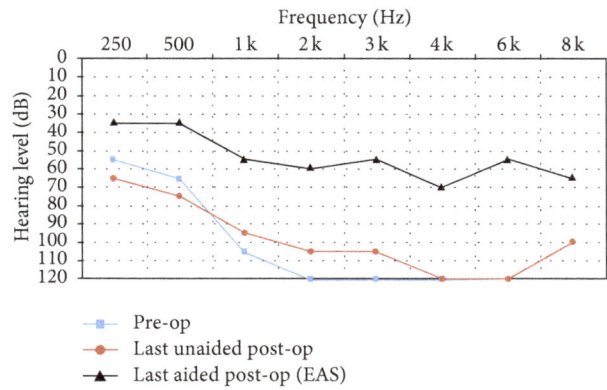

FIGURE 4: Audiometric results for Subject 4.

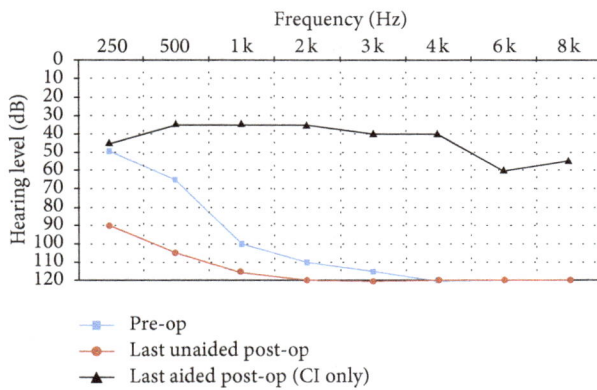

FIGURE 2: Audiometric results for Subject 2.

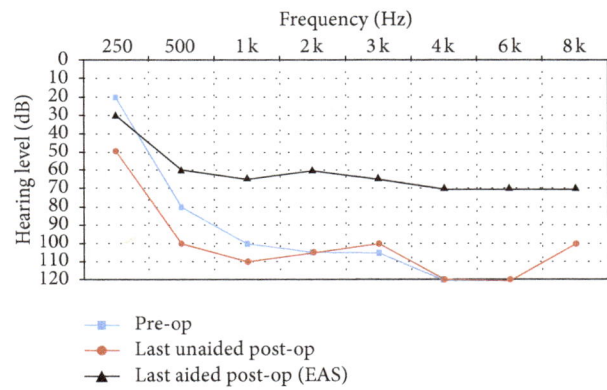

FIGURE 5: Audiometric results for Subject 5.

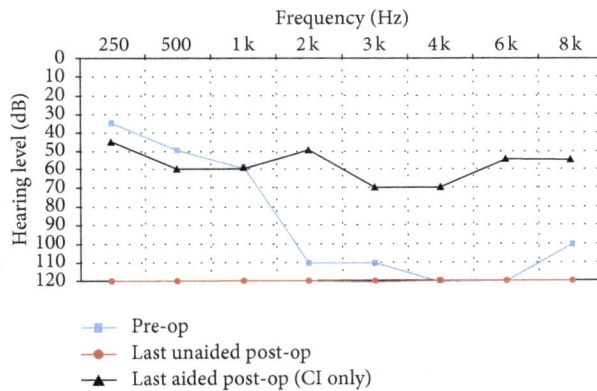

FIGURE 3: Audiometric results for Subject 3.

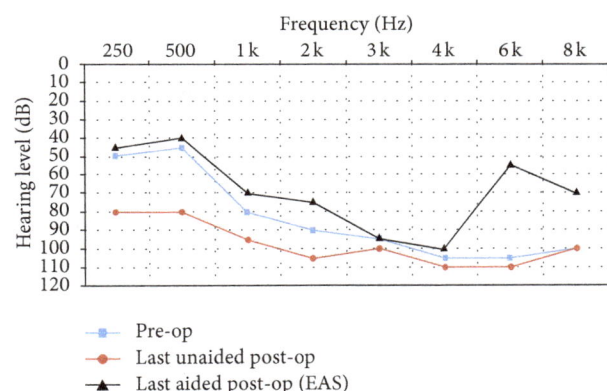

FIGURE 6: Audiometric results for Subject 6.

(17) positioning the ground electrode under the muscle-periosteum flap;

(18) closure with Vicryl 3.0 sutures on the Palva flap planes and subcutaneous tissue; skin closure with Nylon 4.0;

(19) cleaning of the patient and placing an external compressive dressing;

(20) impedance testing, neural response telemetry (NRT), and a transorbital incidence radiograph are done to confirm the position of the intracochlear electrode.

The same surgeon and surgical team performed all six surgeries.

2.4. Audiometric Testing. All subjects had unaided pure-tone audiometry tests at 250, 500, 1000, 2000, 3000, 4000, 6000, and 8000 Hz (Figures 1–6). We used an AC30-SD25 audiometer, calibrated according to ISO 389/64.

To determine subjects' residual hearing, we repeated the unaided pure-tone audiometry tests at 250, 500, 1000, 2000, 3000, 4000, 6000, and 8000 Hz three times: (1) at activation,

TABLE 2: PTA tests of all subjects at all intervals: unaided.

Who	Dates (days since previous test)	250 Hz	500 Hz	1 kHz	2 kHz	3 kHz	4 kHz	6 kHz	8 kHz
Subject 1	Preoperative: 01.06.2010	45	70	80	95	105	120	120	120
	Activation: 22.09.2010	65	90	105	105	105	120	120	120
	Post-op 2: 05.04.2011 (195)	65	95	100	105	110	120	120	120
	Post op-3: 14.12.2011 (253)	65	95	100	105	110	120	120	120
Subject 2	Preoperative: 21.07.2010	50	65	100	110	115	120	120	120
	Activation: 22.09.2010	90	105	115	120	120	120	120	120
	Post-op 2: 13.04.2011 (203)	90	100	110	120	120	120	120	120
	Post op-3: 07.12.2011 (238)	90	105	115	120	120	120	120	120
Subject 3	Preoperative: 22.09.2010	35	50	60	110	110	120	120	100
	Activation: 13.12.2010	115	120	120	120	120	120	120	120
	Post-op 2: 30.06.2011 (198)	120	120	120	120	120	120	120	120
	Post op-3: 11.01.2012 (195)	120	120	120	120	120	120	120	120
Subject 4	Preoperative: 26.04.2011	55	65	105	120	120	120	120	100
	Activation: 17.06.2011	65	75	95	105	120	120	120	120
	Post-op 2: 11.01.2012 (208)	65	70	90	105	120	120	120	120
	Post op-3: 18.09.2012 (251)	65	75	95	105	120	120	120	120
Subject 5	Preoperative: 11.10.2011	20	80	100	105	105	120	120	120
	Activation: 13.12.2011	50	100	110	105	105	120	120	100
	Post-op 2: 25.06.2012 (195)	50	105	110	105	110	120	120	100
	Post op-3: 19.12.2012 (177)	50	100	110	105	105	120	120	100
Subject 6	Preoperative: 18.10.2011	50	45	80	90	95	105	105	100
	Activation: 13.12.2011	80	80	95	105	105	110	110	100
	Post-op 2: 18.07.2012 (218)	85	80	90	105	105	110	105	100
	Post op-3: 08.01.2013 (174)	80	80	95	105	105	110	110	100

(2) 6.5–7 months after activation, and (3) approximately 7 months after their previous test. We defined "residual hearing preservation" in three ways:

(1) "total hearing preservation": a postoperative unaided hearing loss of 0–10 dBs,

(2) "partial hearing preservation": a postoperative unaided hearing loss of >10 dB but leaving the subject with ≤80 dB hearing or better in at least one frequency between 250 and 1000 Hz,

(3) "hearing preservation failure": subject will not benefit from EAS because their unaided postoperative thresholds are >80 dB.

Lastly, to measure efficacy, all subjects had free field warble tone tests with EAS or CI-only (depending on their residual hearing) at the same postoperative intervals as were their unaided tests.

2.5. Speech Perception Tests. Preoperatively, all subjects took a speech perception test the same day as their implantation. We used a speech perception sentence test based on one developed by Bevilacqua et al. from several English language tests [23]. Subjects did the test with their hearing aids on, in a quiet place.

Postoperatively, all subjects repeated the speech perception test after at least 1 year of CI experience. Tests were done in subject's best-aided condition: EAS or CI-only, depending

on their postoperative residual hearing. The same audiologist conducted all the pre- and postoperative tests.

2.6. Subjective Ratings. When the subjects did their postoperative speech tests they were asked to rate the quality of their experience with EAS/a CI over the past year on a Likert scale scored 0 to 10. A score of 0 indicated the user regretted the intervention, would not recommend it to others, and felt he/she had been better off in the past with their hearing aids. A score of 10 indicated the user was completely satisfied with the intervention and would strongly recommend it.

2.7. Ethics. The institutional review board approved this study and all subjects gave written informed consent.

3. Results

All surgeries were uneventful. Although we planned to implant all subjects via their round window, we could not visualize subject 2's round window and had to implant via cochleostomy. All subjects received an implant with a MED-EL FLEX^{EAS} electrode. At no frequency or test interval did any subject's aided or unaided PTA score vary by more than 10 dB from their scores at the same frequency in either of the other 2 tests. For the sake of convenience, the graphs show their PTA scores at their last postoperative test (see Tables 2, 3, and Figure 7).

TABLE 3: PTA tests of all subjects at all intervals: aided (EAS or CI on).

Who	Dates (days since previous test)	250 Hz	500 Hz	1 kHz	2 kHz	3 kHz	4 kHz	6 kHz	8 kHz
Subject 1	Activation: 22.09.2010	35	35	30	25	40	35	35	45
	Post-op 2: 05.04.2011 (195)	30	35	35	20	40	30	30	50
	Post op-3: 14.12.2011 (253)	35	35	30	25	40	35	35	45
Subject 2	Activation: 22.09.2010	45	35	35	35	40	40	60	55
	Post-op 2: 13.04.2011 (203)	40	40	35	40	40	40	55	50
	Post op-3: 07.12.2011 (238)	45	35	35	35	40	40	60	55
Subject 3	Activation: 13.12.2010	45	60	60	50	40	70	55	55
	Post-op 2: 30.06.2011 (198)	40	60	55	50	45	80	65	55
	Post op-3: 11.01.2012 (195)	45	60	60	50	40	70	55	55
Subject 4	Activation: 17.06.2011	55	35	55	60	40	60	55	65
	Post-op 2: 11.01.2012 (208)	65	25	55	65	40	60	55	60
	Post op-3: 18.09.2012 (251)	55	35	55	60	40	70	55	65
Subject 5	Activation: 13.12.2011	30	60	65	60	60	70	55	70
	Post-op 2: 25.06.2012 (195)	30	60	60	55	60	70	60	70
	Post op-3: 19.12.2012 (177)	30	60	65	60	65	70	55	70
Subject 6	Activation: 13.12.2011	45	40	70	75	95	100	55	70
	Post-op 2: 18.07.2012 (218)	40	40	65	75	100	110	55	70
	Post op-3: 08.01.2013 (174)	45	40	70	75	95	100	55	70

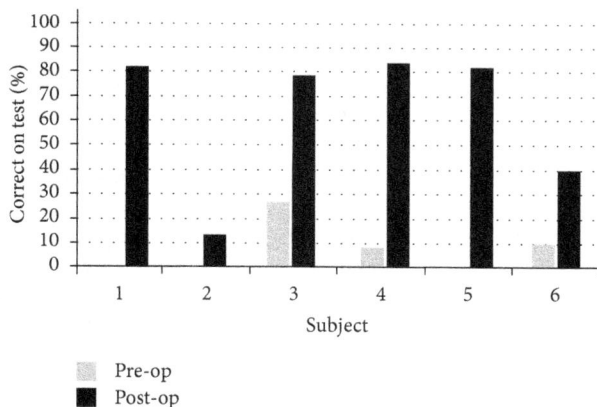

FIGURE 7: Pre- and Postoperative Speech Perception Scores. Note: Subjects 1, 2, and 5 and 0% preoperative scores. *Median speech test results pre-op: 4.0% (range 0% to 28%). **Median speech test results post-op: 80.0% (range 16% to 84%).

All subjects' speech perception was much better after implantation (see Figure 7).

3.1. Subject 1. He had suffered from idiopathic hearing loss for 5 years and had been using hearing aids for 2 years without benefit. He had also been treated with corticosteroids but experienced little improvement. He was fit with EAS with the CI cut-off frequency set at 500 Hz. His preoperative tinnitus was not eliminated by surgery but is now, according to the subject, no longer bothersome.

As you can see from his pre- and postoperative hearing test results, he derived real benefit from implantation. We achieved partial hearing preservation.

His speech perception test score improved from 0% pre-operatively to 82% (with EAS) after 14 months CI experience.

He rated the quality of his experience a 9 on Likert scale, indicating he was very pleased with the intervention.

3.2. Subject 2. He had suffered from idiopathic hearing loss for 10 years and had been using hearing aids for 8 months without benefit. Unlike the other 5 subjects, he was implanted via cochleostomy instead of round window because we could not visualize the round window. The subject was fit with a CI only.

As you can see from his pre- and postoperative hearing test results, he derived real benefit from implantation. We, however, failed to preserve his residual hearing.

His speech test score improved from 0% preoperatively to 16% (with CI-only) after 14 months CI experience. We attribute this relatively poor speaking perception score to the fact that he (1) lost (or had stolen) his external component and so was without CI experience for approximately 11 of the 14.5 months between his activation and post-op speech test and (2) he missed audiological rehabilitation sessions.

He rated the quality of his experience a 6 on the Likert scale, indicating he was mildly pleased with the intervention.

3.3. Subject 3. She had suffered from idiopathic hearing loss for 10 years and had been using hearing aids for the past 6 years, with little benefit. Her preoperative tinnitus and dizziness were eliminated postoperatively. The subject was fit with a CI only.

As you can see from her pre- and postoperative hearing test results, she derived real benefit from implantation. We, however, failed to preserve her residual hearing.

Her speech test score improved from 28% preoperatively to 78% (with CI-only) after 13 months CI experience.

She rated the quality of her experience a 9 on the Likert scale, indicating she was very pleased with the intervention.

3.4. Subject 4. He had suffered from idiopathic hearing loss for 8 years and had been using hearing aids for 4 years in his right ear and 1 year in his left ear, with little benefit. He had also been treated with corticosteroids, with little improvement. The subject was fit with EAS with the CI cut-off frequency set at 700 Hz. His preoperative tinnitus and dizziness were eliminated postoperatively.

As you can see from his pre- and post-op hearing test results, he derived real benefit from implantation. We achieved total residual hearing preservation.

His speech test score improved from 8% preoperatively to 84% (with EAS on) after 15 months CI experience.

He rated the quality of his experience a 10 on the Likert scale, indicating he was extremely pleased with the intervention.

3.5. Subject 5. He had suffered idiopathic hearing loss for 15 years and had using hearing aids for 5 years, with little benefit. The subject was fit with EAS with the CI cut-off frequency set to 350 Hz. His preoperative tinnitus was eliminated postoperatively.

As you can see from the pre- and postoperative data, he derived real benefit from implantation. We achieved partial residual hearing preservation.

His speech test score improved from 0% preoperatively to 82% (with EAS on) after 12 months CI experience.

He rated the quality of his experience a 10 on the Likert scale, indicating he was extremely pleased with the intervention.

3.6. Subject 6. He had suffered from idiopathic hearing loss for 15 years and had been using hearing aids for 5 years, with little benefit. The subject was fit with EAS with the CI cut-off frequency set to 1 kHz.

As you can see from the pre- and postoperative hearing test results, he derived some benefit from implantation. We achieved partial residual hearing preservation.

His speech test score improved from 10% preoperatively to 40% (with EAS) after 13 months CI experience. Despite his relatively poor postoperative speech perception score, the audiologist reports that he is improving.

He rated the quality of his experience an 8 on the Likert scale, indicating he was very pleased with the intervention.

Some benefits of the good outcomes are represented by the individual speech tests of all subjects (Tables 2, 3, and Figure 7).

4. Discussion

Of our 6 subjects, 1 had total residual hearing preservation, 3 had partial residual hearing preservation, and 2 had total residual hearing loss: a residual hearing preservation success rate of 4/6. Looked at another way, postoperatively, 4 subjects will benefit from EAS and 2 subjects (2 and 3) are no longer partially deaf and thus no longer EAS candidates, although they enjoy better hearing from their CI than they had had from their HA before implantation. All subjects who actually had 1-year implant experience had greatly improved postoperative speech perception scores. 3 EAS users (subjects 1, 4, and 5) scored between 82% and 84%, similar to the results of previous studies [8, 24]. Subject 6 scored poorer, only 40% but is said to be improving. Subject 3, who was fitted CI only, improved from 28% pre-op to 78% after 13 months CI experience.

We demonstrated that cochlear implant surgery done with the aim of preserving residual hearing is highly beneficial to the hearing lives of the partially deaf—as evidenced in their extremely positive Likert scale responses—even when we fail to preserve their residual hearing. We, nonetheless, fell short of our lofty goal of 100% residual hearing preservation. We attribute this to 2 primary causes. Firstly, living in and working in Brazil, we have had very few EAS cases and less experience with hearing preservation surgery than do the surgeons whose results are featured in other articles. EAS was developed in Germany as recently as 1999 and, correspondingly, most experts come from Central Europe (Gstoettner, von Ilberg, Lenarz, Skarzynski to name a few).

We (UNICAMP) are the only team in Brazil—a nation of almost 200 million—that does hearing preservation surgeries like this. The surgical technique is difficult and we are confident that with experience, and better-suited cases, we will improve our success rate. Our results should be seen in this context: a regional beginning.

Secondly, we had limited access to suitable EAS candidates. All subjects had idiopathic hearing loss and not all of them were "true" EAS candidates. Subjects 1 and 5 had preoperative scores of 70 dB and 80 db, respectively, at 500 Hz, whereas the maximum indication for EAS is 60 dB at 500 Hz. We implanted them anyway—as other surgical teams have done [25, 26]—because they could still benefit from EAS. If they had been "true" EAS candidates, their postoperative hearing losses of 20–25 dB at 500 Hz might have appeared less severe.

Our residual hearing preservation results were below those of other similar studies. Skarzynski et al. [27] partially or totally preserved the hearing of 39/42 at 3 months and from 34/40 to 36/40 at 13 months after surgery. They used standard or FLEX^{SOFT} electrodes and the hearing preservation round window technique they developed and described in 2007 [15]. Arnoldner et al., achieved 11/11 residual hearing preservation after a mean follow-up of 7.85 months. He used a round window or promontorium technique and FLEX^{EAS} electrodes [16]. Gstoettner et al. reported a success rate of 15/18 after up to 12 months after EAS fitting [8]. They used the Frankfurt surgical technique and MED-EL M-electrode.

Additionally, the provision of a CI decreased subjects' tinnitus and dizziness. 4 subjects (1, 3, 4, and 5) suffered from preoperative tinnitus. Postoperatively, only subject 1 still had tinnitus, but he said it was "not too bad." These results are consistent with past studies [28–31], which found that CI implantation usually eliminates or reduces tinnitus. Subjects 3 and 4's preoperative dizziness disappeared after surgery.

5. Conclusion

We strongly believe that EAS has an important place in the future of otology. While it is entering its teenage years in Central Europe, it is still in its infancy in Brazil. We hope our results will raise the profile of EAS here and hearing preservation surgery and help make it more common. Hopefully, with more experience and sufficient subjects, we—and other new teams—will soon be reporting residual hearing preservation results comparable to those of currently well-established surgeons.

Acknowledgments

The authors would to like to thank all the patients and their families, the UNICAMP cochlear implant group (audiologists, social work, nurse team, psychology, speech therapy and all the staff), their department (ENT, Head and Neck Surgery Department), and everyone at the MED-EL team who helped them.

References

[1] C. von Ilberg, J. Kiefer, J. Tillein et al., "Electric-acoustic stimulation of the auditory system. New technology for severe hearing loss," *Journal for Oto-Rhino-Laryngology and Its Related Specialties*, vol. 61, no. 6, pp. 334–340, 1999.

[2] J. Kiefer, M. Pok, O. Adunka et al., "Combined electric and acoustic stimulation of the auditory system: results of a clinical study," *Audiology and Neurotology*, vol. 10, no. 3, pp. 134–144, 2005.

[3] A. Lorens, M. Polak, A. Piotrowska, and H. Skarzynski, "Outcomes of treatment of partial deafness with cochlear implantation: a DUET study," *Laryngoscope*, vol. 118, no. 2, pp. 288–294, 2008.

[4] W. Gstoettner, S. Helbig, C. Settevendemie, U. Baumann, J. Wagenblast, and C. Arnoldner, "A new electrode for residual hearing preservation in cochlear implantation: first clinical results," *Acta Oto-Laryngologica*, vol. 129, no. 4, pp. 372–379, 2009.

[5] B. J. Gantz and C. W. Turner, "Combining acoustic and electrical hearing," *Laryngoscope*, vol. 113, no. 10, pp. 1726–1730, 2003.

[6] B. J. Gantz, M. R. Hansen, C. W. Turner, J. J. Oleson, L. A. Reiss, and A. J. Parkinson, "Hybrid 10 clinical trial: preliminary results," *Audiology and Neurotology*, vol. 14, supplement 1, pp. 32–38, 2009.

[7] C. W. Turner, B. J. Gantz, C. Vidal, A. Behrens, and B. A. Henry, "Speech recognition in noise for cochlear implant listeners: benefits of residual acoustic hearing," *Journal of the Acoustical Society of America*, vol. 115, no. 4, pp. 1729–1735, 2004.

[8] W. K. Gstoettner, P. van de Heyning, A. O'Connor et al., "Electric acoustic stimulation of the auditory system: results of a multi-centre investigation," *Acta Oto-Laryngologica*, vol. 128, no. 9, pp. 968–975, 2008.

[9] R. H. Gifford, M. F. Dorman, A. J. Spahr, and S. A. McKarns, "Effect of Digital Frequency Compression (DFC) on speech recognition in candidates for combined Electric and Acoustic Stimulation (EAS)," *Journal of Speech, Language, and Hearing Research*, vol. 50, no. 5, pp. 1194–1202, 2007.

[10] T. Lenarz, T. Stöver, A. Buechner, A. Lesinski-Schiedat, J. Patrick, and J. Pesch, "Hearing conservation surgery using the hybrid-L electrode: results from the first clinical trial at the Medical University of Hannover," *Audiology and Neurotology*, vol. 14, supplement 1, pp. 22–31, 2009.

[11] E. Lehnhardt and R. Laszig, "Specific surgical aspects of cochlear implant/soft surgery," in *Advances in Cochlear Implants*, I. J. Hochmair-Desoyer and E. S. Hochmair, Eds., pp. 228–229, Manz, Vienna, Austria, 1994.

[12] J. Kiefer, W. Gstoettner, W. Baumgartner et al., "Conservation of low-frequency hearing in cochlear implantation," *Acta Oto-Laryngologica*, vol. 124, no. 3, pp. 272–280, 2004.

[13] B. J. Gantz, C. W. Turner, K. E. Gfeller, and M. W. Lowder, "Preservation of hearing in cochlear implant surgery: advantages of combined electrical and acoustical speech processing," *Laryngoscope*, vol. 115, no. 5, pp. 796–802, 2005.

[14] W. K. Gstoettner, S. Heibig, N. Maier, J. Kiefer, A. Radeloff, and O. F. Adunka, "Ipsilateral electric acoustic stimulation of the auditory system: results of long-term hearing preservation," *Audiology and Neurotology*, vol. 11, no. 1, pp. 49–56, 2006.

[15] H. Skarzynski, A. Lorens, A. Piotrowska, and I. Anderson, "Preservation of low frequency hearing in partial deafness cochlear implantation (PDCI) using the round window surgical approach," *Acta Oto-Laryngologica*, vol. 127, no. 1, pp. 41–48, 2007.

[16] C. Arnoldner, S. Helbig, J. Wagenblast et al., "Electric acoustic stimulation in patients with postlingual severe high-frequency hearing loss: clinical experience," *Advances in Oto-Rhino-Laryngology*, vol. 67, pp. 116–124, 2010.

[17] O. Adunka, W. Gstoettner, M. Hambek, M. H. Unkelbach, A. Radeloff, and J. Kiefer, "Preservation of basal inner ear structures in cochlear implantation," *Journal for Oto-Rhino-Laryngology and Its Related Specialties*, vol. 66, no. 6, pp. 306–312, 2004.

[18] O. Adunka, J. Kiefer, M. H. Unkelbach, T. Lehnert, and W. Gstoettner, "Development and evaluation of an improved cochlear implant electrode design for electric acoustic stimulation," *Laryngoscope*, vol. 114, no. 7, pp. 1237–1241, 2004.

[19] W. Gstoettner, J. Kiefer, W. D. Baumgartner, S. Pok, S. Peters, and O. Adunka, "Hearing preservation in cochlear implantation for electric acoustic stimulation," *Acta Oto-Laryngologica*, vol. 124, no. 4, pp. 348–352, 2004.

[20] R. J. S. Briggs, M. Tykocinski, K. Stidham, and J. B. Roberson, "Cochleostomy site: implications for electrode placement and hearing preservation," *Acta Oto-Laryngologica*, vol. 125, no. 8, pp. 870–876, 2005.

[21] R. J. S. Briggs, M. Tykocinski, J. Xu et al., "Comparison of round window and cochleostomy approaches with a prototype hearing preservation electrode," *Audiology and Neurotology*, vol. 11, supplement 1, pp. 42–48, 2006.

[22] C. A. von Ilberg, U. Baumann, J. Kiefer, J. Tillein, and O. F. Adunka, "Electric-acoustic stimulation of the auditory system: a review of the first decade," *Audiology and Neurotology*, vol. 16, supplement 2, pp. 1–30, 2011.

[23] M. C. Bevilacqua, M. R. Banhara, E. A. da Costa, A. B. Vignoly, and K. F. Alvarenga, "The Brazilian Portuguese hearing in noise test," *International Journal of Audiology*, vol. 47, no. 6, pp. 364–365, 2008.

[24] S. Helbig, P. van de Heyning, J. Kiefer et al., "Combined electric acoustic stimulation with the PULSARCI[100] implant system using the FLEXEAS electrode array," *Acta Oto-Laryngologica*, vol. 131, no. 6, pp. 585–595, 2011.

[25] S. Helbig, U. Baumann, M. Helbig, N. von Malsen-Waldkirch, and W. Gstoettner, "A new combined speech processor for

electric and acoustic stimulation—eight months experience," *Journal for Oto-Rhino-Laryngology and Its Related Specialties*, vol. 70, no. 6, pp. 359–365, 2008.

[26] C. Arnoldner, W. Gstoettner, D. Riss et al., "Residual hearing preservation using the suprameatal approach for cochlear implantation," *Wiener klinische Wochenschrift*, vol. 123, no. 19-20, pp. 599–602, 2011.

[27] H. Skarzynski, A. Lorens, M. Zgoda, A. Piotrowska, P. H. Skarzynski, and A. Szkielkowska, "Atraumatic round window deep insertion of cochlear electrodes," *Acta Oto-Laryngologica*, vol. 131, no. 7, pp. 740–749, 2011.

[28] T. Pan, R. S. Tyler, H. Ji, C. Coelho, A. K. Gehringer, and S. A. Gogel, "Changes in the tinnitus handicap questionnaire after cochlear implantation," *American Journal of Audiology*, vol. 18, no. 2, pp. 144–151, 2009.

[29] D. M. Baguley, "New insights into tinnitus in cochlear implant recipients," *Cochlear Implants International*, vol. 11, no. 2, pp. 31–36, 2010.

[30] A. Kleine-Punte, K. Vermeire, A. Hofkens, M. de Bodt, D. de Ridder, and P. van de Heyning, "Cochlear implantation as a durable tinnitus treatment in single-sided deafness," *Cochlear Implants International*, vol. 12, supplement 1, pp. 26–29, 2011.

[31] M. Kompis, M. Pelizzone, N. Dillier, J. Allum, N. DeMin, and P. Senn, "Tinnitus before and after 6 months after cochlear implantation," *Audiology and Neurotology*, vol. 17, no. 3, pp. 161–168, 2012.

2

Thirteen Years of Hyoid Suspension Experience in Multilevel OSAHS Surgery: The Short-Term Results of a Bicentric Study

Pietro Canzi,[1] Anna Berardi,[1] Carmine Tinelli,[2] Filippo Montevecchi,[3] Fabio Pagella,[1] Claudio Vicini,[3] and Marco Benazzo[1]

[1] Department of Otorhinolaryngology, University of Pavia and IRCCS Policlinico San Matteo Foundation, Viale Camillo Golgi 19, 27100 Pavia, Italy
[2] Biometrics Unit, University of Pavia and IRCCS Policlinico San Matteo Foundation, Viale Camillo Golgi 19, 27100 Pavia, Italy
[3] ENT Unit, Department of Special Surgery, Morgagni-Pierantoni Hospital, Via Forlanini 34, 47121 Forlì, Italy

Correspondence should be addressed to Pietro Canzi; pcanzio@hotmail.com

Academic Editor: Jeffrey P. Pearson

Aims. To evaluate thirteen years of hyoid suspension experience in multilevel OSAHS surgery, for which hyoidthyroidpexia represented the exclusive hypopharyngeal approach applied. *Materials and Methods.* From 1998 to 2011, a bicentric retrospective study was conducted: all adult patients with a diagnosis of OSAHS were enrolled. Specific eligible criteria were established. Pre-/postoperative data concerning ENT and sleep findings were recorded. Recruited subjects were surveilled for a follow-up range from 6 to 18 months. *Results.* A total of 590 hyoid suspensions were evaluated, but only 140 patients met the specific inclusion criteria. A success rate of 67% was obtained. No intraoperative adverse events or major complications occurred. Excessive daytime sleepiness was observed in 28% of nonresponders. Despite the homogeneous candidate anatomy, ENT awake findings changed differently after surgery. Statistical analysis revealed multilevel surgery to be more effective when AHI < 30. Postoperative AHI was statistically not influenced by preoperative BMI. *Conclusions.* Hyoid suspension in multilevel treatment is effective when short-term results are considered. The necessity of a more valuable anatomic-based diagnostic approach is crucial to guide the patient selection. Long-term followups and randomized prospective trials with case-control series are needed to increase the level of evidence of this surgery.

1. Introduction

Sleep disordered breathing (SDB) surgery has taken its initial steps from the first tracheotomy [1] up to the pioneering applications of robotics in the new millennium [2]. When Sher and colleagues published the unsatisfying results of surgery in patients with hypopharyngeal obstruction, they were probably still not aware that a great number of hypopharyngeal procedures would be developed [3]. Despite the several techniques reported in the literature (e.g., surgical reduction of the tongue base, tongue base stabilization, genioglossus advancement, mortised genioplasty, tongue radiofrequency treatment, hyoepiglottoplasty, and hyoid suspension), many of them should be critically analyzed anyway because they are extremely invasive. The idea of restoring the retrolingual space acting on the hyoid bone was codified by Riley et al.

in 1986 [4], but a few years before experimental attempts in animal models had already been demonstrated [5, 6]. Since then, hyoid suspension has been adopted by many authors finally turning into a stepping stone in SDB surgical management [7].

We conducted a bicentric retrospective study to evaluate thirteen years of hyoid suspension experience in multilevel surgery, for which hyoidthyroidpexia represented the exclusive hypopharyngeal approach applied.

2. Materials and Methods

2.1. Study Design and Patient Selection. From 1998 to 2011, a bicentric retrospective study was conducted at the Otorhinolaryngology Department of the University of Pavia and the Otorhinolaryngology Unit of the Morgagni-Pierantoni

Hospital of Forlì. All adult patients (over 18 years of age) with a diagnosis of obstructive sleep apnea hypopnea syndrome (OSAHS) and no other SDB affection were enrolled. This happened after they had accomplished a 6-month or longer lasting CPAP treatment and only after they refused it, in accordance with Mickelson's principles [8]. Eligible criteria also included a multilevel pharyngeal obstruction, for which hyoid suspension represented the exclusive hypopharyngeal surgical approach applied. Institutional review board informed consent was preoperatively obtained from all participants. Recruited subjects were surveilled for a follow-up range from 6 to 18 months.

2.2. Clinical and Diagnostic Assessment. A sleep medical diagnosis was executed using a nocturnal, complete, and fully attended polysomnography according to the Associazione Italiana di Medicina del Sonno (Italian Association of Sleep Medicine) Guidelines [9]. OSAHS evidence and CPAP therapy were defined by sleep medicine specialists. Daytime sleepiness was measured using the Epworth Sleepiness Scale (ESS). Weight and height were recorded, and the body mass index (BMI) was calculated. Otorhinolaryngoiatric examination consisted of complete traditional ENT evaluation, upper airway endoscopy using Müller's manoeuvre with the patient in supine position, X-ray cephalometry, and drug-induced sleep endoscopy as previously reported [10]. Patients were staged following the "Nose Oropharynx Hypopharynx" (NOH) classification system introduced, in clinical practice, by the authors since 1999 [11, 12]. Grade and patterns of upper airways collapse were evaluated at the nasal cavities (nose = N), retropalatal space (oropharynx = O), and hypopharyngeal region (hypopharynx = H). The minimal sectional area during Müller's manoeuvre was staged in the following 4 obstructing grades:

Grade I: <25% collapse;

Grade II: between 25% and 50% collapse;

Grade III: between 51% and 75% collapse;

Grade IV: >75% collapse.

Identification of the obstructing pattern—patient in a supine position—was evaluated according to the shape of the dynamic collapse: anterior-posterior (ap), concentric (c), and transversal (t).

2.3. Notes on Hyoid Suspension Technique. The hyoid suspension type II (hyoidthyroidpexia) according to Riley et al.'s modification of 1994 [13] was carried out by the same surgical team (M. Benazzo, F. Pagella, F. Montevecchi, and C. Vicini) on all patients. Key steps in hypopharyngeal reconstruction were the following.

(i) Anti-Trendelenburg position with neck hyperextension.

(ii) Natural skin crease incision between the hyoid inferior body and the thyroid notch.

(iii) Median strap muscle dissection between two imaginary parasagittal planes crossing the lesser cornu of the hyoid bone.

(iv) Hyoid bone mobilizing test in anteroinferior direction.

(v) Exposure of the thyroid cartilage (thyroid notch and superior border of thyroid lamina).

(vi) Four stitches (2 on each side) between the hyoid bone and the thyroid notch with reabsorbable sutures (after having reduced neck hyperextension).

(vii) Carry out permanent hyoid fixation after having tested the correct position of the thyroid cartilage below the hyoid bone, following fixed steps which are as follows:

(a) double stitching of the anterior parts—hyoid bone, thyroid cartilage—simultaneously,

(b) double stitching of the lateral parts—hyoid bone, thyroid cartilage—simultaneously,

(c) to achieve an optimal result, the tension of the lateral stitches should be lower than the tension of the anterior ones, in order to avoid hyoid bone fractures.

2.4. Postoperative Followup. As part of the standard postoperative protocol, a nasopharyngolaryngoscopic assessment by Müller's manoeuvre was carried out and another polysomnography was performed in all patients from six months onwards after surgery. The apnea hypopnea index (AHI), ESS, NOH, and BMI were assessed during the follow-up period. Responder patients were defined by AHI postoperative values <10 ev/h (recovered) or between 10 ev/h and 20 ev/h (cardiovascular prevention). Nonresponder group was composed of postoperative AHI > 20 ev/h but inferior to preoperative AHI (improved), postoperative AHI = preoperative AHI (unchanged), and postoperative AHI > preoperative AHI (worsened).

2.5. Statistical Analysis. The Shapiro-Wilk test was used to test the normal distribution of quantitative variable. If they were normally distributed, mean and standard deviation were used to summarize them and Student's t-test for dependent samples was used for comparisons between preoperative and postoperative values. If data were not distributed normally, we used median and interquartile range (IQR; 25° and 75° percentile), and nonparametric tests were used to compare data. The χ^2 test or Fisher's exact test, as appropriate, was used to determine whether observed differences in proportions between study groups were statistically significant. $P < 0.05$ was considered statistically significant. All tests were two-sided. Statistica 6.0 (StatSoft, Inc., 2006, Tulsa, OK, USA) was used for statistical computations.

3. Results

A total of 590 hyoid suspensions were evaluated, but only 140 patients (128 men and 12 women) aged 32–76 years (mean 50.7, median 51) met the specific inclusion criteria. Analyzed data were not distributed normally; therefore, median and interquartile ranges were adopted. Sleep endoscopy findings

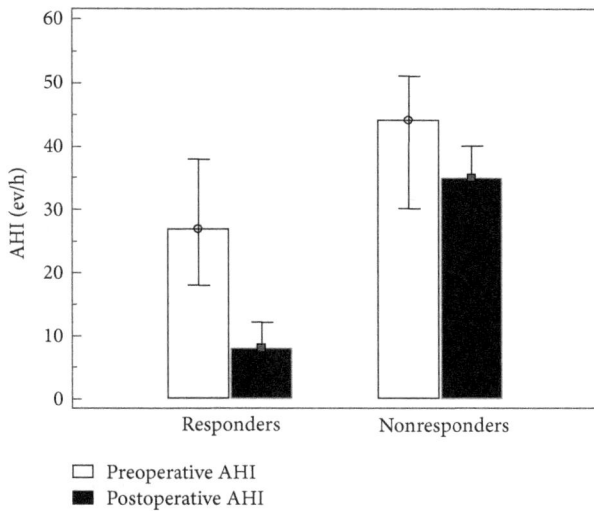

FIGURE 1: Comparison of pre-/postoperative AHI reduction between responder and nonresponder groups.

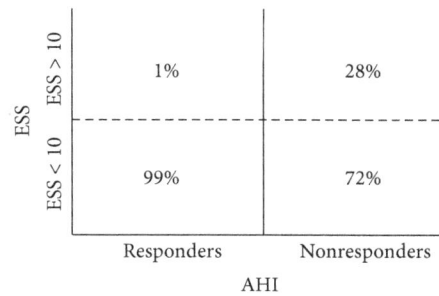

FIGURE 2: Comparison between postoperative ESS and postoperative AHI.

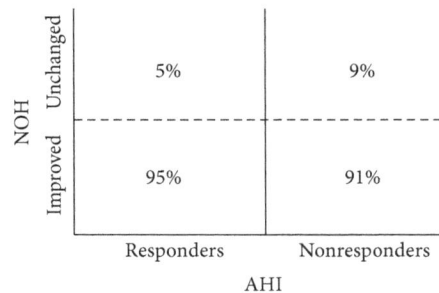

FIGURE 3: Comparison between postoperative NOH and postoperative AHI.

could not be incorporated in our review due to the lack of a statistical significance in the included population.

None of the patients had a reduction in the posterior airway space or changes in skeletal measurements at the lateral cephalometric radiograph performed preoperatively.

We always adopted a single-staged multilevel surgery. Among 140 hyoidthyroidpexia procedures, hyoid suspension was combined as follows:

(i) nasal + palatal + hyoid surgery = 117 cases,

(ii) nasal + hyoid surgery = 2 cases,

(iii) palatal + hyoid surgery = 21 cases.

Rhinosurgical procedures were carried out in 119 subjects (septoplasty ± turbinoplasty) and 138 patients needed a palatal approach (128 uvulopalatopharyngoplasties with 80 tonsillectomies, 8 laser assisted uvulopalatoplasties, and 2 uvulopalatal flaps). Twenty-three patients previously underwent surgery elsewhere (21 nasal surgery and 2 palatal surgery). No intraoperative adverse events occurred. Major complications were not reported. Two cases of neck seroma, one hyoid bone fracture and one keloid scar development, were noticed without any further significant effects.

Detailed pre-/postoperative data are abstracted in Table 1.

Before surgery, 15% of the patients had mild OSAHS (AHI = 5–15 ev/h), 33% moderate (AHI = 16–30 ev/h), and 52% severe (AHI > 30 ev/h), according to the American Sleep Association [14]. Overall, OSAHS level decreased after surgery from a median preoperative AHI value of 31 ev/h (IQR 21 ev/h–44 ev/h) to a median postoperative AHI value of 12 ev/h (IQR 6 ev/h–25 ev/h) with a difference (gain) of −19 ev/h ($P < 0.05$). The responses to multilevel treatment are summarized in Table 2, indicating a success rate of 67% ($P < 0.05$). Comparison of pre-/postoperative AHI reduction between responder and non-responder groups is shown in Figure 1.

Excessive daytime sleepiness, also defined as pathological ESS (ESS > 10), characterized the untreated population in 66% of the cases. Hypersomnolence improved significantly after hyoid suspension from a median preoperative ESS of 10 (IQR 8–12) to a median postoperative ESS of 8 (IQR 6–9; gain −2; $P < 0.05$). ESS > 10 was observed in 10% of the postoperative population. The non-responder group included 28% of pathological ESS (Figure 2).

According to the NOH staging system, the median preoperative finding was N3O4cH3t (IQR N2O3cH2t-N3O4cH3t), thus underlining a homogeneous population with multilevel nose, palate, and hypopharyngeal collapse. The identified pattern of obstruction was typically concentric and transversal in the retropalatal and hypopharyngeal region, respectively. The median postoperative NOH score was N0O1cH1t (IQR N0O0H0-N0O1cH1t; gain −N3O3cH2t; $P < 0.05$) with only 6% (8 patients) of the 140 patients showing no NOH changes postoperatively and 9% of non-responders (4 patients) showing no NOH changes (Figure 3).

The BMI outcome did not change after surgery (difference between pre-/postoperative BMI = 0; $P > 0.05$), and postoperative AHI was statistically not influenced by preoperative BMI (Figure 4). Median followup lasted 9 months (IQR 7 months–14 months).

4. Discussion

Many questions still remain unanswered concerning the SDB physiopathology, but currently it is generally accepted that pharyngeal airflow obstruction is the consequence of

TABLE 1: Pre-/postoperative statistical data.

	Median		Lower quartile		Upper quartile		Gain
	Preoperative	Postoperative	Preoperative	Postoperative	Preoperative	Postoperative	
AHI (ev/h)	31	12	21	6	44	25	−19 ($P < 0.05$)
ESS	10	8	8	6	12	9	−2 ($P < 0.05$)
NOH	N3O4cH3t	N0O1cH1t	N2O3cH2t	N0O0H0	N3O4cH3t	N0O1cH1t	−N3O3cH2t ($P < 0.05$)
BMI (Kg/m^2)	27.8	27.5	26.5	26.0	29.4	29.0	0 ($P > 0.05$)
Followup (mo)	9 mo		7 mo		14 mo		/

Gain: median postoperative value − median preoperative value. mo: months.

TABLE 2: Multilevel treatment response rates.

	Responders			Nonresponders	
	Recovered (postoperative AHI < 10)	Cardiovascular prevention (10 < postoperative AHI < 20)	Improved (postoperative AHI < preoperative AHI, but postoperative AHI > 20)	Unchanged (postoperative AHI = preoperative AHI)	Worsened (postoperative AHI > preoperative AHI)
Percentage	44%	23%	18%	7%	8%
Total	67%			33%	

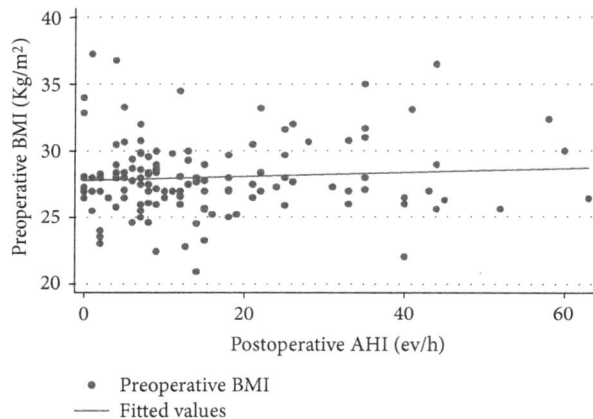

FIGURE 4: Statistical correlation between preoperative BMI and postoperative AHI.

a complex interaction between anatomical and functional factors. Because there is more than one variable involved, it is difficult to define a precise and direct relationship between surgery (cause) and clinical effectiveness (effect). Actually, in order to achieve clinical effectiveness, surgery needs to work on the structural features; in other words, it must act reconstructing the airway wall anatomy. Anatomy is not only different among apneic and nonapneic patients, but it also shows a high individual variability in the OSAHS population. That is why accurate knowledge of the structural defects is crucial in allowing the design of a surgery exactly tailored to each patient [15]. To do this, it is first of all necessary to understand whether a patient is suitable for surgery or not. The selection criteria are, indeed, essential key points to guide surgical treatment decision making. Historically,

Fujita developed a specific classification of the airway collapse levels and more recently, Friedman's staging was introduced to increase the surgical response [16, 17]. In 1996 Sher et al. highlighted the hypopharyngeal role, reporting a success rate of 5.3% in all patients belonging to type II-III Fujita's system [3]. Since then, many surgical procedures have developed in order to reshape the hypopharyngeal region.

The hyoid is a u-shaped bone located in the anterior neck midline, at the centre of three force vectors directed, respectively, towards the mandible, sternum, and mastoid process. It gives insertion to the middle constrictor muscles, which form the lateral wall of the hypopharynx. The suspension of this bone to the thyroid cartilage restores the transversal collapse caused by the decreased tone of the middle constrictor muscles in OSAHS patients [13, 18]. Currently, only three clinical trials have been written to investigate the effect of an isolated hyoid suspension for OSAHS, which have reported a response rate ranging from 40% to 53% [13, 19, 20]. A recent MEDLINE meta-analysis proved hyoid suspension to be better recommended in the context of a multilevel surgery in OSAHS patients with retrolingual and hypopharyngeal obstruction (grade of recommendation B) [21]. When genioglossus advancement is associated with hyoid suspension, the success rate reported is apparently not higher than the one after hyoid suspension as the sole procedure to treat hypopharyngeal collapse [22]. Despite the increasing number of reports about hyoidthyroidpexia, there is still insufficient evidence to recommend one suspension technique over another [23]. Nevertheless, as far as we could experience and in accordance with the literature, hyoidthyroidpexia has been shown to be a safe procedure without any major complications [24].

During thirteen years of SDB surgical experience, 590 patients were submitted to hyoid suspension but only 140 of them were evaluated. Many factors caused the numeric reduction of our study which are as follows:

(i) the limited selection criteria,

(ii) the statistical need of a homogeneous population,

(iii) the relatively recent introduction in our hospitals of a patient data recording system enables to prevent the loss of information,

(iv) lost patients at followup or dropouts.

To the best of our knowledge, we documented the largest cohort of patients submitted to a multilevel surgery, for which hyoidthyroidpexia represents the exclusive hypopharyngeal approach applied. Our success rate of 67% cannot be directly compared with the results reported in the literature because the authors' modalities are different when analyzing response to surgery. In 2006, Kezirian and Goldberg published an evidence-based medicine review collecting all hyoid suspension results and defined as the main surgical goal an AHI reduction of 50% or more and an AHI of less than 20 ev/h [22]. The studies taken into consideration showed a success rate ranging from 17% to 78% of the cases. Borrowing Sher et al.'s criteria [3], we obtained 59% of success rate ($P < 0.05$), in accordance with the results published in the literature. Following our own experience, over and above an accurate identification of the obstructing sites, the successful outcome benefits also from a preoperative AHI. Comparison of pre-/postoperative AHI reduction between responders and non-responders revealed multilevel surgery to be more effective when AHI scored <30 ev/h ($P < 0.05$) (Figure 1).

Despite the homogeneous anatomy of the enrolled candidates, NOH findings changed differently after surgery as shown in Figure 3. Our results support the necessity of a more valuable anatomic-based diagnostic approach, crucial to guiding surgical treatment decision making. Concerning this matter, drug-induced sleep endoscopy could represent a useful additional instrument in detecting any occult obstruction site, not only during the preoperative assessment but also during the analysis of treatment failures, in order to establish a further salvage therapy [25]. Treatment of the non-responders becomes even harder when clinical aspects are taken into account (Figure 2). The subjective ESS improvement in 72% of the non-responders is surprising and underlines the difficulties in persuading these subjects to continue a therapeutic plan.

There was no functional correlation between BMI observed before surgery and postoperative AHI, that appeared independent, due to the lack of statistically significant percentage of obese patients (BMI > 30) among the preoperative subjects.

Although this is the widest cohort study ever published, it is not free from certain limitations. The absence of a long-term followup and of a randomized prospective design with a case-control series has weakened the strength of our work. The relatively recent introduction of drug-induced sleep endoscopy in our ENT diagnostic equipment did not allow a statistically significant amount of sleep findings in the included population. The awake condition may differ, indeed, quite dramatically from the sleep-breathing one,

leading to inaccurate information and limiting the ability to predict upper airway changes during sleep. The adoption of a more complete clinical classification able to record all the patients' features (e.g., NOHL system) could overcome this methodological bias and allow a better patients' selection [12].

5. Conclusions

Hyoid suspension in multilevel treatment is effective when short-term results are considered. The necessity of a more valuable anatomic-based diagnostic approach is crucial to guide the patient selection. Long-term follow-ups and randomized prospective trials with case-control series are needed to increase the level of evidence of this surgery.

Conflict of Interests

The authors declare that they have no conflict of interests.

References

[1] W. Kuhlo, E. Doll, and M. C. Franck, "Successful management of Pickwickian syndrome using long-term tracheostomy," Deutsche Medizinische Wochenschrift, vol. 94, no. 24, pp. 1286–1290, 1969.

[2] C. Vicini, I. Dallan, P. Canzi, S. Frassineti, M. G. La Pietra, and F. Montevecchi, "Transoral robotic tongue base resection in obstructive sleep apnoea-hypopnoea syndrome: a preliminary report," ORL Journal of Otorhinolaryngology and Its Related Specialties, vol. 72, no. 1, pp. 22–27, 2010.

[3] A. E. Sher, K. B. Schechtman, and J. F. Piccirillo, "The efficacy of surgical modifications of the upper airway in adults with obstructive sleep apnea syndrome," Sleep, vol. 19, no. 2, pp. 156–177, 1996.

[4] R. W. Riley, N. B. Powell, and C. Guilleminault, "Inferior sagittal osteotomy of the mandible with hyoid myotomy-suspension: a new procedure for obstructive sleep apnea," Otolaryngology, vol. 94, no. 5, pp. 589–593, 1986.

[5] T. J. Patton, S. E. Thawley, R. C. Water, P. J. Vandermeer, and J. H. Ogura, "Expansion hyoidplasty: a potential surgical procedure designed for selected patients with obstructive sleep apnea syndrome. Experimental canine results," Laryngoscope, vol. 93, no. 11 I, pp. 1387–1396, 1983.

[6] W. B. van de Graaff, S. B. Gottfried, J. Mitra, E. van Lunteren, N. S. Cherniack, and K. P. Strohl, "Respiratory function of hyoid muscles and hyoid arch," Journal of Applied Physiology Respiratory Environmental and Exercise Physiology, vol. 57, no. 1, pp. 197–204, 1984.

[7] T. Verse, A. Baisch, J. T. Maurer, B. A. Stuck, and K. Hörmann, "Multilevel surgery for obstructive sleep apnea: short-term results," Otolaryngology, vol. 134, no. 4, pp. 571–577, 2006.

[8] S. A. Mickelson, "Preoperative and postoperative management of obstructive sleep apnea patients," Otolaryngologic Clinics of North America, vol. 40, no. 4, pp. 877–889, 2007.

[9] Commissione Paritetica AIPO-AIMS, "Linee guida di procedura diagnostica nella sindrome delle apnee ostruttive dell'adulto," Rassegna di Patologia dell'Apparato Respiratorio, vol. 16, pp. 278–280, 2001.

[10] A. Campanini, P. Canzi, A. de Vito, I. Dallan, F. Montevecchi, and C. Vicini, "Awake versus sleep endoscopy: personal

experience in 250 OSAHS patients," *Acta Otorhinolaryngologica Italica*, vol. 30, no. 2, pp. 73–77, 2010.

[11] S. Frassineti, C. Vicini, and I. Dallan, "Fibroscopia e sistema NOH," in *Chirurgia Della Roncopatia*, C. Vicini, Ed., pp. 253–259, Eureka S.r.l., Lucca, Italy, 2007.

[12] C. Vicini, A. De Vito, M. Benazzo et al., "The nose oropharynx hypopharynx and larynx (NOHL) classification: a new system of diagnostic standardized examination for OSAHS patients," *European Archives of Oto-Rhino-Laryngology*, vol. 269, no. 4, pp. 1297–1300, 2012.

[13] R. W. Riley, N. B. Powell, and C. Guilleminault, "Obstructive sleep apnea and the hyoid: a revised surgical procedure," *Otolaryngology*, vol. 111, no. 6, pp. 717–721, 1994.

[14] A. Oack, K. Strohl, J. Wheatley et al., "Sleep-related breathing disorders in adults: recommendations for syndrome definition and measurement techniques in clinical research," *Sleep*, vol. 22, no. 5, pp. 667–689, 1999.

[15] B. Tucker Woodson, "Non-Pressure therapies for obstructive sleep apnea: surgery and oral appliances," *Respiratory Care*, vol. 55, no. 10, pp. 1314–1320, 2010.

[16] S. Fujita, "Pharyngeal surgery for obstructive sleep apnea and snoring," in *Snoring and Obstructive Sleep Apnea*, D. N. F. Fairbanks, Ed., pp. 101–128, Raven Press, New York, NY, USA, 1987.

[17] M. Friedman, H. Tanyeri, M. La Rosa et al., "Clinical predictors of obstructive sleep apnea," *Laryngoscope*, vol. 109, no. 12, pp. 1901–1907, 1999.

[18] D. P. White, "Pathophysiology of obstructive sleep apnoea," *Thorax*, vol. 50, no. 7, pp. 797–804, 1995.

[19] B. A. Stuck, W. Neff, K. Hörmann et al., "Anatomic changes after hyoid suspension for obstructive sleep apnea: an MRI study," *Otolaryngology*, vol. 133, no. 3, pp. 397–402, 2005.

[20] C. Den Herder, H. Van Tinteren, and N. De Vries, "Hyoidthyroidpexia: a surgical treatment for sleep apnea syndrome," *Laryngoscope*, vol. 115, no. 4, pp. 740–745, 2005.

[21] W. J. Randerath, J. Verbraecken, S. Andreas et al., "Non-CPAP therapies in obstructive sleep apnoea," *European Respiratory Journal*, vol. 37, no. 5, pp. 1000–1028, 2011.

[22] E. J. Kezirian and A. N. Goldberg, "Hypopharyngeal surgery in obstructive sleep apnea: an evidence-based medicine review," *Archives of Otolaryngology*, vol. 132, no. 2, pp. 206–213, 2006.

[23] J. K. M. Chau and R. L. Goode, "Are hyoid procedures a reasonable choice in the surgical treatment of obstructive sleep apnea?" *Laryngoscope*, vol. 120, no. 2, pp. 221–222, 2010.

[24] W. Richard, F. Timmer, H. Van Tinteren, and N. De Vries, "Complications of hyoid suspension in the treatment of obstructive sleep apnea syndrome," *European Archives of Oto-Rhino-Laryngology*, vol. 268, no. 4, pp. 631–635, 2011.

[25] E. J. Kezirian, "Nonresponders to pharyngeal surgery for obstructive sleep apnea: insights from drug-induced sleep endoscopy," *Laryngoscope*, vol. 121, no. 6, pp. 1320–1326, 2011.

3

Aural Foreign Bodies: Descriptive Study of 224 Patients in Al-Fallujah General Hospital, Iraq

Ahmad Nasrat Al-juboori

Ibn Sina College of Medicine, Al-Iraqia University, Baghdad, Iraq

Correspondence should be addressed to Ahmad Nasrat Al-juboori; ahmednas2005@yahoo.com

Academic Editor: Charles Monroe Myer

Foreign bodies (FB) in the external auditory canal are relative medical emergency. The objective of this study was to describe the types of FB and their complications and to highlight on new FB not seen before which was the bluetooth devices that were used for cheating during high school examination in Al-Fallujah city. This was a two-year hospital-based descriptive study performed in the Department of Ear, Nose and Throat (ENT), Al-Fallujah General Hospital, from June 2011 to May 2013; during this period, 224 FB had been extracted from 224 patients. Beads were extracted from 68 patients (30.4%), cotton tips were extracted from 50 patients (22.3%), seeds and garlic were extracted from 31 patients (13.8%), papers were extracted from 27 patients (12.1%), insects were extracted from 24 patients (10.7%), button batteries were extracted from 13 patients (5.8%), and bluetooth devices were extracted from 7 patients (3.1%). Most of the cases did not develop complications (87.5%) during extraction. The main complications were canal abrasion (4.5%). Proper instrumentation allows the uncomplicated removal of many FB. The use of general anesthesia is preferred in very young children. Bluetooth device objects should be considered as new aural FB, especially in our territory.

1. Introduction

Foreign bodies (FB) in the external auditory meatus are most commonly seen in children who have inserted them into their own ears. Children may present asymptomatically, or with pain or a discharge caused by otitis externa. Adults are often seen with cotton wool or broken matchsticks which have been used to clean or scratch the ear canal [1]. Live insects in the ear, commonly small cockroaches [2], are annoying due to discomfort created by loud noise and movement. FB in the ear is relatively common in emergency medicine. However, attempts of removal made outside the healthcare setting by untrained persons can result in complications of varying degrees [3]. An aural FB can involve damage to tympanic membrane or middle ear by itself or by improper management during removal. The etiology of FB in the ear has been ascribed to general curiosity and a whim to explore orifices in children, playful insertion of FB into others' body parts, accidental entry of foreign body, preexisting disease in ear causing irritation, and habitual cleaning of ear and nose with objects like ear buds [4, 5]. FB in ear can be classified in many ways like organic-inorganic, animate-inanimate, metallic-nonmetallic, hygroscopic-nonhygroscopic, regular or irregular, soft or hard, and so forth, according to their nature [6]. The method of removal usually depends on the type of FB, its position, and cooperation of the patient [7, 8]. Based on criteria used by American Family Physician (with Strength of Recommendation Taxonomy (SORT) grade C), all ear FB cases should be referred to ENT specialty for removal except for only those which are directly visible and "graspable" [9].

The objective of this study was to describe the types of FB and their complications and to highlight on new FB not seen before which was the bluetooth devices that were used for cheating during high school examination in Al-Fallujah city.

2. Materials and Methods

This was a two-year hospital-based prospective descriptive study performed in the Department of Ear, Nose and Throat (ENT), Al-Fallujah General Hospital, from June 2011 to May

TABLE 1: Age and sex distribution.

Age (years)	Male	Female	Total (%)
<1–10	37	20	57 (25.5)
11–20	31	13	44 (19.6)
21–30	19	18	37 (16.5)
31–40	20	16	36 (16.1)
41–50	21	10	31 (13.8)
51–>60	11	8	19 (8.5)
Total	139	85	224 (100)

TABLE 2: Types of aural foreign bodies extracted from 224 patients.

Types of foreign body	Number	Percentage
Beads	68	30.4
Cotton tips	50	22.3
Seeds and garlic	31	13.8
Paper	27	12.1
Insects	24	10.7
Button batteries	13	5.8
Bluetooth device	7	3.1
Miscellaneous*	4	1.8
Total	224	100

*Matchstick, eraser, and stone.

TABLE 3: Complications of aural foreign body extraction from 224 patients.

Complications	Number	Percentage
No complications	196	87.5
Canal abrasion	10	4.5
Canal laceration and/or bleeding	8	3.6
Otitis externa	7	3.1
Tympanic membrane perforation	2	0.9
Otitis media	1	0.4
Total	224	100

2013; during this period, 224 FB had been extracted from 224 patients. History and patients data included age, sex and presenting symptoms had been taken as well as ear, nose and throat examination was performed. All patients with suggestive history of FB entry into ear were included. Those patients with no suggestive history but were found to have the FB are also included in the study. Patients with complications arising out of FB, whose extraction was done at a different centre, are excluded. The use of aural syringing, vacuum suction, and manual instrumentation by the use of Jobson Horne's probe or hook and forceps may be indicated. In a very limited number of patients, especially in children, general anesthesia was used because of poor cooperation. After extraction of FB, reexamination of the affected ear was performed immediately and after three days to exclude the possible complications.

3. Results

The total number of patients with FB was 224 patients; they ranged from below one year to above 60 years old, and the mean age with standard deviation was 19 years ±2.1 years. They were 139 male patients and 85 patients were females, with male to female ratio of 1.6 : 1 as shown in Table 1. The onset of presentation was noticed mainly in the first 24 hours of the injury; 180 of such patients presented in the first 24 hours, 25 patients presented in the second 24 hours, and 13 patients presented between 48 and 72 hours of the onset, while the remaining six patients presented after 72 hours.

The types of 224 aural FB extracted from the patients are shown in Table 2 in order of frequency. Beads extracted from 68 patients (30.4%), cotton tips extracted from 50 patients (22.3%), seeds in different types and garlic extracted from 31 patients (13.8%), papers extracted from 27 patients (12.1%), insects extracted from 24 patients (10.7%), button batteries extracted from 13 patients (5.8%), bluetooth devices extracted from 7 patients (3.1%), and miscellaneous types of FB including matchstick, eraser, and stone are shown in Table 2.

Bluetooth device objects were used in cheating during students' examinations, especially college and secondary school students, where the concealed mobile device was used and bluetooth metallic pieces were applied in contact with tympanic membrane, with the help of another person present outside the examination hall test for the purpose of the solving questions. Those aural foreign bodies were not seen before.

Here, the insertion of these magnetic bluetooth device objects done by someone else, who inserted them inside the ear canal (Figure 2), and after the end of the examination, they could not get rid of them; that is, they could not extract these objects from the ear canal, so that they consulted ENT clinic for extraction.

The complications which happened were observed due to presence of FB and/or during and after the extraction shown in Table 3. Most of the cases did not develop complications (87.5%). The main complications were canal abrasion (4.5%), canal laceration and/or bleeding (3.6%), otitis externa (3.1%), tympanic membrane perforation (0.9%), and otitis media (0.4%).

4. Discussion

Foreign body insertion into the ear in children is becoming increasingly common in developing countries. Children tend to be curious and exploratory; hence, the easily accessible orifices tend to be at risk of this form of injury [10]. In our study, the main age group below 10 years of age, representing 25.5%, was mostly affected; this was consistent with other studies. [3, 11]. A total of 480 cases were presented with ear FB during the study of Chai et al. The highest incidence of ear FB occurred in 0–5 years of age which consisted of 232 (48.3%) cases. This was followed by children between 6 and 10 years [12]. Most of the cases presented in the first 24 hours of the FB insertion, as in our study; this was also observed in other studies [3, 13]. There were wide variations

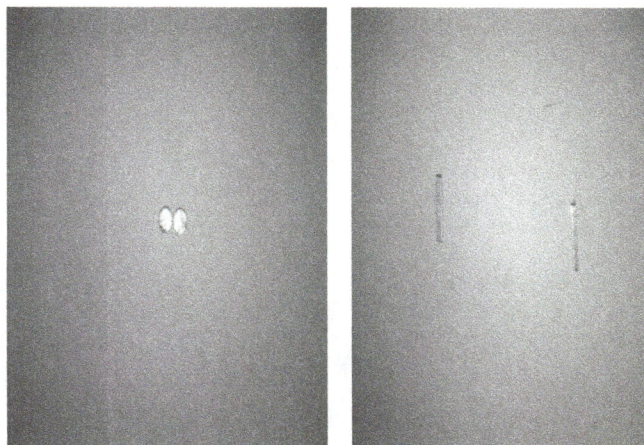

FIGURE 1: Different types of bluetooth devices extracted from the external auditory canal.

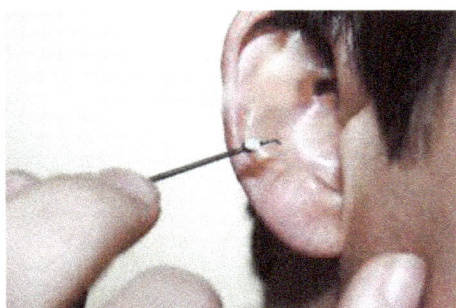

FIGURE 2: The method of inserting the bluetooth device in the external auditory canal.

regarding the type of the aural FB; in Chai et al. study, seeds or nuts were the commonest ear FB encountered which consisted of 226 (47.1%) cases; this was followed by plastic toys or beads [12]. In Ologe et al. study grains and seeds (27.9%), beads (19.7%), cotton wool (13.6%), paper (8.8%), and eraser (8.2%) formed the bulk of the aural FB [14], but this differed from our results in which beads and cotton tips were common as compared to seeds; this was consistent with other studies [15]. In our study, garlic was encountered as an animate FB because it was used traditionally for the relief of earache. Bluetooth device objects were small pieces of magnetic property (Figure 1) used with the aid of mobile for cheating during final examinations in high school; this was one of the figures of corruption; this metallic piece was introduced through the ear canal and applied in contact with the tympanic membrane (Figure 2). Here, there was a person outside the examination hall answering the key questions and sending the solution to the examiner; this type of FB was not recorded or mentioned before, but we recorded seven cases after the insertion of those small objects in the external auditory canal (EAC).

Complication due to presence of FB or the extraction was uncommon; no complications were recorded in 87.5% of the cases in contrast to Singh et al. study which recorded

77% complication rate [16]. Adequate immobilization and proper instrumentation allow the uncomplicated removal of many EAC foreign bodies in the pediatric population. The use of general anesthesia is preferred in very young children and in children of any age with aural FB whose contour, composition, or location predispose to traumatic removal in the ambulatory setting [17].

5. Conclusion

Proper instrumentation allows the uncomplicated removal of many EAC foreign bodies. The use of general anesthesia is preferred in very young children and the uncooperative. Bluetooth device objects should be considered as new aural FB, especially in our territory.

Disclosure

This study was conducted by Department of Ear, Nose and Throat, Al-Fallujah General Hospital, Al-Anbar Health Directorate, Republic of Iraq, and approved by the research and ethical committee of the hospital.

Conflict of Interests

The author had no conflicting interests and is not supported or funded by any drug company.

References

[1] G. R. Kroukamp and J. W. Loock, "Foreign bodies in the ear," in Scott-Brown's Otorhinolaryngology, Head and Neck Surgery, M. Gleeson, G. G. Browning, M. J. Burton et al., Eds., vol. 3, pp. 3370–3372, Hodder Arnold, New York, NY, USA, 7th edition, 2008.

[2] G. Kroukamp and J. G. H. Londt, "Ear-invading arthropods: a South African survey," South African Medical Journal, vol. 96, no. 4, pp. 290–292, 2006.

[3] T. G. Olajide, F. E. Ologe, and O. O. Arigbede, "Management of foreign bodies in the ear: a retrospective review of 123 cases

in Nigeria," *Ear, Nose and Throat Journal*, vol. 90, no. 11, p. E16, 2011.

[4] S. K. Das, "Aetiological evaluation of foreign bodies in the ear and nose (a clinical study)," *Journal of Laryngology and Otology*, vol. 98, no. 10, pp. 989–991, 1984.

[5] A. Kalan and M. Tariq, "Foreign bodies in the nasal cavities: a comprehensive review of the aetiology, diagnostic pointers, and therapeutic measures," *Postgraduate Medical Journal*, vol. 76, no. 898, pp. 484–487, 2000.

[6] S. L. Schulze, J. Kerschner, and D. Beste, "Pediatric external auditory canal foreign bodies: a review of 698 cases," *Otolaryngology—Head and Neck Surgery*, vol. 127, no. 1, pp. 73–78, 2002.

[7] A. P. S. Balbani, T. G. Sanchez, O. Butugan et al., "Ear and nose foreign body removal in children," *International Journal of Pediatric Otorhinolaryngology*, vol. 46, no. 1-2, pp. 37–42, 1998.

[8] S. K. Thompson, R. O. Wein, and P. O. Dutcher, "External auditory canal foreign body removal: management practices and outcomes," *Laryngoscope*, vol. 113, no. 11, pp. 1912–1915, 2003.

[9] I. Mohamad, "Ear foreign body: tackling the uncommons," *Medical Journal of Malaysia*, vol. 67, no. 3, p. 53, 2012.

[10] M. Ibekwe, L. Onotai, and B. Otaigbe, "Foreign body in the ear, nose and throat in children: a five year review in Niger delta," *African Journal of Paediatric Surgery*, vol. 9, no. 1, pp. 3–7, 2012.

[11] I. Wada, Y. Kase, and T. Iinuma, "Statistical study on the case of aural foreign bodies," *Journal of Otolaryngology of Japan*, vol. 106, no. 6, pp. 678–684, 2003.

[12] C. K. Chai, I. P. Tang, T. Y. Tan, and D. E. Y. H. Jong, "A review of ear, nose and throat foreign bodies in Sarawak General Hospital. A five year experience," *Medical Journal of Malaysia*, vol. 67, no. 1, pp. 17–20, 2012.

[13] S. K. Hon, T. M. Izam, C. B. Koay, and A. Razi, "A prospective evaluation of foreign bodies presenting to the Ear, Nose and Throat Clinic, Hospital Kuala Lumpur," *Medical Journal of Malaysia*, vol. 56, no. 4, pp. 463–470, 2001.

[14] F. E. Ologe, A. D. Dunmade, and O. A. Afolabi, "Aural foreign bodies in children," *Indian Journal of Pediatrics*, vol. 74, no. 8, pp. 755–758, 2007.

[15] C. Ryan, A. Ghosh, B. Wilson-Boyd, D. Smit, and S. O'Leary, "Presentation and management of aural foreign bodies in two Australian emergency departments," *Emergency Medicine Australasia*, vol. 18, no. 4, pp. 372–378, 2006.

[16] G. B. Singh, T. S. Sidhu, A. Sharma, R. Dhawan, S. K. Jha, and N. Singh, "Management of aural foreign body: an evaluative study in 738 consecutive cases," *American Journal of Otolaryngology*, vol. 28, no. 2, pp. 87–90, 2007.

[17] J. F. Ansley and M. J. Cunningham, "Treatment of aural foreign bodies in children," *Pediatrics*, vol. 101, no. 4, pp. 638–641, 1998.

4

Contralateral Ear Occlusion for Improving the Reliability of Otoacoustic Emission Screening Tests

Emily Papsin,[1] Adrienne L. Harrison,[1] Mattia Carraro,[1,2] and Robert V. Harrison[1,2,3]

[1] *Auditory Science Laboratory, Neuroscience and Mental Health Program, The Hospital for Sick Children, 555 University Avenue, Toronto, ON, Canada M5G 1X8*
[2] *Institute of Biomaterials and Biomedical Engineering, University of Toronto, Toronto, ON, Canada M5S 1A1*
[3] *Department of Otolaryngology-Head and Neck Surgery, University of Toronto, 190 Elizabeth Street, Toronto, ON, Canada M5G 2N2*

Correspondence should be addressed to Robert V. Harrison; rvh@sickkids.ca

Academic Editor: Charles Monroe Myer

Newborn hearing screening is an established healthcare standard in many countries and testing is feasible using otoacoustic emission (OAE) recording. It is well documented that OAEs can be suppressed by acoustic stimulation of the ear contralateral to the test ear. In clinical otoacoustic emission testing carried out in a sound attenuating booth, ambient noise levels are low such that the efferent system is not activated. However in newborn hearing screening, OAEs are often recorded in hospital or clinic environments, where ambient noise levels can be 60–70 dB SPL. Thus, results in the test ear can be influenced by ambient noise stimulating the opposite ear. Surprisingly, in hearing screening protocols there are no recommendations for avoiding contralateral suppression, that is, protecting the opposite ear from noise by blocking the ear canal. In the present study we have compared transient evoked and distortion product OAEs measured with and without contralateral ear plugging, in environmental settings with ambient noise levels <25 dB SPL, 45 dB SPL, and 55 dB SPL. We found out that without contralateral ear occlusion, ambient noise levels above 55 dB SPL can significantly attenuate OAE signals. We strongly suggest contralateral ear occlusion in OAE based hearing screening in noisy environments.

1. Introduction

Audiometric testing in general is best carried out in a low noise environment. Indeed most clinical testing is done in sound attenuating booths, where background noise levels are typically below 20 dB SPL (for frequencies of audiometric interest). For performing behavioral (pure tone and speech audiometry) and physiological tests (auditory evoked potentials and OAEs) the focus has been on maintaining a good signal to noise ratio for the test signals presented. The issue addressed in the present study pertains not to the test ear but to the contralateral ear that may or may not be occluded. In neonatal or newborn hearing screening with OAEs most protocols do not specify any occlusion or plugging of the nontest ear (e.g., [1–11]). However, such screening tests are routinely carried out in a noisy hospital or clinic environments. Newborn babies may be screened in patient's rooms, clinical areas, or a neonatal intensive care

unit (NICU), where ambient sound levels can be as high as 60–70 dB SPL (e.g., [12–16]). The American Academy of Pediatrics recommends that sound levels in an NICU should not exceed 45 dB, but most often this is not the case. Indeed a review by Konkani and Oakley reveals that ambient noise levels in typical NICUs can exceed 80 dB SPL [16].

It is now well established that OAEs—discovered by Kemp in 1978 [17]—are suppressed or modulated by acoustic signals presented to the contralateral ear. The role of the olivocochlear neural efferent system in inhibiting outer hair cell activity is well understood [18–24]. The consequent modulation of the outer hair cell mechanics and their contribution to OAE generation are the basis of clinical tests of the contralateral OAE suppression reflex [25–36].

The question posed in the present study is do ambient noise levels, typical of OAE screening environments, suppress OAEs in the test ear by stimulation of the contralateral, nonoccluded ear? In a sense the answer is already known

Differences in TEOAE with contralateral ear plugged or unplugged

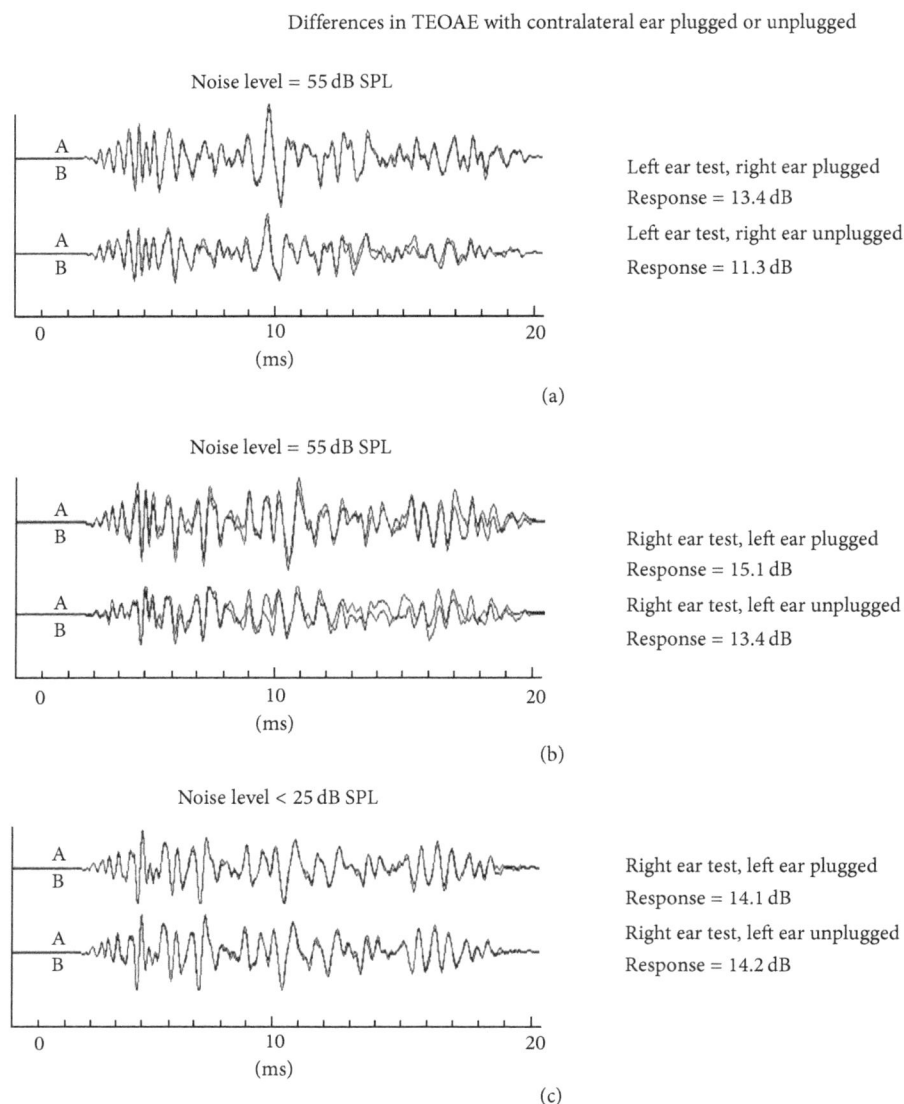

Noise level = 55 dB SPL

Left ear test, right ear plugged
Response = 13.4 dB

Left ear test, right ear unplugged
Response = 11.3 dB

(a)

Noise level = 55 dB SPL

Right ear test, left ear plugged
Response = 15.1 dB

Right ear test, left ear unplugged
Response = 13.4 dB

(b)

Noise level < 25 dB SPL

Right ear test, left ear plugged
Response = 14.1 dB

Right ear test, left ear unplugged
Response = 14.2 dB

(c)

FIGURE 1: Differences in TEOAE wave forms (ILO88 format) measured with contralateral ear canal plugged or open, in 55 dB SPL ambient noise level ((a) and (b)) versus noise levels <25 dB SPL (c). Data shown are from one subject.

in that numerous studies (as referenced above) have utilized contralateral sound stimuli to enable OAE suppression, which have stimulus levels that are similar to those of ambient noise. Furthermore, work including that by our own group [35] has clearly shown that OAE suppression is not a reflex with a defined threshold response. The efferent system enables OAE suppression with contralateral stimuli over a wide range of stimulus intensities. In other words acoustic signal levels constantly influence the system. We have chosen to "model" the situation of hearing screening testing in environments with different level of ambient noise.

2. Materials and Methods

2.1. Subjects and OAE Measurements. We tested 6 young adult females (18–24 yrs.) with normal audiograms and

robust OAEs (signals above noise, in the normal range and repeatable). OAE recordings were made in each individual ear ($N = 12$). Two OAE measurement methods were used. Transient evoked (TE) OAEs (ILO88 Otodynamics, Hatfield, UK) and distortion product (DP) OAEs (Vivo 600DPR; Vivosonic, Toronto, Canada). In each of the 4 acoustic environments (described below) TEOAE and DPOAE measures were repeated 3 times with and without occlusion of the contralateral ear. The ear canal was occluded with a standard memory foam earplug, and a circumaural headphone shell was also worn to achieve a combined attenuation greater than 40 dB. We measured TEOAEs to click stimuli (ILO88 default mode) and quantified using the average dB response. DPOAEs were measured in the form of a DPgram; $2f1\text{-}f2$ signal levels as a function of $f2$ frequency (0.25–6 kHz; e.g., Figure 3). These DPgrams were quantified by simple average of emission levels at all test frequencies.

TABLE 1: TEOAE data from six subjects comparing OAE levels with contralateral ear occluded versus open. *P* values of paired Student's *t*-test results and significance are indicated.

Subject	TEOAE (dB) contra ear plugged	TEOAE (dB) contra ear open	Difference (dB)	*P* value	Significance
		Noise level <25 dB SPL			
PAP	14.21	14.11	0.1	0.42	NO
ALL	9.42	9.3	0.12	0.629	NO
GLU	13.1	13.4	−0.3	0.471	NO
LAR	10.35	10.05	0.3	0.46	NO
HAR	5.08	4.86	0.21	0.15	NO
SKL	13.2	13.18	0.016	0.6109	NO
		Noise level c. 45 dB SPL			
PAP	14.59	13.62	0.96	0.003	**YES**
ALL	9.6	8.35	1.25	0.044	**YES**
GLU	13.22	12.28	0.93	0.112	NO
LAR	9.12	8.72	0.4	0.093	NO
HAR	5.75	5.6	0.13	0.604	NO
SKL	12.12	11.65	0.46	0.0004	**YES**
		Noise level 55 dB SPL			
PAP	13.98	12.88	1.1	<0.0001	**YES**
ALL	8.55	7.7	1.05	0.0085	**YES**
GLU	13.55	11.9	1.65	<0.0001	**YES**
LAR	8.78	7.9	0.88	0.151	NO
HAR	5.75	5.0	0.21	0.021	**YES**
SKL	12.28	11.92	0.366	0.0197	**YES**
		Babble level 55 dB SPL			
PAP	13.63	12.62	1.02	0.0113	**YES**
ALL	9.47	8.41	1.057	0.0036	**YES**
GLU	13.55	12.15	1.4	0.0002	**YES**
LAR	9.43	8.33	1.1	0.009	**YES**
HAR	5.95	5.38	0.56	0.035	**YES**
SKL	13.35	12.95	0.4	0.0015	**YES**

2.2. Acoustic Environments. (i) Control experiments were carried out in a sound attenuated booth (single wall ACO) with ambient sound levels below 25 dB SPL (100 Hz–16 kHz). (ii) Experiments were also made in the open laboratory environment, where ambient noise level was approximately 45 dB SPL. (iii) A study was made in noise-augmented environment in which white noise generation was adjusted to give an overall ambient noise level of 55 dB SPL. (iv) A recorded babble/shopping mall sound sample was used to provide a 55 dB SPL ambient noise that was more dynamic in character than the white noise augmented environment. In other words this background noise had significant temporal and spectral fluctuations. All acoustic signal levels were measured in free field at the level of the subject's head using a calibrated (B&K 4230, 94 dB 1 kHz) sound meter (Larson Davis 831) with half-inch condenser microphone (PCB Piezotronics). We used a linear (nonweighted) mode with a 100 Hz–16 kHz bandwidth.

2.3. Data Analysis. For each acoustic condition, TEOAE and DPOAE signals with and without plugging of contralateral ear are compared with a two tailed, paired Student's *t*-test, after confirmation of normal data distribution with Kolmogorov and Smirnov analysis.

3. Results

3.1. TEOAE Results. Figure 1 illustrates OAE waveforms evoked by broadband click stimuli in the ILO88 (Otodynamics) format; results are from one subject. Each data pair is a record made with and without contralateral ear plugging. The upper two data records were made in the environment with a 55 dB SPL ambient noise level. Note the attenuation of the wave forms in the nonplugged ear canal condition. In both cases the TEOAE response is decreased by almost 2 dB. The lower traces show control records in the sound booth; contralateral ear occlusion does not alter TEOAE response.

Table 1 lists, for all 6 subjects, the TEOAE levels (average of 3 repeat recordings) for the contralateral ear plugged and nonplugged conditions. The upper panel shows records made in the sound booth with ambient noise levels <25 dB SPL.

TEOAE with contralateral ear plugged versus open

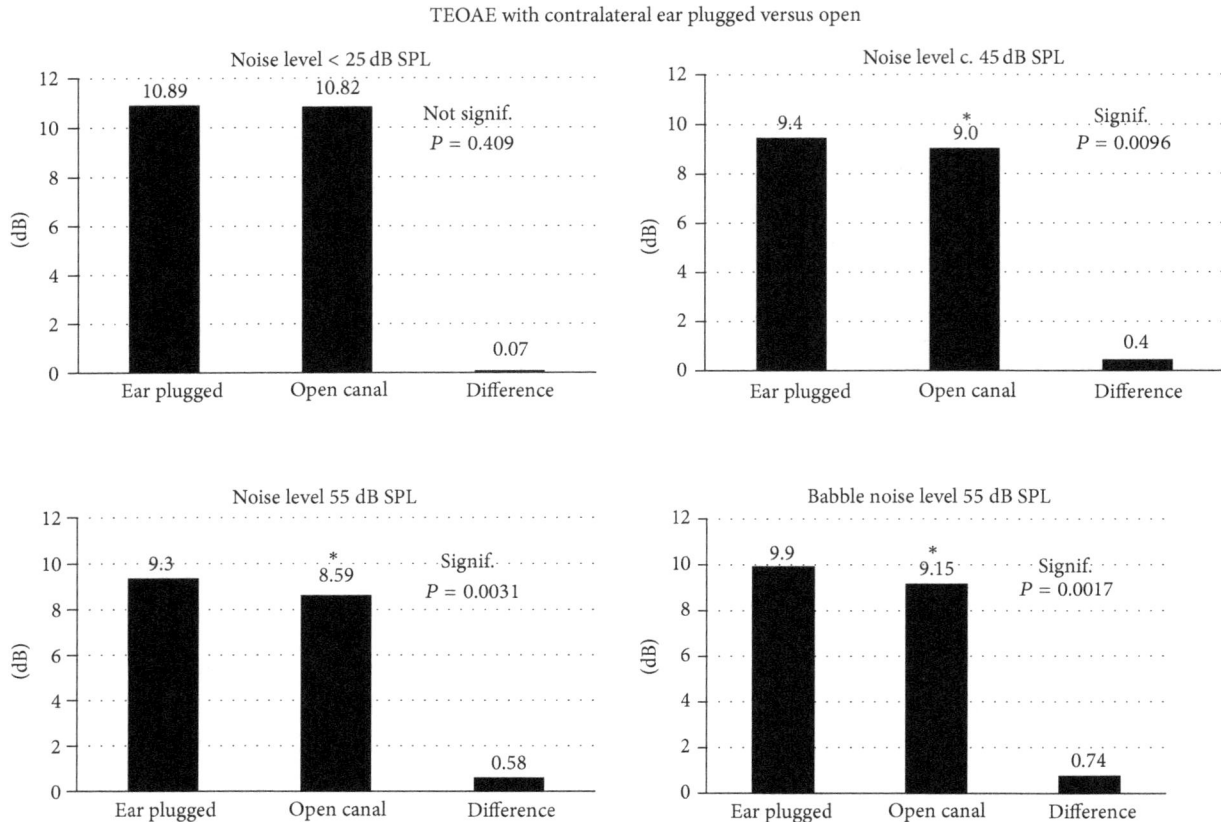

FIGURE 2: Plots of average DPOAE levels and the difference recoded with contralateral ear occluded or open ($N = 6$ subjects). Significance of the difference (paired Student's t-test) is indicated.

There are no significant differences between contralateral ear plugged versus open ear canal conditions. Significance and P values of paired t-test results are listed. The lower panels show comparisons in sound environments with noise levels at 45 dB SPL and in (white) noise and babble noise augmented environments (55 dB SPL). In the 45 dB SPL environment three subjects have statistically significant differences in OAE level with versus without opposite ear plugging. In the 55 dB SPL ambient noise environments all but one subject show significant differences between TEOAE levels with and without opposite ear occlusion. Figure 2 shows pooled subject data for each sound environment. Overall there is a significant difference in TEOAE levels for environments with ambient noise levels of 45 dB and above.

3.2. DPOAE Results. Figure 3 shows DPgrams for two subjects measured in an environment with ambient noise at 55 dB SPL. In each case the solid lines indicate DPOAE level measured with contralateral ears plugged versus unplugged (dashed lines). Note the suppression caused by the environmental noise, especially between 0.5 and 1 kHz, where the decrease in DPOAE level amounted up to 3 dB. Table 2 shows data from all 6 subjects. The 55 dB ambient environmental noise results in a significant contralateral suppression in only some subjects. However, it will be noted that the subjects with a significant suppression effect are those with an initially

higher level DPOAE (subject list in Table 2 is ordered according to DPOAE level). Furthermore, the P values for the paired t-test are mainly low hinting of an effect. Indeed an analysis of pooled results graphed in Figure 4 shows a very significant effect ($P < 0.0001$) of the 55 dB SPL environmental noise.

4. Discussion

There has been some considerable attention paid to the issue of ambient noise in environments in which OAE screening tests are carried out. The main concerns however have related to the test ear rather than the contralateral ear. Thus there is concern about the signal-to-noise ratio in the test ear that has to be high for getting a valid OAE response [37, 38]. The authors are unaware of studies that have considered the effects of ambient noise on the contralateral ear. As previously mentioned, there are no provisions or recommendations to use occlusion of the contra lateral ears in screening testing, and thus the contralateral suppression effects on test ear OAEs is an issue. The effects of contralateral acoustic stimulation on OAEs have been extensively documented in experimental studies, animal models, and clinical research. It is surprising therefore that these effects have not been seriously considered in newborn hearing screening protocols that employ OAE measures.

Average DPOAE grams with and without plugging of contralateral ear

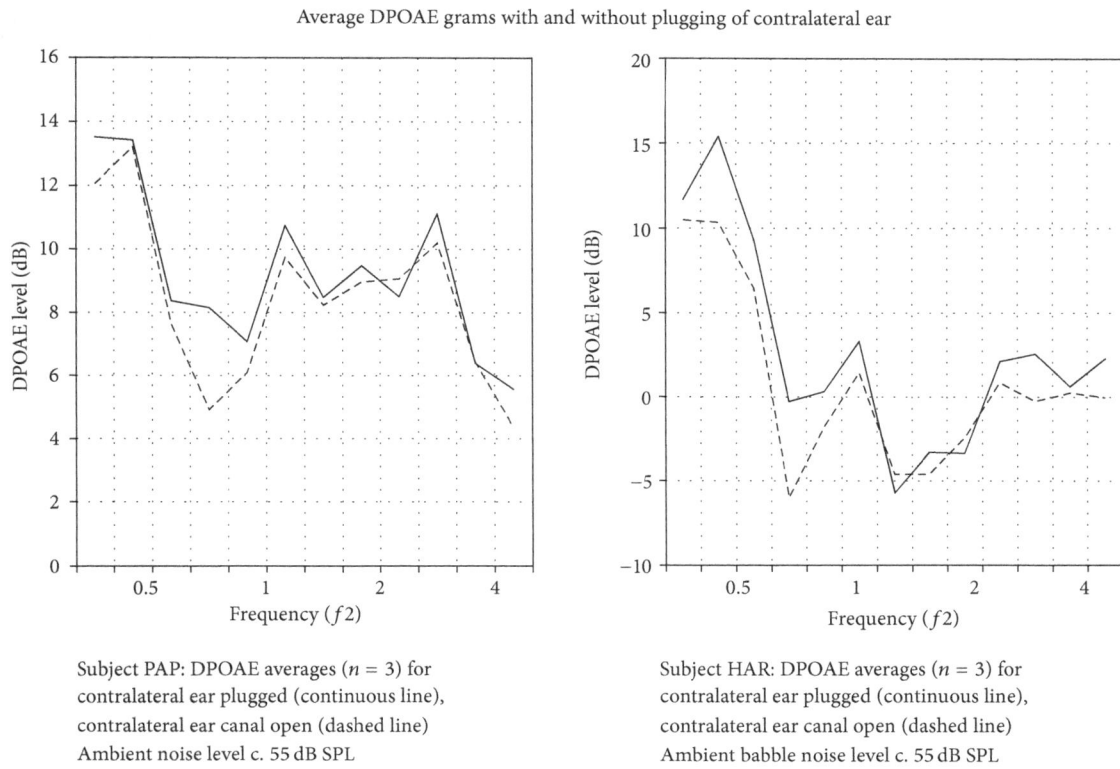

Subject PAP: DPOAE averages ($n = 3$) for
contralateral ear plugged (continuous line),
contralateral ear canal open (dashed line)
Ambient noise level c. 55 dB SPL

Subject HAR: DPOAE averages ($n = 3$) for
contralateral ear plugged (continuous line),
contralateral ear canal open (dashed line)
Ambient babble noise level c. 55 dB SPL

FIGURE 3: Example DPOAE ($2f1$-$f2$) versus frequency ($f2$) plots, DPgrams, for two subjects measured with (solid lines) and without (dashed curves) contralateral ear canal occlusion. Measurements were made in an environment with an ambient noise level of 55 dB SPL. DP grams shown are an average of three sequential recordings.

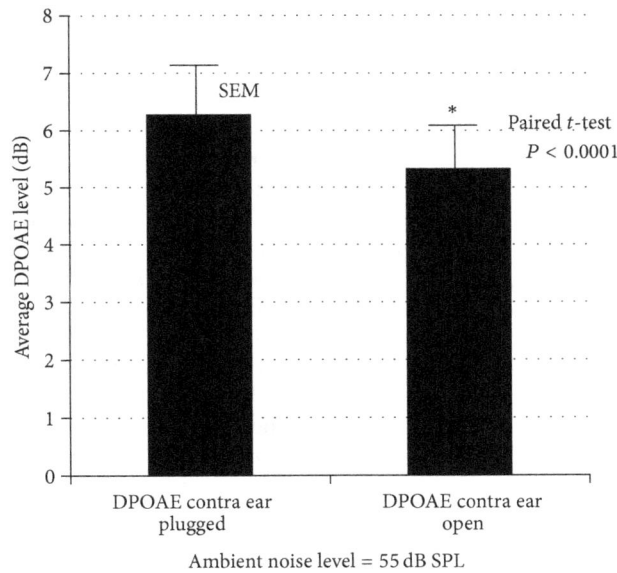

Ambient noise level = 55 dB SPL

FIGURE 4: Average DPOAE level changes between contralateral ear open versus occluded conditions, measured in an environment with an ambient noise level of 55 dB SPL. Significant difference as indicated by paired Student's t-test.

TABLE 2: DPOAE data from six subjects indicating OAE level recorded with and without occlusion of the contralateral ear in four different ambient sound environments. Results of Student's t-test are indicated.

Subject	DPOAE (dB) contra ear plugged	DPOAE (dB) contra ear open	Difference	P value	Significance
		Noise level <25 dB SPL			
PAP	10.76	10.77	−0.014	0.937	NO
DAV	9.73	9.66	0.07	0.88	NO
LAR	6.9	6.59	0.3	0.378	NO
ALL	4.38	4.3	0.087	0.625	NO
HAR	3.94	3.62	0.32	0.234	NO
GLU	2.8	1.64	1.165	0.105	NO
		Noise level c. 45 dB SPL			
DAV	12.56	12.39	0.168	0.457	NO
PAP	8.78	8.56	0.23	0.467	NO
LAR	6.9	6.37	0.53	0.351	NO
HAR	5.48	4.97	0.51	0.66	NO
ALL	5.21	4.58	0.63	0.323	NO
GLU	2.32	2.18	0.148	0.805	NO
		Noise level 55 dB SPL			
DAV	10.96	10.22	0.74	0.0861	**almost**
PAP	8.73	7.95	0.777	0.0995	**almost**
LAR	7.5	6.02	1.48	0.001	**YES**
HAR	5.68	4.37	1.31	0.153	NO
ALL	4.14	3.21	0.92	0.117	NO
GLU	3.23	2.39	0.84	0.2537	NO
		Babble level 55 dB SPL			
PAP	10.12	9.13	0.99	0.0061	**YES**
LAR	7.27	5.7	1.56	0.0481	**YES**
DAV	6.96	5.5	1.46	0.0054	**YES**
HAR	4.49	4.03	0.45	0.417	NO
ALL	4.62	3.39	1.23	0.165	NO
GLU	1.62	1.96	−0.34	0.627	NO

In the present study, we have tested the hypothesis that moderate levels of environmental noise can suppress OAE responses by activation of the olivocochlear efferent system. In the present study a level of 55 dB SPL has a significant effect. Given that most hospital ward and clinic environments have ambient noise levels higher than 55 dB SPL we conclude that, unless the untested ear is occluded, there will almost certainly be a suppression effect. It should be noted that clinical diagnostic OAE testing is almost always carried out in a low noise environment, typically in a sound attenuating booth. Here the problem of contralateral ear stimulation is negligible. However, in neonatal hearing OAE screening the availability of a sound booth or even a quiet environment is not a reality. It has been suggested that the olivocochlear efferent system is not fully matured or operational in a neonatal human subject, and therefore the precaution of occluding the contralateral ear is unnecessary. It has been reported that in some species efferent innervation is one of the final stages of cochlear maturation [39–41]. In the mouse, an altricious species, efferents do not fully connect with outer hair cells until postnatal day 20 [42]. However, the human is a precocious species with a much more mature peripheral auditory system at birth. There is some evidence that continued maturation of contralateral OAE suppression continues for some weeks after term birth [43]. However, a number of authors report that OAE suppression reflexes can be recorded in at term [36, 44, 45].

The results of this present study indicate that with a 55 dB ambient noise OAE levels can be attenuated by as much as 3 dB. It could be argued that such small attenuations will be of little significance in a screening test. However, it should be noted that this level of ambient noise is very low compared with that in a typical NICU or hospital clinic environment. Furthermore, 3 dB is a significant level change when the original OAE signal level may be of a similar order of magnitude. Will small OAE attenuations make a difference in a pass/refer (fail) screening paradigm? We suggest that it will definitely lead to more false positive results, and that means increasing parent anxiety and further healthcare costs.

5. Conclusion

In OAE screening tests, a nonoccluded contralateral ear will be stimulated by ambient environmental noise. Noise levels above 55 dB SPL can significantly suppress OAEs in the test ear and lead to false positive results. Such inaccuracy can be avoided by occlusion of the contralateral ear canal.

Conflict of Interests

The authors declare that there is no conflict of interests regarding the publication of this paper.

Acknowledgment

The Canadian Institutes of Health Research (CIHR) funded this study.

References

[1] American Academy of Pediatrics, Joint Committee on Infant Hearing, "Year 2007 position statement: principles and guidelines for early hearing detection and intervention programs," *Pediatrics*, vol. 120, no. 4, pp. 898–921, 2007.

[2] H. D. Nelson, C. Bougatsos, and P. Nygren, "Universal newborn hearing screening: systematic review to update the 2001 US preventive services task force recommendation," *Pediatrics*, vol. 122, no. 1, pp. e266–e276, 2008.

[3] W. D. Eiserman, D. M. Hartel, L. Shisler, J. Buhrmann, K. R. White, and T. Foust, "Using otoacoustic emissions to screen for hearing loss in early childhood care settings," *International Journal of Pediatric Otorhinolaryngology*, vol. 72, no. 4, pp. 475–482, 2008.

[4] T. Foust, W. Eiserman, L. Shisler, and A. Geroso, "Using otoacoustic emissions to screen young children for hearing loss in primary care settings," *Pediatrics*, vol. 132, no. 1, pp. 118–123, 2013.

[5] M. J. Barker, E. K. Hughes, and M. Wake, "NICU-only versus universal screening for newborn hearing loss: population audit," *Journal of Paediatrics and Child Health*, vol. 49, no. 1, pp. E74–E79, 2013.

[6] V. S. de Freitas, K. de Freitas Alvarenga, M. C. Bevilacqua, M. A. N. Martinez, and O. A. Costa, "Critical analysis of three newborn hearing screening protocols," *Pro-Fono*, vol. 21, no. 3, pp. 201–206, 2009.

[7] S. Hatzopoulos, J. Petruccelli, A. Ciorba, and A. Martini, "Optimizing otoacoustic emission protocols for a UNHS program," *Audiology and Neurotology*, vol. 14, no. 1, pp. 7–16, 2008.

[8] M. Ptok, "Fundamentals of hearing screening in neonates (standard of care)," *Zeitschrift fur Geburtshilfe und Neonatologie*, vol. 207, no. 5, pp. 194–196, 2003.

[9] S. Bansal, A. Gupta, and A. Nagarkar, "Transient evoked otoacoustic emissions in hearing screening programs-Protocol for developing countries," *International Journal of Pediatric Otorhinolaryngology*, vol. 72, no. 7, pp. 1059–1063, 2008.

[10] G. Pastorino, P. Sergi, M. Mastrangelo et al., "The Milan Project: a newborn hearing screening programme," *Acta Paediatrica*, vol. 94, no. 4, pp. 458–463, 2005.

[11] D. J. MacKenzie and L. G. U. Galbrun, "Noise levels and noise sources in acute care hospital wards," *Building Services Engineering Research and Technology*, vol. 28, no. 2, pp. 117–131, 2007.

[12] E. McLaren and C. Maxwell-Armstrong, "Noise pollution on an acute surgical ward," *Annals of the Royal College of Surgeons of England*, vol. 90, no. 2, pp. 136–139, 2008.

[13] W. B. Carvalho, M. L. G. Pedreira, and M. A. L. De Aguiar, "Noise level in a pediatric intensive care unit," *Jornal de Pediatria*, vol. 81, no. 6, pp. 495–498, 2005.

[14] J. L. Darbyshire and J. D. Young, "An investigation of sound levels on intensive care units with reference to the WHO guidelines," *Critical Care*, vol. 17, no. 5, p. R187, 2013.

[15] C. Tegnestedt, A. Günther, A. Reichard et al., "Levels and sources of sound in the intensive care unit—an observational study of three room types," *Acta Anaesthesiologica Scandinavica*, vol. 57, no. 8, pp. 1041–1050, 2013.

[16] A. Konkani and B. Oakley, "Noise in hospital intensive care units—a critical review of a critical topic," *Journal of Critical Care*, vol. 27, no. 5, pp. 522.e1–522.e9, 2012.

[17] D. T. Kemp, "Stimulated acoustic emissions from within the human auditory system," *Journal of the Acoustical Society of America*, vol. 64, no. 5, pp. 1386–1391, 1978.

[18] J. H. Siegel and D. O. Kim, "Effect neural control of cochlear mechanics? Olivocochlear bundle stimulation affects cochlear biomechanical nonlinearity," *Hearing Research*, vol. 6, no. 2, pp. 171–182, 1982.

[19] M. C. Liberman, "Rapid assessment of sound-evoked olivocochlear feedback: suppression of compound action potentials by contralateral sound," *Hearing Research*, vol. 38, no. 1-2, pp. 47–56, 1989.

[20] E. H. Warren III and M. C. Liberman, "Effects of contralateral sound on auditory-nerve responses. I. Contributions of cochlear efferents," *Hearing Research*, vol. 37, no. 2, pp. 89–104, 1989.

[21] M. C. Liberman, S. Puria, and J. J. Guinan Jr., "The ipsilaterally evoked olivocochlear reflex causes rapid adaptation of the 2f1-f2 distortion product otoacoustic emission," *Journal of the Acoustical Society of America*, vol. 99, no. 6, pp. 3572–3584, 1996.

[22] J. J. Guinan Jr., "Olivocochlear efferents: anatomy, physiology, function, and the measurement of efferent effects in humans," *Ear and Hearing*, vol. 27, no. 6, pp. 589–607, 2006.

[23] A. L. James, R. V. Harrison, M. Pienkowski, H. R. Dajani, and R. J. Mount, "Dynamics of real time DPOAE contralateral suppression in chinchillas and humans," *International Journal of Audiology*, vol. 44, no. 2, pp. 118–129, 2005.

[24] J. B. Mott, S. J. Norton, S. T. Neely, and W. B. Warr, "Changes in spontaneous otoacoustic emissions produced by acoustic stimulation of the contralateral ear," *Hearing Research*, vol. 38, no. 3, pp. 229–242, 1989.

[25] L. Collet, D. T. Kemp, E. Veuillet, R. Duclaux, A. Moulin, and A. Morgon, "Effect of contralateral auditory stimuli on active cochlear micro-mechanical properties in human subjects," *Hearing Research*, vol. 43, no. 2-3, pp. 251–261, 1990.

[26] J.-L. Puel and G. Rebillard, "Effect of contralateral sound stimulation on the distortion product 2F1-F2: evidence that the medial efferent system is involved," *Journal of the Acoustical Society of America*, vol. 87, no. 4, pp. 1630–1635, 1990.

[27] E. Veuillet, L. Collet, and R. Duclaux, "Effect of contralateral acoustic stimulation on active cochlear micromechanical properties in human subjects: dependence on stimulus variables," *Journal of Neurophysiology*, vol. 65, no. 3, pp. 724–735, 1991.

[28] A. Moulin, L. Collet, and R. Duclaux, "Contralateral auditory stimulation alters acoustic distortion products in humans," *Hearing Research*, vol. 65, no. 1-2, pp. 193–210, 1993.

[29] C. I. Berlin, L. J. Hood, A. Hurley, and H. Wen, "Contralateral suppression of otoacoustic emissions: an index of the function of the medial olivocochlear system," *Otolaryngology—Head and Neck Surgery*, vol. 110, no. 1, pp. 3–21, 1994.

[30] D. M. Williams and A. M. Brown, "The effect of contralateral broad-band noise on acoustic distortion products from the human ear," *Hearing Research*, vol. 104, no. 1-2, pp. 127–146, 1997.

[31] A. L. Giraud, J. Wable, A. Chays, L. Collet, and S. Chéry-Croze, "Influence of contralateral noise on distortion product latency in humans: is the medial olivocochlear efferent system involved?" *Journal of the Acoustical Society of America*, vol. 102, no. 4, pp. 2219–2227, 1997.

[32] S. Maison, C. Micheyl, G. Andéol, S. Gallégo, and L. Collet, "Activation of medial olivocochlear efferent system in humans: influence of stimulus bandwidth," *Hearing Research*, vol. 140, no. 1-2, pp. 111–125, 2000.

[33] A. L. James, R. J. Mount, and R. V. Harrison, "Contralateral suppression of DPOAE measured in real time," *Clinical Otolaryngology and Allied Sciences*, vol. 27, no. 2, pp. 106–112, 2002.

[34] J. J. Guinan Jr., B. C. Backus, W. Lilaonitkul, and V. Aharonson, "Medial olivocochlear efferent reflex in humans: otoacoustic emission (OAE) measurement issues and the advantages of stimulus frequency OAEs," *Journal of the Association for Research in Otolaryngology*, vol. 4, no. 4, pp. 521–540, 2003.

[35] R. V. Harrison, A. Sharma, T. Brown, S. Jiwani, and A. L. James, "Amplitude modulation of DPOAEs by acoustic stimulation of the contralateral ear," *Acta Oto-Laryngologica*, vol. 128, no. 4, pp. 404–407, 2008.

[36] A. L. James, "The assessment of olivocochlear function in neonates with real-time distortion product otoacoustic emissions," *Laryngoscope*, vol. 121, no. 1, pp. 202–213, 2011.

[37] J. T. Jacobson, "The effects of noise in transient EOAE newborn hearing screening," *International Journal of Pediatric Otorhinolaryngology*, vol. 29, no. 3, pp. 235–248, 1994.

[38] B. O. Olusanya, "Ambient noise levels and infant hearing screening programs in developing countries: an observational report," *International Journal of Audiology*, vol. 49, no. 8, pp. 535–541, 2010.

[39] A. Shnerson, C. Devigne, and R. Pujol, "Age-related changes in the C57BL/6J mouse cochlea. II. Ultrastructural findings," *Brain Research*, vol. 254, no. 1, pp. 77–88, 1981.

[40] D. D. Simmons, "Development of the inner ear efferent system across vertebrate species," *Journal of Neurobiology*, vol. 53, no. 2, pp. 228–250, 2002.

[41] A. V. Bulankina and T. Moser, "Neural circuit development in the mammalian cochlea," *Physiology*, vol. 27, no. 2, pp. 100–112, 2012.

[42] Y. Narui, A. Minekawa, T. Iizuka et al., "Development of distortion product otoacoustic emissions in C57BL/6J mice," *International Journal of Audiology*, vol. 48, no. 8, pp. 576–581, 2009.

[43] R. Chabert, M. J. Guitton, D. Amram et al., "Early maturation of evoked otoacoustic emissions and medial olivocochlear reflex in preterm neonates," *Pediatric Research*, vol. 59, no. 2, pp. 305–308, 2006.

[44] C. Abdala, E. Ma, and Y. S. Sininger, "Maturation of medial efferent system function in humans," *Journal of the Acoustical Society of America*, vol. 105, no. 4, pp. 2392–2402, 1999.

[45] T. Morlet, A. Hamburger, J. Kuint et al., "Assessment of medial olivocochlear system function in pre-term and full-term newborns using a rapid test of transient otoacoustic emissions," *Clinical Otolaryngology and Allied Sciences*, vol. 29, no. 2, pp. 183–190, 2004.

5

Sinus Fungus Ball in the Japanese Population: Clinical and Imaging Characteristics of 104 Cases

Kazuhiro Nomura,[1,2] **Daiya Asaka,**[1] **Tsuguhisa Nakayama,**[1] **Tetsushi Okushi,**[1] **Yoshinori Matsuwaki,**[1] **Tsuyoshi Yoshimura,**[1] **Mamoru Yoshikawa,**[1] **Nobuyoshi Otori,**[1] **Toshimitsu Kobayashi,**[2] **and Hiroshi Moriyama**[1]

[1] *Department of Otorhinolaryngology, Jikei University School of Medicine, 3-25-8 Nishishinbashi, Minato-ku, Tokyo 105-8461, Japan*
[2] *Department of Otolaryngology-Head and Neck Surgery, Tohoku University Graduate School of Medicine, 1-1 Seiryo-cho, Aoba-ku, Sendai, Miyagi 980-8574, Japan*

Correspondence should be addressed to Kazuhiro Nomura; kazuhiroe@gmail.com

Academic Editor: Jeffrey P. Pearson

Sinus fungus ball is defined as noninvasive chronic fungal rhinosinusitis occurring in immunocompetent patients with regional characteristics. The clinical and imaging characteristics of paranasal sinus fungus ball were retrospectively investigated in 104 Japanese patients. All patients underwent endoscopic sinus surgery. Preoperative computed tomography (CT), magnetic resonance (MR) imaging, age, sex, chief complaint, causative fungus, and clinical outcome were analyzed. Patients were aged from 25 to 79 years (mean 58.8 years). Female predominance was noted (58.7%). Most common symptoms were nasal discharge and facial pain. CT showed high density area in 82.0% of the cases (82/100), whereas T2-weighted MR imaging showed low intensity area in 100% of the cases (32/32). Histological examination showed that most causative agents were *Aspergillus* species (94.2% (98/104)). Culture test was positive for 16.7% (11/66). Recurrence was found in 3.2% (3/94). Older age and female predominance were consistent with previous reports. MR imaging is recommended to confirm the diagnosis.

1. Introduction

Fungal rhinosinusitis is encountered in about 10% of patients requiring surgery for diseases of the nose and sinuses, and fungal or mixed fungal and bacterial infections are responsible for 13.5% to 28.5% of all cases of maxillary sinusitis [1, 2]. Sinus fungus ball is a form of fungal sinusitis defined as noninvasive chronic fungal sinusitis without inspissated allergic mucin and occurs in immunocompetent hosts. The clinical condition now defined as "fungus ball" was previously called "mycetoma," "aspergillosis," or "aspergilloma," but better understanding of its pathophysiology has led to an update of terminology by recommending the use of the term "fungus ball" [1, 2]. Surgical treatment with the endoscope usually results in good outcome.

Several case series have been reported [2–6], but none in the Japanese population. Fungal infection is reported to have regional characteristics. Only 30 of 109 patients lived in urban areas with a population greater than 50,000 [5]. A study of the composition of the ambient air showed different fungus species present in France and the USA [7]. This study analyzed cases of sinus fungus ball in the Japanese population.

2. Materials and Methods

We retrospectively reviewed the clinical records of patients diagnosed with sinus fungus ball who underwent surgery at the Department of Otorhinolaryngology, Jikei University Hospital, Tokyo, Japan, between April 2005 and November 2010. The diagnosis was based on histological examination of the surgically removed material. Patients diagnosed with invasive fungal sinusitis or allergic fungal sinusitis (AFS) were excluded. We analyzed age, sex, chief complaint, location of the fungus ball, presence of high density area on computed

TABLE 1: Chief complaint.

Symptoms	N	(%)
Purulent nasal discharge	37	(35.6)
Facial pain	25	(24.0)
Post nasal drip	14	(13.5)
Facial discomfort	9	(8.7)
Nasal obstruction	4	(3.8)

TABLE 2: CT and MR imaging findings.

	N (%)
High density area on CT	82/100 (82%)
Low intensity area on T2-weighted MR imaging	32/32 (100%)

TABLE 3: Paranasal sinus localizations.

	N	(%)
Maxillary sinus	86	(82.7)
Sphenoid sinus	11	(10.6)
Maxillary sinus and ethmoid sinus	5	(4.8)
Maxillary sinus and sphenoid sinus	1	(1.0)
Ethmoid sinus	1	(1.0)
Total	104	(100)

TABLE 4: Histological examination of fungus ball.

	N	(%)
Aspergillus	98	(94.2)
Candida	3	(2.9)
Actinomycetes	1	(1.0)
Unable to differentiate	2	(1.9)
Total	104	(100)

TABLE 5: Culture study of fungus ball.

	N	(%)
Aspergillus sp.	10	(15.2)
Aspergillus sp. + Candida sp.	1	(1.5)
Negative	55	(83.3)
Total	66	(100)

The paranasal sinus localizations of fungus ball in the 104 patients are shown in Table 3. The most commonly involved sinus was the maxillary sinus (86/104, 82.7%) followed by the sphenoid sinus (11/104, 10.6%). Two patients had bilateral fungus ball in maxillary sinuses. Three patients with a history of transsphenoidal excision of pituitary macroadenoma had sphenoid fungus ball (3/11, 27.3%). Histological examination found that most of the fungus balls consisted of Aspergillus species (98/104, 94.2%) (Table 4). The sensitivity of culture study was low (11/66, 16.7%) (Table 5).

All cases were treated with endoscopic sinus surgery. The affected sinus was widely opened and the mass was meticulously removed. Edematous mucosa of the affected sinus was curetted leaving the basal membrane intact. The sinus was irrigated with normal saline according to the surgeon's preference.

Patients were instructed to perform nasal lavage with normal saline two times per day. The nasal cavity was examined with a rigid endoscope and secretions and crusts were cleaned at the outpatient department. Any small pieces of fungus ball in the operated sinus were removed immediately. Recurrence with occlusion of the operated sinus occurred in 3 (3.2%) of 94 patients who visited the outpatient clinic at least once.

4. Discussion

Sinus fungus ball is the most common form of fungal sinusitis. Fungal sinusitis is classified into two major categories, noninvasive fungal sinusitis and invasive fungal sinusitis [1, 8, 9]. Non-invasive fungal sinusitis is defined as absence of the fungal hyphae in the mucosa of the sinus and occurs in immunocompetent patients. This subtype is divided into fungus ball and AFS. Diagnosis of AFS is based on the detection of inspissated allergic mucin grossly at surgery. And histologically, the allergic mucin must be positive for fungal hyphae on fungal staining [10]. Invasive fungal sinusitis is defined as fungal sinusitis with mucosal infiltration of mycotic organisms and can be classified into three categories, granulomatous, acute fulminant, and chronic invasive, depending on the histological features [11, 12]. Invasive fungal sinusitis occurs in immunocompromised hosts or patients with diabetes mellitus, and the outcome is poor, especially for patients with the acute fulminant type.

Sinus fungus ball is mostly encountered in older individuals with the average age at presentation of 49 years ($n = 173$, France) [3], 52.7 years ($n = 160$, Italy) [2], and 61.1 years ($n = 90$, Taiwan) [6]. In our Japanese patients, the average age was 58.8 years ($n = 104$) with a range from 25 to 79 years. Female predominance has been consistent. The ratio of females is

tomography (CT), presence of low intensity area on T2-weighted magnetic resonance (MR) imaging, causative fungus, and surgical outcome. Good outcome is defined as opening of the operated sinus. Patients were followed up for 6 months postoperatively. The institutional review board of Jikei University School of Medicine approved the study.

3. Results

One hundred four patients aged 25 to 79 years (mean 58.8 years) were diagnosed with sinus fungus ball based on the histological findings. Female dominance was seen with 61 female patients (58.7%) and 43 male patients (41.3%). Major presenting symptom was purulent nasal discharge (35.6%) and facial pain (24.0%) (Table 1). CT was performed preoperatively for all cases, but complete data were available for only 100 cases. High density area in the affected sinus was seen in 82 cases (82%) (Table 2). Preoperative T2-weighted MR imaging was performed for 32 cases and showed low intensity area in the involved sinuses in all cases (100%) (Table 2).

(a)

(b)

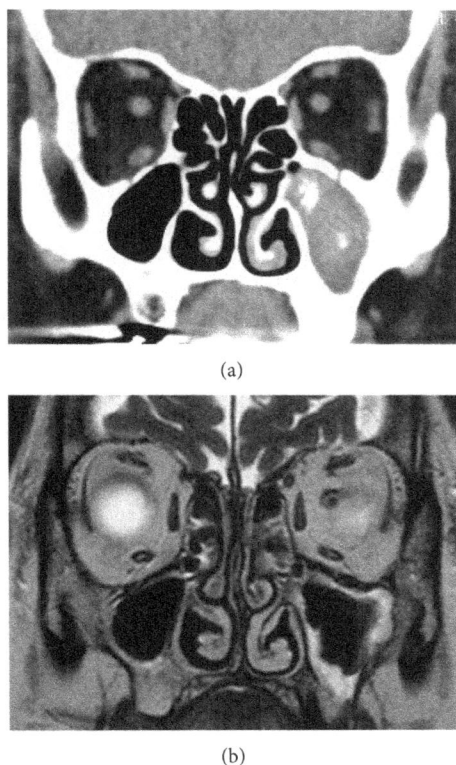

Figure 1: Typical neuroimaging findings of maxillary fungus ball. (a) Coronal CT scan with soft tissue density. Left maxillary sinus is completely filled with material. High density spots are seen. (b) Coronal T2-weighted MR image. Extremely low signal intensity to signal void indicates the presence of fungus ball. Peripheral high intensity area indicates edematous mucosa.

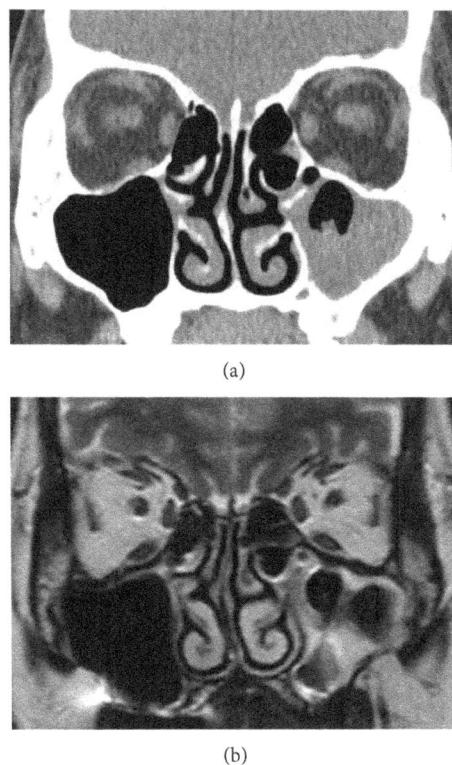

(a)

(b)

Figure 2: Representative case of fungus ball identifiable only on MR imaging. (a) Coronal CT scan with soft tissue density. Left maxillary sinus is filled with material. Irregular surface of the material suggests the possibility of fungus ball. High density spot is not seen. (b) Coronal T2-weighted MR image. Extremely low signal intensity to signal void indicates the presence of fungus ball.

60.1% (n = 173, France) [7], 66.1% (n = 109, France) [5], 73.8% (n = 160, Italy) [2], and 76.7% (n = 90, Taiwan) [6]. In this study, the ratio was 58.7%. The cause of female predominance remains unexplained but one possible reason is that fungus balls are more common in the older population and older women outnumber older men [13]. The life expectancy in the Japanese population was 79.6 years for males and 86.4 years for females in 2009 (http://www.mhlw.go.jp/toukei/saikin/hw/life/life09/sankou02.html). However, the numbers of male and female patients aged under 60 years in our series were the same (26 males and 26 females), so this idea is very plausible.

Common CT findings include the following: ipsilateral involvement; bony thickening of the diseased sinus wall; and hyperdense area within the lesion (Figure 1). This high density is the consequence of the high content of heavy metals (iron and manganese) and calcium within the fungal hyphae and is extremely specific but lacks sensitivity [14, 15]. In our series, CT showed high density mass in 82% of cases. Heavy metals and calcium appear as a very low signal intensity to signal void on T2-weighted MR imaging (Figure 2). In our series, sensitivity was 100% (n = 32). In contrast to the specificity of high density on CT, low signal intensity on T2-weighted MR imaging is not specific to fungus ball.

The signal patterns of eosinophilic mucin are similar to those of fungus ball. To distinguish fungus ball from eosinophilic chronic rhinosinusitis and AFS, the localization of the disease should be considered. Fungus ball is mostly isolated and unilateral, whereas eosinophilic chronic rhinosinusitis and AFS are diffuse and often associated with nasal polyp [14, 15]. Since the sensitivity of MR imaging was 100% in our series, we suggest that MR imaging is performed if CT demonstrates isolated and unilateral lesion without apparent calcification area.

In this study, the most common localizations were the maxillary sinus (82.7%) and the sphenoid sinus (10.6%) as in previous studies [2, 3, 5, 6]. The reason for this remains unexplained. Aerogenic theory suggests that the inhaled fungal spores are deposited in the sinuses, commonly the ethmoid sinus, and become pathogenic when the sinus begins to be anaerobic [2]. Fungal sinusitis may be regarded as a special form or complication of chronic recurring sinusitis [16]. However, ostiomeatal complex obstruction is not correlated with the growth of maxillary fungus ball which contradicts these hypotheses [17].

The causative fungus was mainly *Aspergillus* species, as shown by both histological examination and culture study as previously reported [2, 5, 7]. However, culture survey had extremely low sensitivity of 16.7%, as seen in previous studies ranging from 20.3% to 31.0% [2, 5, 7]. This difficulty in getting fungi to grow can be attributed to lack of viability of the fungus ball [13]. On the other hand, *Aspergillus* is a ubiquitous fungus found in nature. Culture of meticulously irrigated solutions of the noses of healthy people detected fungi in 100% of cases [18]. The value of culture study for the identification of fungus ball remains unclear.

The prognosis for sinus fungus ball is favorable. The reported recurrence rates are 0% ($n = 160$) [2], 0.6% ($n = 173$) [3], and 3.7% ($n = 109$) [5]. In our series, 3 of 94 patients (3.2%) had recurrence at 3, 5, and 6 months after operation. The recurrence was accompanied with occlusion of the operated sinus. Meticulous removal of the fungus ball, widening the drainage pathway, nasal irrigation at and after operation, and outpatient followup with endoscopic examination are necessary.

In conclusion, MR imaging provides high sensitivity but poor specificity for the identification of sinus fungus ball but is valuable for the investigation of undiagnosed cases detected with paranasal CT. The prognosis for fungus ball is very good, but recurrence is possible. Wide opening of the affected sinus and complete removal of the fungus ball are essential.

Conflict of Interests

There is no conflict of interests.

References

[1] P. Grosjean and R. Weber, "Fungus balls of the paranasal sinuses: a review," *European Archives of Oto-Rhino-Laryngology*, vol. 264, no. 5, pp. 461–470, 2007.

[2] P. Nicolai, D. Lombardi, D. Tomenzoli et al., "Fungus ball of the paranasal sinuses: experience in 160 patients treated with endoscopic surgery," *Laryngoscope*, vol. 119, no. 11, pp. 2275–2279, 2009.

[3] X. Dufour, C. Kauffmann-Lacroix, J. C. Ferrie, J. M. Goujon, M. H. Rodier, and J. M. Klossek, "Paranasal sinus fungus ball: epidemiology, clinical features and diagnosis. A retrospective analysis of 173 cases from a single medical center in France, 1989–2002," *Medical Mycology*, vol. 44, no. 1, pp. 61–67, 2006.

[4] J. A. Ferreiro, B. A. Carlson, and D. T. Cody III, "Paranasal sinus fungus balls," *Head and Neck*, vol. 19, no. 6, pp. 481–486, 1997.

[5] J.-M. Klossek, E. Serrano, L. Péloquin, J. Percodani, J.-P. Fontanel, and J.-J. Pessey, "Functional endoscopic sinus surgery and 109 mycetomas of paranasal sinuses," *Laryngoscope*, vol. 107, no. 1, pp. 112–117, 1997.

[6] J.-C. Lai, H.-S. Lee, M.-K. Chen, and Y.-L. Tsai, "Patient satisfaction and treatment outcome of fungus ball rhinosinusitis treated by functional endoscopic sinus surgery," *European Archives of Oto-Rhino-Laryngology*, vol. 268, no. 2, pp. 227–230, 2011.

[7] X. Dufour, C. Kauffmann-Lacroix, J.-C. Ferrie et al., "Paranasal sinus fungus ball and surgery: a review of 175 cases," *Rhinology*, vol. 43, no. 1, pp. 34–39, 2005.

[8] R. D. DeShazo, M. O'Brien, K. Chapin et al., "Criteria for the diagnosis of sinus mycetoma," *Journal of Allergy and Clinical Immunology*, vol. 99, no. 4, pp. 475–485, 1997.

[9] M. S. Schubert, "Fungal rhinosinusitis: diagnosis and therapy," *Current Allergy and Asthma Reports*, vol. 1, no. 3, pp. 268–276, 2001.

[10] M. S. Schubert, "Allergic fungal sinusitis: pathophysiology, diagnosis and management," *Medical Mycology*, vol. 47, supplement 1, pp. S324–S330, 2009.

[11] R. D. Deshazo, M. O'Brien, K. Chapin, M. Soto-Aguilar, L. Gardner, and R. Swain, "A new classification and diagnostic criteria for invasive fungal sinusitis," *Archives of Otolaryngology*, vol. 123, no. 11, pp. 1181–1188, 1997.

[12] K. Nakaya, T. Oshima, T. Kudo et al., "New treatment for invasive fungal sinusitis: three cases of chronic invasive fungal sinusitis treated with surgery and voriconazole," *Auris Nasus Larynx*, vol. 37, no. 2, pp. 244–249, 2010.

[13] B. J. Ferguson, "Fungus balls of the paranasal sinuses," *Otolaryngologic Clinics of North America*, vol. 33, no. 2, pp. 389–398, 2000.

[14] H.-J. Dhong, J.-Y. Jung, and J. H. Park, "Diagnostic accuracy in sinus fungus balls: CT scan and operative findings," *American Journal of Rhinology*, vol. 14, no. 4, pp. 227–231, 2000.

[15] R. Maroldi and P. Nicolai, Eds., *Imaging in Treatment Planning For Sinonasal Diseases*, Springer, Berlin, Germany, 2005.

[16] H. Stammberger, "Endoscopic surgery for mycotic and chronic recurring sinusitis," *The Annals of Otology, Rhinology & Laryngology*, vol. 119, pp. 1–11, 1985.

[17] T.-L. Tsai, Y.-C. Guo, C.-Y. Ho, and C.-Z. Lin, "The role of ostiomeatal complex obstruction in maxillary fungus ball," *Otolaryngology*, vol. 134, no. 3, pp. 494–498, 2006.

[18] J. U. Ponikau, D. A. Sherris, E. B. Kern et al., "The diagnosis and incidence of allergic fungal sinusitis," *Mayo Clinic Proceedings*, vol. 74, no. 9, pp. 877–884, 1999.

6

Internal Nasal Valve Incompetence Is Effectively Treated Using Batten Graft Functional Rhinoplasty

J. C. Bewick, M. A. Buchanan, and A. C. Frosh

Department of ENT, East and North Hertfordshire NHS Trust, Lister Hospital, Corey's Mill Lane, Stevenage SG1 4AB, UK

Correspondence should be addressed to A. C. Frosh; a.frosh@btinternet.com

Academic Editor: Angela Faga

Introduction. Internal nasal valve incompetence (INVI) has been treated with various surgical methods. Large, single surgeon case series are lacking, meaning that the evidence supporting a particular technique has been deficient. We present a case series using alar batten grafts to reconstruct the internal nasal valve, all performed by the senior author. *Methods.* Over a 7-year period, 107 patients with nasal obstruction caused by INVI underwent alar batten grafting. Preoperative assessment included the use of nasal strips to evaluate symptom improvement. Visual analogue scale (VAS) assessment of nasal blockage (NB) and quality of life (QOL) both pre- and postoperatively were performed and analysed with the Wilcoxon signed rank test. *Results.* Sixty-seven patients responded to both pre- and postoperative questionnaires. Ninety-one percent reported an improvement in NB and 88% an improvement in QOL. The greatest improvement was seen at 6 months (median VAS 15 mm and 88 mm resp., with a P value of <0.05 for both). Nasal strips were used preoperatively and are a useful tool in predicting patient operative success in both NB and QOL (odds ratio 2.15 and 2.58, resp.). *Conclusions.* Alar batten graft insertion as a single technique is a valid technique in treating INVI and produces good outcomes.

1. Introduction

Internal nasal valve incompetence (INVI) is an often overlooked cause of nasal obstruction which in turn can mistakenly be attributed to other anatomical variations such as septal deviation and turbinate hypertrophy. It is characterised by the collapse during inspiration of the upper lateral cartilages; a narrowing of the angle between the dorsal septum and upper laterals can also contribute but to a lesser extent. Functional rhinoplasty procedures for INVI have evolved over the past decade. A wide range of techniques exists in which surgeons use alar batten and/or spreader grafts, butterfly grafts, lateral crural strut grafts, alar rim grafts [1], and lateral suspension sutures. Alar batten grafts were first shown by Toriumi et al. [2] as an effective technique for correction of internal nasal valve collapse. Since then they have been widely used, but a reliable case series has yet to be published.

Case-based series assessing specific techniques are not widely available. When single-technique series are published, they often concentrate on the cosmetic outcomes. Series are usually small [3] and involve several operating surgeons [4] without specific outcomes. Recent papers have called for a single technique by a single operating surgeon to be assessed [5].

Predictors of which patients will benefit from alar batten graft functional rhinoplasty are also not well described. Without actively examining for INVI, a clinician may not identify the cause of symptoms which many patients find to have a considerable impact on their quality of life. Various scoring systems such as the NOSE scale do not specifically relate to the symptoms of INVI [6]. While clinicians could carry out rhinomanometry to assess the severity of INVI, how this relates to symptom improvement following an invasive procedure is not clear. As functional rhinoplasty procedures continue to grow, there is a need for a simple yet effective method for assessing patients preoperatively. We present a large case series of one specific technique, alar batten grafts, to treat INVI; this includes the use of nasal strips as a positive predictor in the success of surgery. All procedures were performed by the senior author with long-term followup.

2. Methods

One hundred and seven consecutive patients with INVI seen in the routine Ear, Nose, and Throat clinics of the East and North Hertfordshire NHS Trust district were included in this prospective study over a seven-year period. All patients were assessed pre-operatively by the senior author for clinical confirmation of INVI. This assessment included verification of nasal airflow restriction, worse on inspiration, in either newly presenting patients or those not previously improved by other surgical procedure(s). Patients were assessed for a positive Cottle's manoeuvre for evidence of INVI on inspiration. They were also assessed for airflow improvement after decongestion with xylometazoline 0.1% spray whereby those cases with nasal congestion secondary to inferior turbinate hypertrophy who improved with decongestion were excluded. Patients were asked to complete a pre-operative questionnaire detailing previous procedures, nasal trauma, and the use of nasal strips during pre-operative assessment.

All patients were asked to try adhesive nasal strips prior to surgery and asked if the strips had improved nasal breathing. This was not compulsory and therefore not all patients took part in this intervention.

Visual analogue scales (VAS) (0–100 mm) were used to assess the degree of nasal blockage (where 0 is the least possible blockage and 100 the worst possible) and quality of life (where 0 is "severe impact on quality of life" and 100 "excellent quality of life"). The scales were marked with the extreme of symptoms but not a numbered scale. This was completed at pre-operative assessment and then postoperatively at the appropriate follow-up appointments, at 1 week, 6 weeks, 6 months, and 12 months. Patients were seen at varying intervals depending on clinical need.

Pre- and post-operative VAS scores were evaluated. The Wilcoxon signed-rank test was used to assess the nonparametric data at the post-operative time intervals indicated above. Some patients were followed up for longer periods of time with the VAS but numbers were too low to be clinically relevant.

2.1. Operative Technique. It was the senior author's practice to use batten grafts only as the single method for correction of INVI. The aim of this technique was to strengthen the lateral walls, thus preventing internal nasal valve collapse, rather than increasing the cross-sectional space or reconstructing the external nasal valve. All patients were consented for functional rhinoplasty with graft harvesting from septal or auricular cartilage.

2.2. Preparation. Following preparation of the nose with Moffat's solution, a Killian's incision was made. Subsequent raising of the submucoperichondrial flaps allowed access to

the quadrilateral cartilage. If septal deviation was present, a septoplasty was performed to improve nasal patency. Cartilage was harvested via a standard submucous resection technique. The cartilage was assessed for size and quality intraoperatively and kept in 0.9% saline solution until required. If the amount of septal cartilage harvested was deemed insufficient in amount and/or quality, auricular cartilage was harvested instead. Conchal cartilage was obtained following marking the antihelical fold through the posterior aspect of the pinna with Bonney's blue ink applied with a 16 G gauge (green) needle. An incision was made on the posterior surface of the pinna along the line of the blue marks, conchal cartilage harvested, and the incision closed with dissolvable sutures.

2.3. Alar Batten Graft Insertion. Grafts were fashioned in strips from the harvested cartilage, measuring 12–20 mm by 6–8 mm. This was dependent on the dimension of the lateral nasal wall as evaluated by the senior author and also partially related to the quality of quadrilateral cartilage available. To raise pockets for graft insertion, an incision was made at the dorsal edge of the septum at the junction of the upper lateral cartilages (ULCs). The caudal edges of the ULCs were dissected just to the edge of the piriform aperture and a pocket fashioned. Following this, the cartilage grafts were adjusted to fit the dissected pockets within the "scroll" area between the ULCs and lateral crura of the lower lateral cartilages (see Figure 1). The scroll area itself is left intact with the graft laying cephalic to the s-shaped scroll. Once inserted, the grafts were secured with 5/0 Ethilon to the septum to prevent migration. The Killian's incision was closed with dissolvable sutures.

3. Results

One hundred and seven patients underwent functional rhinoplasty to treat INVI. Sixty-two patients were females.

Ninety-four patients (87.9%) responded to a pre-operative questionnaire. Eighty-five patients (79.4%) responded to post-operative questionnaires reevaluation of their symptoms using the exact VAS assessment tool used preoperatively. Post-operative followup (and repeat of VAS assessment) was performed according to patient clinical need, and hence patients were assessed at different post-operative time points. For those patients who completed both pre- and post-operative questionnaires (67 patients), 91% of patients reported long-term improvement in nasal blockage on VAS using the Wilcoxon signed-rank test; P values for this test can be seen in Table 1.

3.1. Improvement over Time. Nasal breathing: prior to surgery, the median VAS of nasal blockage (0 mm = no blockage, 100 mm = full blockage) was 73.5 (range 18–100). Post-operatively, this improved to 32 mm, 17 mm, 15 mm, 19 mm, and 25 mm for 1-week, 6-week, 6-month, 12-month and 18-month periods respectively (see Table 1 for ranges). This is displayed in Figure 2, and 3 patients felt there was a decline in nasal patency following surgery; 2 patients

TABLE 1: Nasal blockage and quality of life VAS scores with Wilcoxon signed-rank test P values. Eleven patients completed the questionnaire at both 6 and 12 months.

	Median nasal blockage VAS score in mm (range)	Nasal blockage P-value	Median overall quality of life VAS score in mm (range)	Quality of life P value (Wilcoxon signed-rank test)
Preoperatively ($n = 85$)	73.5 (18–100)		31 (3–87)	
1 week ($n = 18$)	32 (5–90)	<0.005	78 (4–96)	<0.005
6 weeks ($n = 53$)	17 (1–94)	<0.005	85 (3–100)	<0.005
6 months ($n = 29$)	15 (0–90)	<0.005	88 (16–100)	<0.005
12 months ($n = 27$)	19 (2–100)	<0.005	80 (20–100)	<0.005

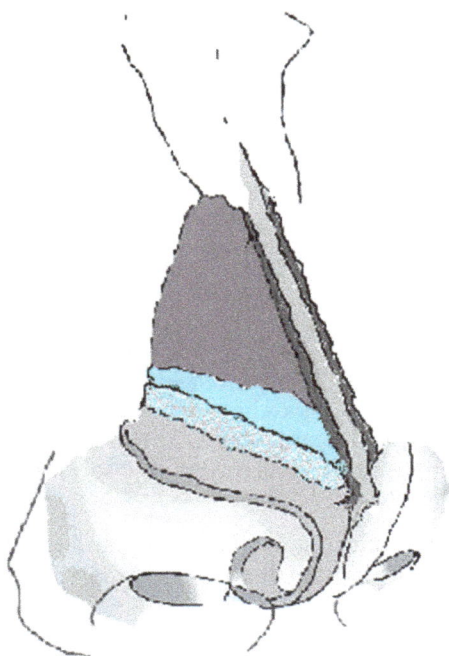

FIGURE 1: Alar batten graft insertion. The graft can be seen superficial and cephalic to the upper lateral cartilage thereby supporting the upper lateral cartilage and preventing collapse.

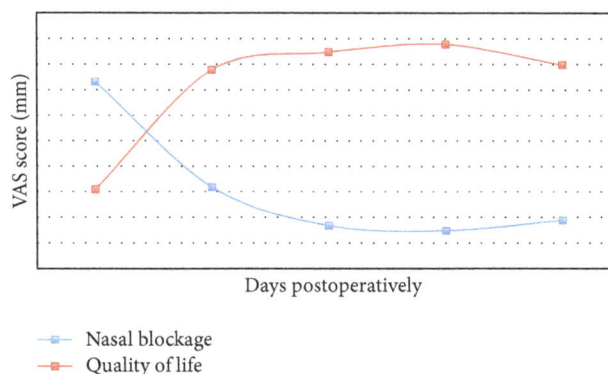

FIGURE 2: Median nasal breathing scores over time in months (0 = no patency, 100 = full patency) and quality of life scores over time (0 = severe impact on quality of life, 100 = no impact on quality of life).

experienced an initial improvement then decline. One patient experienced no change in symptoms.

Quality of life scores: similar to nasal patency scores, quality of life scores also improved post-operatively (albeit based on a slightly lower figure of 59 patients, 88%). The largest improvement was seen within the first 6 months following surgery. Two patients felt there was no improvement in QOL following surgery, 3 patients felt there was a decline, and 3 patients felt an initial improvement followed by decline.

3.2. Postoperative Complications. Of the 107 patients initially included in the study, one patient developed unsightly nostril asymmetry as a result of inadvertent hitching of the graft to the lower lateral cartilage necessitating a subsequent cosmetic surgical treatment. One patient developed a post-operative infection characterised by persistent pain and redness. This

settled with oral antibiotics. In 5 cases, the graft was seen to have resorbed significantly necessitating further surgery using auricular cartilage graft replacement for the original septal batten grafts; revision grafting was successful in all occasions. One patient required removal of the graft at a second procedure as the initial procedure had failed to improve nasal airflow and the graft was deemed unsightly.

3.3. Do Nasal Strips Predict Future Surgical Success? Following initial examination, patients were asked to try nasal strips prior to surgery. Fifty-four patients did so and of them 46 patients found that the nasal strips improved their symptoms. Following surgery, 49 patients within this group had improvement in post-operative "nasal blockage" scores (odds ratio 2.152 (95% confidence interval 0.303–4.001)). This was similar to "quality of life scores" with odds ratio of 2.580 (95% confidence interval 0.566–4.594).

4. Discussion

Alar batten grafting as a single procedure is a useful technique for treating INVI. The technique concentrates on improving the structural integrity of the internal nasal valve rather than increasing its cross-sectional area. This is thought to be the key in treating this condition [7] and probably accounts for the improvements in nasal obstruction score experienced by patients. Symptomatic INVI is due to significant collapse of the ULCs during nasal inspiration either during exercise or at rest. Alar batten grafts improve the rigidity of the ULCs preventing collapse during negative upper airway pressure during inspiration (with septoplasty where necessary, although all patients have undergone a degree of submucous resection for graft harvesting or during previous septal surgery at a separate date). As collapse of the internal nasal valve is a dynamic process, the alar batten graft is not required to improve the overall nasal patency.

Our study has provided evidence that the procedure is helpful to patients not only for short-term 6 weeks but also for longer periods of time. It is difficult within a busy NHS department (from which the majority of patients were recruited) to follow up NHS patients a long term due to a variety of factors the most important of which are demanding on-clinic follow-up slots, frequent change in clinical staff and patient migration to other areas. We readily admit that longer followup would be desirable but we feel that the current data as presented is at least useful. Another area for criticism is the use of a VAS to assess quality of life; while not recognised as a specific health utility to assess this aspect of surgical outcome, it does provide a useful insight into patient satisfaction in regard to their nasal surgery with minimal time input for the user. We felt that just assessing nasal blockage as the sole outcome would be too biased opinion in the technique and we wanted a more holistic view of outcomes but appreciated that patients did not always have time to complete lengthy questionnaires.

INVI has been treated with a range of different techniques. Several different types of grafts have been used such as lateral crural strut grafts and spreader grafts [1], sometimes in combination with alar batten grafts [8]. It is difficult to assess the effectiveness of alar batten graft placement alone. This paper allows evaluation of this single technique. The assessment of a single technique for purely functional reasons is not widely available. Graft insertion is often combined with other procedures such as inferior turbinate reduction [9] and can concentrate on cosmetic outcome rather than functional results [10] or the correction of external nasal valve correction. Further INVI surgery is often performed by several surgeons within an institution [11]. This case series adds valuable data to previously published work [5] and is one of the only case series performed by one operating surgeon. This provides consistency in technique unlike other series published.

Many patients presenting with INVI have had previous nasal surgery with unsuccessful results/outcomes. We feel that this is often due to mis-diagnosis leading to unsatisfactory outcomes following routine nasal procedures. We would advise clinicians to include Cottle's manoeuvre when performing routine examination of the nose for nasal obstruction although it should only be used in quiet inspiration as applicable to routine respiration. We would advise this during general inspection of the nose and prior to decongestion with xylometazoline spray. In our experience, patients with INVI often find immediate relief during this manoeuvre although it can be nonspecific and should not be used as the sole basis for recommending surgery for INVI.

Nasal strips are a useful positive predictor of those who will benefit from alar batten grafts. By using nasal strips in pre-operative assessment, the clinician can identify those patients who will improve both in terms of nasal obstruction and in quality of life (odds ratio 2.15 and 2.58, resp.). Ideally all patients in our study would have used the strips but as these are not provided on the NHS and come therefore at the patients' own cost, we did not insist on patients' participation. Gruber et al. have documented the use of nasal strips to evaluate "inspiratory nasal function" [12] but to our knowledge the relationship between this and post-operative outcomes has not previously been documented. With such a simple, noninvasive test, clinicians now have an excellent diagnostic tool in the investigation of such patients.

5. Conclusions

(i) Clinicians should use Cottle's manoeuvre to examine all patients with nasal obstruction prior to application of nasal decongestants but must recognise that its results are user dependent and that oversupporting the upper lateral cartilages will give a false impression of possible surgical outcomes.

(ii) Alar batten graft to provide structural integrity of the internal nasal valve is a reliable technique with good outcomes in both nasal patency and quality of life scores. This technique has been refined by the senior author and shows that alar batten grafts alone (rather than in combination with spreader grafts) are adequate.

(iii) Improvement in nasal patency with nasal strips is a good predictor of those patients who will benefit from alar batten grafting.

References

[1] D. W. Kim and K. Rodriguez-Bruno, "Functional rhinoplasty," *Facial Plastic Surgery Clinics of North America*, vol. 17, no. 1, pp. 115–131, 2009.

[2] D. M. Toriumi, J. Josen, M. Weinberger, and M. E. Tardy Jr., "Use of alar batten grafts for correction of nasal valve collapse," *Archives of Otolaryngology*, vol. 123, no. 8, pp. 802–808, 1997.

[3] B. Millman, "Alar batten grafting for management of the collapsed nasal valve," *Laryngoscope*, vol. 112, no. 3, pp. 574–579, 2002.

[4] J. S. Rhee, D. M. Poetker, T. L. Smith, A. Bustillo, M. Burzynski, and R. E. Davis, "Nasal valve surgery improves disease-specific quality of life," *Laryngoscope*, vol. 115, no. 3, pp. 437–440, 2005.

[5] P. M. Spielmann, P. S. White, and S. S. M. Hussain, "Surgical techniques for the treatment of nasal valve collapse: a systematic review," *Laryngoscope*, vol. 119, no. 7, pp. 1281–1290, 2009.

[6] M. G. Stewart, D. L. Witsell, T. L. Smith, E. M. Weaver, B. Yueh, and M. T. Hannley, "Development and validation of the Nasal Obstruction Symptom Evaluation (NOSE) scale," *Otolaryngology*, vol. 130, no. 2, pp. 157–163, 2004.

[7] S. M. Weber and S. R. Baker, "Alar cartilage grafts," *Clinics in Plastic Surgery*, vol. 37, no. 2, pp. 253–264, 2010.

[8] M. M. Khosh, A. Jen, C. Honrado, and S. J. Pearlman, "Nasal valve reconstruction: experience in 53 consecutive patients," *Archives of Facial Plastic Surgery*, vol. 6, no. 3, pp. 167–171, 2004.

[9] S. P. Most, "Analysis of outcomes after functional rhinoplasty using a disease-specific quality-of-life instrument," *Archives of Facial Plastic Surgery*, vol. 8, no. 5, pp. 306–309, 2006.

[10] D. R. Byrd, C. C. Otley, and T. H. Nguyen, "Alar batten cartilage grafting in nasal reconstruction: functional and cosmetic results," *Journal of the American Academy of Dermatology*, vol. 43, no. 5, part 1, pp. 833–836, 2000.

[11] V. Cervelli, D. Spallone, J. D. Bottini et al., "Alar batten cartilage graft: treatment of internal and external nasal valve collapse," *Aesthetic Plastic Surgery*, vol. 33, no. 4, pp. 625–634, 2009.

[12] R. P. Gruber, A. Y. Lin, and T. Richards, "Nasal strips for evaluating and classifying valvular nasal obstruction," *Aesthetic Plastic Surgery*, vol. 35, no. 2, pp. 211–215, 2011.

7

HPV Prevalence and Prognostic Value in a Prospective Cohort of 255 Patients with Locally Advanced HNSCC: A Single-Centre Experience

E. Thibaudeau,[1] B. Fortin,[2] F. Coutlée,[3] P. Nguyen-Tan,[4] X. Weng,[5] M.-L. Audet,[5] O. Abboud,[1] L. Guertin,[1] A. Christopoulos,[1] J. Tabet,[1] and D. Soulières[5,6]

[1] Department of Head and Neck Surgery, Centre Hospitalier de l'Université de Montréal, Hôpital Notre-Dame, 1560 Sherbrooke Est, Montreal (Quebec), Canada H2L 4M1

[2] Department of Radiation Oncology, Hôpital Maisonneuve-Rosemont, 5415 Boulevard de l'Assomption, Montréal (Quebec), Canada H1T 2M4

[3] Department of Microbiology, Centre Hospitalier de l'Université de Montréal, Hôpital Notre-Dame, 1560 Sherbrooke Est, Montreal (Quebec), Canada H2L 4M1

[4] Department of Radiation Oncology, Centre Hospitalier de l'Université de Montréal, Hôpital Notre-Dame, 1560 Sherbrooke Est, Montreal (Quebec), Canada H2L 4M1

[5] Department of Haematology and Medical Oncology, Centre Hospitalier de l'Université de Montréal, Hôpital Notre-Dame, 1560 Sherbrooke Est, Montreal (Quebec), Canada H2L 4M1

[6] Laboratoire de Biologie Moléculaire et Hématologie Spéciale, Département d'Hématologie, Hématologue et Oncologue Médical, Centre Hospitalier de l'Université de Montréal, Hôpital Notre-Dame, 1560 Sherbrooke Est, Montreal (Quebec), Canada H2L 4M1

Correspondence should be addressed to D. Soulières; denis.soulieres.chum@ssss.gouv.qc.ca

Academic Editor: David W. Eisele

Background. HPV is a positive prognostic factor in HNSCC. We studied the prevalence and prognostic impact of HPV on survival parameters and treatment toxicity in patients with locally advanced HNSCC treated with concomitant chemoradiation therapy. *Methods.* Data on efficacy and toxicity were available for 560 patients. HPV was detected by PCR. Analysis was performed using Kaplan-Meier survival curves, Fisher's test for categorical data, and log-rank statistics for failure times. *Results.* Median follow-up was 4.7 years. DNA extraction was successful in 255 cases. HPV prevalence was 68.6%, and 53.3% for HPV 16. For HPV+ and HPV−, median LRC was 8.9 and 2.2 years ($P = 0.0002$), median DFS was 8.9 and 2.1 years ($P = 0.0014$), and median OS was 8.9 and 3.1 years ($P = 0.0002$). Survival was different based on HPV genotype, stage, treatment period, and chemotherapy regimen. COX adjusted analysis for T, N, age, and treatment remained significant ($P = 0.004$). *Conclusions.* Oropharyngeal cancer is increasingly linked to HPV. This study confirms that HPV status is associated with improved prognosis among H&N cancer patients receiving CRT and should be a stratification factor for clinical trials including H&N cases. Toxicity of CRT is not modified for the HPV population.

1. Introduction

Tobacco and alcohol consumption has long been known as the major risk factor for HNSCC. However, HPV has recently been recognised to play a role in the pathogenesis of a subset of clinically and molecularly distinct HNSCC, most often located in the oropharynx and associated with wild-type p53 and downregulation of cyclin D and retinoblastoma protein pRb [1–5], and in which viral oncoproteins E6 and E7 play a crucial part [6].

HPV prevalence in HNSCC has been increasing significantly in the past few decades [5, 7]; it is estimated at 25% in HNSCC [8], but reaches up to 70% or more in tonsillar SCCs [9–11]. Unlike the HPV-negative oropharyngeal cancers, the HPV-positive subset is not associated with tobacco or alcohol use, but with certain types of sexual behaviours [12, 13]. The HPV 16 subtype is present in up to 90% of HPV-related oropharyngeal cancers, while HPVs 18, 31, and 33 have been identified in the remainder [14, 15]. HPV has recently been recognised as a good prognostic factor in head and neck (H&N) cancer [5, 16–26], which has been attributed to several mechanisms, including absence of field cancerisation and increased sensitivity to chemoradiation therapy [5, 16, 20, 22–24, 26].

Most of the available data is derived from small randomised trials with different treatment options or small heterogeneous cohorts; moreover, data were often collected retrospectively. Even though one prospective clinical trial concluded with the same prognostic advantage [16], other favourable prognostic factors associated with HPV positivity, such as younger age or early tumour stages, could not be ruled out entirely. The study presented here evaluates the prevalence and prognostic impact of HPV on overall survival (OS), disease-free survival (DFS), local-regional control (LRC), and treatment toxicity, in a large cohort of consecutive patients with locally advanced HNSCC, treated with concomitant platinum-based chemoradiation therapy (CRT) and followed prospectively. A more specific focus is placed on oropharyngeal squamous cell carcinoma, as previous literature has demonstrated that the prognostic impact of HPV is most important in this subsite, which also represents the largest group in our HNSCC population.

2. Materials and Methods

2.1. Study Design and Eligibility. The present series comprises cases from patients participating in an ongoing tumor bank of patients treated for HNSCC at CHUM Hôpital-Notre-Dame since 1998. Eligibility criteria included locally advanced HNSCC and treatment with primary chemoradiation and with a minimal followup of three years. Surgical treatment preceding chemoradiation was the main exclusion criterion. Data were collected prospectively from a regular assessment of outcome variables such as response rates, local or regional recurrences, and survival rates by means of regular clinical and radiological evaluations. All patients had histological confirmation of SCC based on histological features in hematoxylin and eosin-stained tissue sections diagnosed by a pathologist experienced in head and neck pathology. Staging was performed according to the TNM classification system from clinical and radiological assessment.

2.2. Patient Population. All patients with locally advanced HNSCC stage III-IVA-IVB treated with radical radiation therapy (min 7000cGY standard fractionation or altered fractionation) and concurrent chemotherapy (Cisplatin 100 mg/m^2 q 3 weeks × 3 or Carboplatin 70 mg/m^2 d1-4 + 5-FU 600 mg/m^2 d1-4 q 3 weeks × 3 or Cisplatin 6 mg/m^2 daily or Carboplatin 25 mg/m^2 daily) were included in this analysis. Patients were secondarily selected based on the availability of tumor samples (cf. Table 1).

2.3. Sample Preparation. Three to eight sections of 10 μm were obtained from each tumor. To avoid cross-contamination during sectioning, disposable microtome blades were used, and the microtome was cleaned after cutting each specimen. Biopsy specimens were fixed in 10% formalin solution and processed according to conventional methods for paraffin-embedded histological sections for routine diagnosis.

2.4. Overview. Prior to HPV detection, samples underwent PCR for detection of β-globin using the PCO4/GH2O method (268-base pair primers) to control for DNA integrity and for the absence of competing inhibitors.

Samples were then tested for the presence of HPV DNA using the Roche Linear Array detection method (LA-HPV) (primers 450 bp).

Samples that tested negative for HPV-DNA with the LA-HPV technique were tested using the GP5+/GP6+ PCR detection method (primers 150 bp).

Samples that tested negative for both HPV-DNA and β-globin with the LA-HPV detection method, and also negative for HPV DNA using the GP5+/GP6+ technique, were also tested for the presence of β-globin using PCO3/PCO4 probes (110 bp) to ensure that negative results were not caused by excessive DNA fragmentation due to extended preservation in paraffin.

2.5. DNA Extraction. Paraffin-embedded samples were heated to 72°C and washed with xylene for two minutes, four times. The samples were then submitted to four one-minute washes with ethanol 100% and four one-minute washes with ethanol 95%. Remaining tissue was then incubated in 200 μL lysis buffer (10 mM tris-HCl, pH 8.0, 1 mM EDTA, pH 8.0, and 20 mM NaCl) containing 0.2 mg/mL proteinase K for 2 hours at 55°C. The mixture was then heated at 96°C for 5 minutes in order to inactivate proteinase K. Optic density was calculated for the supernate after having centrifuged the mixture at 12000 G for 20 minutes. Tubes were then stored at −4°C.

2.6. PCO4/GH2O PCR. Amplification of a β-globin gene fragment was performed by the use of PCO4 and GH2O primers to control for target DNA integrity.

PCR products were separated by electrophoresis on a 2% ethidium-stained agarose gel and visualised on a UV transilluminator. Samples generating a visible 268-base pair band were judged suitable for detection of HPV DNA using the LA-HPV method [27], which includes detection of β-globin using the PCO4/GH2O method.

2.7. LA-HPV. As previously described [28] PCR was performed in a final reaction volume of 100 μL with 5 μL of sample material and 95 μL of kit working master mix (containing MgCl$_2$, KCl, AmpliTaq, gold DNA polymerase (AmpliTaq; Perkin-Elmer; Foster City, CA), uracil-N-glycosylase, dATP, dCTP, dGTP, dUTP, dTTP, and biotinylated PGMY primers and β-globin primers GH2O and PCO4). Test tubes were incubated in a TC 9700 thermal cycler set at maximum ramp

TABLE 1: Patient characteristics according to HPV status.

Patient characteristic	Number of patients			
	HPV+	HPV−	P	Total
Number of patients	175	80		
Age (years)				
Median	55.42	59.56	t-test $P = 0.0086$	57.00
Range	25.25–75.03	39.64–78.72		25.25–78.72
T ($n = 255$)				
T1	36 (20.57%)	7 (8.75%)		43 (16.86%)
T2	39 (22.29%)	17 (21.25%)		56 (21.96%)
T3	48 (27.43%)	26 (32.50%)	Fisher $P = 0.0203$	74 (29.02%)
T4	51 (29.14%)	25 (31.25%)		76 (29.80%)
TX	0	1 (1.25%)		1 (0.39%)
Recurrence	1 (0.57%)	4 (5.00%)		5 (1.96%)
N ($n = 254$)*				
N0	15 (8.62%)	11 (13.75%)		26 (10.24%)
N1	25 (14.37%)	10 (12.50%)		35 (13.78%)
N2	0	1 (1.25%)		1 (0.39%)
N2a	27 (15.52%)	10 (12.50%)	Fisher $P > 0.1$	37 (14.57%)
N2b	42 (24.14%)	16 (20.00%)		58 (22.83%)
N2c	36 (20.69%)	22 (27.50%)		58 (22.83%)
N3	29 (16.67%)	10 (12.50%)		39 (15.35%)
TNM stage ($n = 255$)				
I	0	0		0 (0%)
II	0	2 (2.5%)		2 (0.78%)
III	24 (13.71%)	11 (13.75%)	Fisher $P > 0.1$	35 (13.73%)
IVa	117 (68.86%)	49 (61.25%)		166 (65.10%)
IVb	30 (17.14%)	14 (17.50%)		44 (17.25%)
Recurrence	4 (2.29%)	4 (5.00%)		8 (3.14%)
KPS ($n = 212$)*				
60	1 (0.67%)	0		1 (0.47%)
70	3 (2.00%)	1 (1.61%)		4 (1.89%)
80	30 (20.00%)	11 (17.74%)	Fisher $P = 0.1$	41 (19.34%)
90	99 (66.00%)	49 (79.03%)		148 (69.81%)
100	17 (11.33%)	1 (1.61%)		18 (8.49%)
Chemotherapy ($n = 254$)*				
Daily Carboplatin or Cisplatin	17 (9.71%)	10 (12.66%)		27 (10.63%)
Daily Carboplatin + 5FU	113 (64.57%)	33 (41.77%)	Fisher $P = 0.00061$	146 (57.48%)
Cisplatin q 1 week or q 3 weeks	45 (25.71%)	36 (45.57%)		81 (31.89%)
Radiotherapy ($n = 254$)*				
Conventional	143 (82.18%)	77 (96.25%)	Fisher $P = 0.0017$	220 (86.28%)
IMRT	31 (17.82%)	3 (3.75%)		34 (13.33%)
Primary ($n = 255$)				
Oropharynx	137 (78.29%)	32 (40.00%)		169 (66.27%)
Larynx	14 (8.00%)	18 (22.50%)		32 (12.54%)
Oral cavity	9 (5.14%)	16 (20.00%)		25 (9.80%)
Hypopharynx	6 (3.43%)	9 (11.25%)	Fisher $P < 0.0001$	15 (5.88%)
Nasopharynx	6 (3.43%)	2 (2.50%)		8 (3.14%)
Paranasal sinuses	2 (1.14%)	1 (1.25%)		3 (1.18%)
Nose	1 (0.57%)	1 (1.25%)		2 (0.78%)
Unknown	0	1 (1.25%)		1 (0.39%)

*Indicates missing data.

speed for 2 minutes at 50°C and 9 minutes at 95°C, followed by 40 cycles of 30 seconds at 95°C, 1 minute at 55°C, and 1 minute at 72°C, with a final extension at 72°C (ramp set at 50%) for 5 minutes.

Negative and positive controls were included for each reaction.

Amplicons were denatured in 0.4 N NaOH and hybridise to an immobilised probe array containing probes for 37 HPV genotypes (according to the protocol provided by Roche Molecular Systems).

Following the hybridization reaction, Linear Array HPV Genotyping Strips were stringently washed to remove unbound material, and positive hybridization reactions were detected by streptavidin-horseradish peroxidase-mediated color precipitation on the membrane at the probe line.

The probe for detection of HPV 52 amplicons was a cross-reactive probe that also hybridised with types 33, 35, and 58; samples positive with the HPV 52 probe and containing at least one of those types were thus also tested with a real-time PCR assay specific for HPV 52 (see below). Only samples positive for HPV 52 with real-time PCR were considered HPV 52 positive.

2.8. Real-Time PCR Assay for HPV 52. As described previously [28], $20\,\mu L$ reaction mixtures contained 10 mM tris-HCl; pH 8.0; 50 mM KCl; a $200\,\mu M$ concentration of (each) ATP, dGTP, and dCTP; $400\,\mu M$ dUTP; $0.05\,\mu M$ of TaqMan probe 52-TM (CGTGCAGGGTCCGGGGTC); 0.3 pmol each of primers 52JA-3 (GAACACAGTGTAGCTAACGCACG) and 52JA-4 (GCATGACGTTACACTTGGGTCA) (targeting the E6 gene); 2.0 mM $MgCl_2$; and 5 units of Ampli*Taq* gold DNA polymerase. Capillaries were placed in a LightCycler system (Roche Molecular Systems; Branchburg, NJ, USA) and amplified at 95°C for 10 minutes, followed by 50 cycles at 95°C for 15 seconds and 60°C for 60 seconds. Ten copies of an HPV 52-expressing plasmid in 500 ng of cellular DNA served as a weak positive control.

2.9. GP5+/GP6+ PCR. The primers used for HPV PCR were a single pair of consensus GP5+/GP6+ (150 bp), as previously described [4]. PCR was carried out in a reaction volume of $50\,\mu L$ containing 50 mM KCl, 10 mM Tris HCl (pH 8.3), $200\,\mu M$ each deoxynucleoside triphosphate, 3.5 mM $MgCl_2$, 1 unit of thermostable DNA polymerase (Ampli*Taq*; Perkin-Elmer; Foster City, CA), and 50 pmol each of the GP5+ (5′-TTTGTTACTGTGGTAGATACTAC-3′) and GP6+ (3′-CTTATACTAAATGTCAAATAAAAAG-5′) primers. Samples were denatured for 4 minutes at 94°C and then underwent 40 cycles of amplification with a PCR processor (PE9600; Perkin-Elmer). Each cycle consisted of a denaturation step (1 minute at 94°C), a primer annealing step (2 minutes at 40°C), and a chain elongation step (1.5 minute at 72°C). Complete extension of amplified DNA was ensured by prolongation of the final elongation step by 4 minutes [29].

Negative and positive controls were included for each reaction.

PCR products were layered on 1.5% agarose gel and transferred onto positively charged nylon membranes (Qiabrane; Westburg) by diffusion blotting in 0.5 N NaOH-0.6 M NaCl.

DNA purification by gel extraction was done for samples that tested weakly positive.

A BLAST search was performed to assign sequences to known HPV types.

2.10. Gel Extraction Protocol. Gel extraction was performed with the QIAquick Gel Extraction Kit (Qiagen Inc., Valencia, CA), according to the supplied protocol. Briefly, DNA fragments were excised from the agarose gel with a clean, sharp scalpel. Gel slices were weighed in a colorless tube, and 3 volumes of buffer QG were added to 1 volume of gel. Gel was then dissolved via incubation at 50°C for 10 minutes. DNA was bound to the supplied column by centrifugation for 1 minute followed by discarding of flow-through. 0.5 of buffer QG was added to each sample, and flow-through discarded once more after centrifugation for 1 minute. 0.75 mL of buffer PE was added to the column and flow-through discarded after centrifugation for further washing. Columns were centrifuged again at 17,900 ×g and DNA was eluded by addition of $50\,\mu L$ of elution buffer (10 mM tris-Cl, pH 8.5) to the central membrane of the column followed by centrifugation for 1 minute.

2.11. Statistical Analysis. Locoregional control (LRC) was defined as time elapsed between initial diagnosis and development of recurrent locoregional disease. Overall survival (OS) was defined as time elapsed between diagnosis and death from any cause, and disease-free survival was defined as time from initial diagnosis to tumour recurrence.

Statistical analysis was performed using Fisher's test for categorical data and Kaplan-Meier's curves and log-rank statistics for disease-free survival, overall survival and locoregional control according to HPV status (and HPV genotype), treatment period, chemotherapy regimen, TNM stage, tumour site, and patient age. Multivariate analysis using COX models was used to adjust for imbalances in the aforementioned prognostic factors between groups. Fisher's exact test was also performed to determine the difference in acute toxicities (cutaneous toxicity, mucitis, nausea, and vomiting, as well as grade 3-4 neutropenia) according to HPV status.

Smoking status was excluded from our analyses because the data were inconsistently recorded in our database.

This protocol was approved by our institution's ethics committee.

3. Results

3.1. Patient Characteristics. Prospective data on efficacy and toxicity was available for 560 patients treated with concomitant CRT. All patients had histological confirmation of SCC based on histological features in hematoxilin and eosin-stained tissue sections diagnosed by a pathologist experienced in head and neck pathology. From these 560 patients, 270 fixed and paraffin-embedded specimens were collected. Sufficient tissue for DNA extraction was present in 255 samples.

Of these 255 patients, 79.61% ($n = 203$) were male and 20.39% ($n = 52$) female. Patient characteristics are listed in

Table 1. Two hundred and ten (82.25%) initially presented with stage IV cancers. Primary tumour sites are listed in Table 1; the oropharynx was the most common primary site, comprising 66.27% of cases. HPV prevalence was 68.6% and 53.3% for HPV 16 specifically in our patient population.

Median followup was 4.69 years.

3.2. HPV Testing. Prior to HPV DNA detection, 26 samples underwent PCR for detection of β-globin using the PCO_4/GH_2O method (also included in the LA-HPV Detection kit) to ensure that DNA suitable for detection with the LA-HPV method was present, and to control for the absence of competing inhibitors. 24 samples tested positive for β-globin.

Combining the results of HPV DNA detection with the LA-HPV and GP5+/GP6+ detection methods, 175 samples (68.63%) tested positive for HPV DNA. HPV 16 was identified in 138 samples (78.86%).

255 samples were tested for the presence of HPV DNA using the LA-HPV detection method. Of these, 127 samples tested positive for the presence of HPV DNA. HPV 16 was the only genotype in 109 samples; coinfection was found in 6 samples. Among theses, coinfection with HPV 16 and HPV 18 was present in 3 cases; the others were co-infected with HPV 16 and HPV 84 ($n = 1$), HPV 16 and HPV 11 ($n = 1$), and HPV 33 and HPV 35 ($n = 1$). The other genotypes detected were HPV 18 ($n = 4$), HPV 33 ($n = 3$), HPV 35 ($n = 3$), HPV 26 ($n = 1$), and HPV 58 ($n = 1$).

The 128 samples that tested negative for HPV DNA with the LA method were tested for the presence of HPV DNA using the GP5+/GP6+ detection method, using a set of shorter primers (150 bp), to ensure that negative results were not caused by excessive DNA fragmentation due to prolonged preservation in paraffin. 48 samples tested positive for the presence of HPV DNA. DNA was present in sufficient amounts to be submitted for sequencing in 24 samples, for which a BLAST search was performed to assign sequences to known HPV types. HPV 16 was identified as the single genotype present in all 24 samples.

Among the 128 samples that tested negative for HPV DNA using the LA-HPV detection method, 27 were judged invalid as β-globin was not detected by the test, suggesting that the samples did not contain DNA suitable for analysis. Of these 27 samples, 16 also tested negative for HPV DNA using the GP5+/GP6+ detection method; these samples were tested for the presence of β-globin using PCO_3/PCO_4 probes (110 bp). All 16 tested positive for β-globin, confirming that negative results were unlikely to result from excessive DNA fragmentation.

3.3. Survival According to TNM Stage. Overall survival was statistically significantly different based on TNM (log-rank $P = 0.0017$; cf. Figure 1); OS was also statistically significant according to T (log-rank $P < 0.0001$) and N (log-rank $P = 0.0112$) separately.

DFS and LRC were also significantly different according to TNM ($P = 0.0046$ and $P = 0.0150$, resp.).

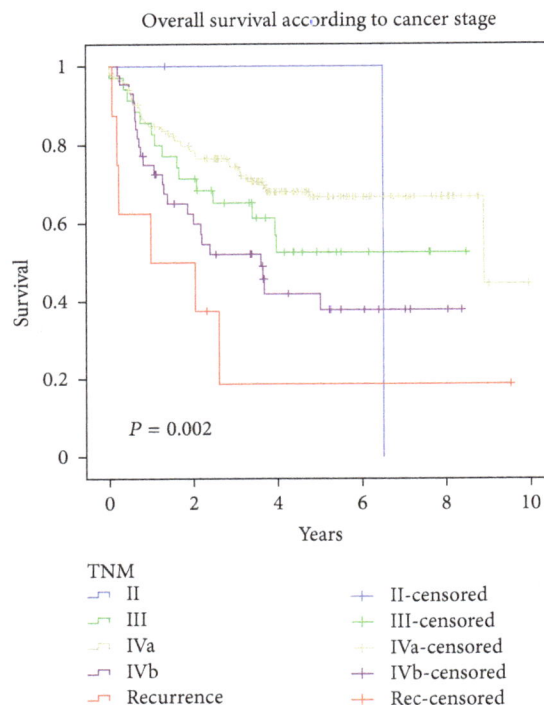

FIGURE 1: Overall survival according to TNM.

3.4. Survival According to HPV by Primary Subsite. Overall survival was not statistically significantly different according to primary site ($P = 0.187$; cf. Figure 2), nor was LRC ($P = 0.0651$). This is probably related to the fact that many cancer subsites were rare in our population. We therefore decided not to conduct a statistical analysis of interaction using the terms "primary site * HPV status." However, within the largest subgroup of patients suffering from oropharyngeal HNSCC, survival was significantly different according to HPV positivity ($P = 0.002$). Patients with HPV− oropharyngeal SCC had a median overall survival of 2.46 years, while median survival was not reached at a minimum of 4.63 years of followup for HPV-positive patients (cf. Figure 3).

3.5. Efficacy Parameters According to HPV Status. For HPV+ and HPV− cases, respectively, median overall survival was 8.89 and 3.09 years ($P = 0.0002$) (cf. Figure 4). This trend was also observed, and statistically significant, for HPV 16+ versus HPV 16− cases (log-rank $P = 0.0005$). Since there were statistically significant differences between the HPV+ and HPV− populations, a COX analysis adjusting for age, T, N, and treatment period (i.e., before and after 2001) and regimen was conducted and showed that the difference in overall survival remained significant (HR = 0.45; 95%CI = [0.289, 0.701]; $P = 0.0004$).

Disease-free survival (DFS) for HPV+ and HPV− cases was 8.89 years and 2.10 years, respectively (log-rank $P = 0.0014$). For HPV 16+ cases specifically and HPV 16− cases, respectively, median DFS was 8.89 and 3.53 years (log-rank $P = 0.0010$).

HPV Prevalence and Prognostic Value in a Prospective Cohort of 255 Patients with Locally Advanced...

41

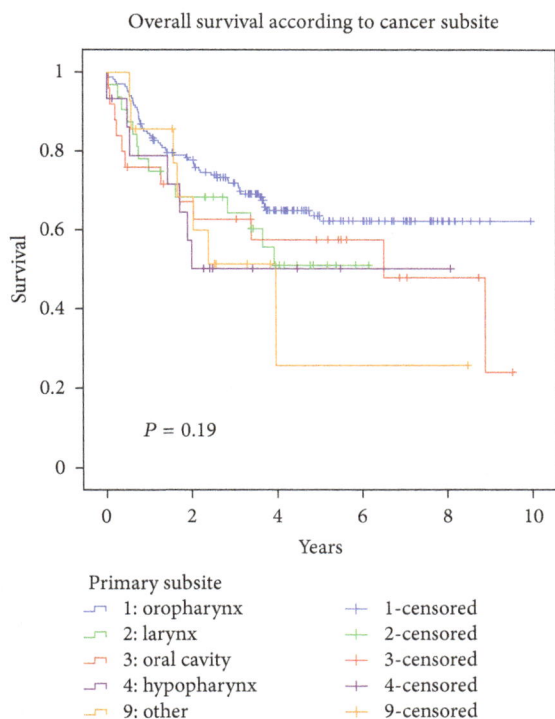

FIGURE 2: Overall survival according to primary subsite.

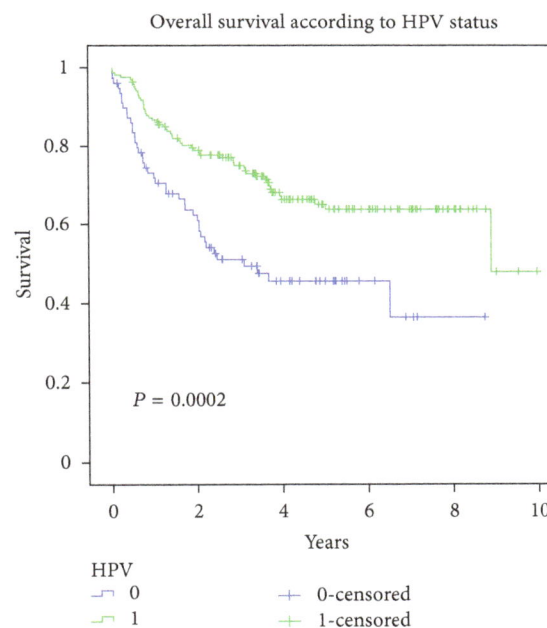

FIGURE 3: Overall survival for oropharyngeal primaries according to HPV status.

As for OS, the difference in DFS remained significant after adjustment for T, N, age, and treatment period and regimen (HR = 0.52; 95% CI = [0.333, 0.818]; P = 0.0048).

LRC for HPV-negative and HPV-positive cases was 2.17 years and 8.89 years, respectively (P = 0.0002). For HPV 16-negative cases, median LRC was 3.09 years, while it was not reached for HPV 16-positive cases (P = 0.0001). This persisted on multivariate analysis (HR = 0.44; 95% CI = [0.289, 0.679]; P = 0.0002).

There was no statistically significant difference in acute treatment-related toxicity between the two groups in the thirty days following treatment (data not shown). Toxic effects that were evaluated included cutaneous toxicities, mucitis, nausea and vomiting, need for gavage, grade 3-4 neutropenia, per-treatment hospitalisation, and per-treatment deaths.

3.6. Survival Based on HPV Genotype. Overall survival, DFS, and LRC were statistically significantly different based on HPV genotype (log-rank P = 0.0013, P = 0.0061, and P = 0.0008, resp.; cf. Figure 5) but this was essentially driven by the large differences between the HPV16 positive group compared to the HPV-negative group, with the other subgroups being small.

3.7. Survival According to Chemotherapy Regimen. Overall survival was statistically significantly different based on chemotherapy regimen (P < 0.0001; cf. Figure 6).

For patients receiving high-dose chemotherapy, that is, concurrent chemotherapy (Cisplatin 100 mg/m^2 q 3 weeks × 3

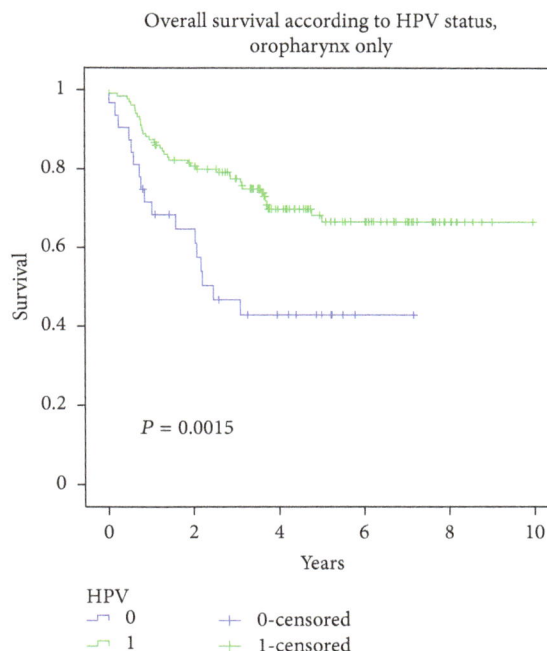

FIGURE 4: Overall survival according to HPV status.

or Carboplatin 70 mg/m^2 d1-4 + 5-FU 600 mg/m^2 d1-4 q 3 weeks × 3) median overall survival was 8.89 years; while median OS was 2.04 years for patient receiving low-dose (Cisplatin 6 mg/m^2 daily or Carboplatin 25 mg/m^2 daily), chemotherapy.

Overall survival according to HPV genotype

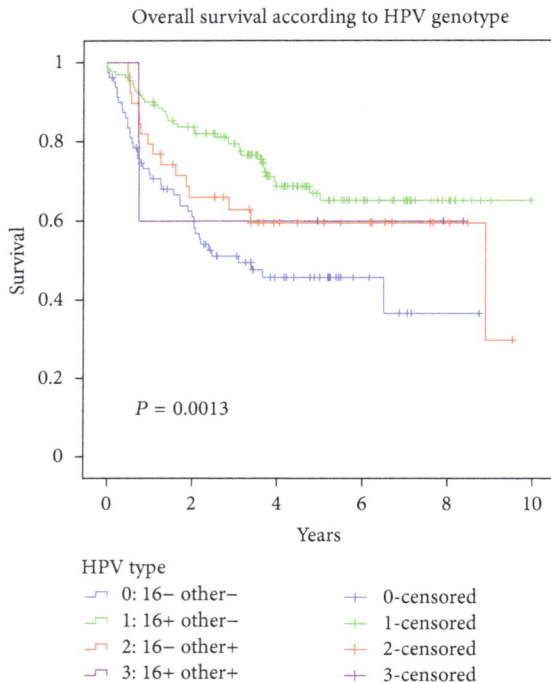

$P = 0.0013$

HPV type
- 0: 16– other–
- 1: 16+ other–
- 2: 16– other+
- 3: 16+ other+
- 0-censored
- 1-censored
- 2-censored
- 3-censored

FIGURE 5: Overall survival according to HPV genotype.

Overall survival according to chemotherapy intensity

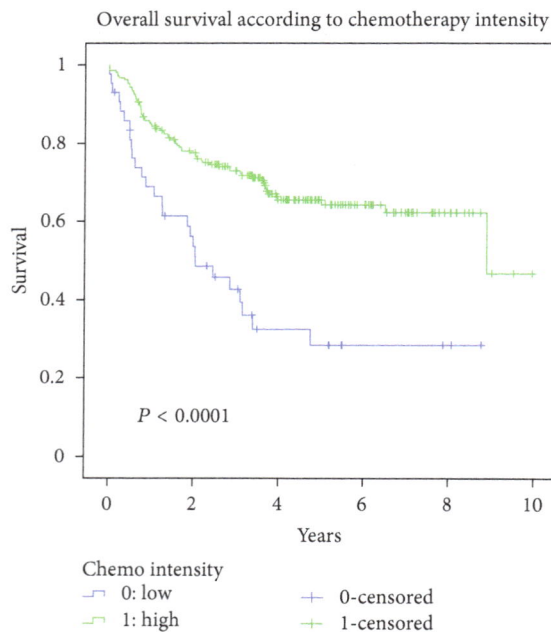

$P < 0.0001$

Chemo intensity
- 0: low
- 1: high
- 0-censored
- 1-censored

FIGURE 6: Overall survival according to chemotherapy regimen.

DFS was also 8.89 years for patients receiving high-dose chemotherapy and 1.63 years for patients receiving low-dose chemotherapy ($P = 0.0001$).

Median LRC was 8.89 years and 1.92 years for patients receiving high- and low-dose chemotherapy, respectively ($P < 0.0001$).

HPV subgroup remains a statistically significant predictor of survival even in the high-dose chemotherapy group (which includes most of the cohort) with a median OS of 6.5 years in the high-dose chemotherapy HPV-negative group compared to a median OS not reached in the high-dose chemotherapy HPV-positive subgroup ($P = 0.0006$). This effect was present although not statistically significant in the low-dose chemotherapy, probably due to the small number of patients in that subgroup ($n = 43$).

Treatment regimen was modified from low-dose chemotherapy to high-dose chemotherapy in 2001; our results also show that OS, DFS, and LRC are statistically significantly different according to treatment period, that is, before and after 2001 (data not shown).

4. Discussion

Previous studies have reported improved outcomes in HPV-associated oropharyngeal cancer [5, 18, 30, 31], but need to be interpreted with caution as samples were often small, comprised patients who were not treated in a uniform fashion, and data were often collected retrospectively. Our data confirm the improved outcomes in terms of OS, DFS, and LRC for patients with HPV-positive HNSCC observed in retrospective studies. Moreover, our analysis confirms the prognostic impact of HPV positivity because treatment was similar for all patients in our cohort. HPV can thus be seen as strong positive prognostic factor even though no specific mechanism has been identified to explain higher rates of response to chemoradiation in spite of genetically distinct characteristics [32]. HPV-positive HNSCC patients seem to experience greater local-regional control; this could be due to a higher intrinsic sensitivity to radiation or better radiosensitisation with cisplatin. However, HPV-positive HNSCCs demonstrate a favourable prognosis regardless of treatment modality (surgery, radiation therapy, concurrent chemoradiation as in this study, or induction chemotherapy plus concurrent chemoradiation therapy) [5, 6, 22–24, 33]. This is consistent with the theory that HPV-positive and -negative tumours are different biological entities [34].

HPV prevalence may have been underestimated in our trial because of the reduced sensitivity of PCR in FFPE samples [35]. However, previous studies have demonstrated that a higher sensitivity was achieved by using PCR for HPV detections than that with other methods such as ISH or p16 immunohistochemistry [25, 36], though the gold standard for defining a tumour as being associated with HPV remains the detection of expression of HPV oncogenes E6 and E7 [32, 37].

Other studies have suggested that the biological behaviour of HPV-positive tumours may be altered by tobacco use [3, 4], possibly because these tumours are at higher risk for both local recurrence and distant metastases [38]. Indeed, genetic mutations induced by tobacco-related carcinogens may render HPV-positive tumours less responsive to therapy [39]. Previous studies have also demonstrated that tobacco smoking was associated with overall survival, and progression-free survival, with risks of death and cancer recurrence increasing for each additional pack-year of tobacco smoking; this effect has been shown to be similar for patients with HPV-positive and HPV-negative cancers [26]. These data were however excluded from our study as smoking status was inconsistently recorded in our database.

An increasing proportion of oropharyngeal cancer is linked to HPV, which, along with tobacco use, is the strongest independent determinant of OS in OSCC patients treated with chemoradiotherapy [26, 39]. Though our results are consistent with an increased response to chemoradiation therapy in HPV-positive HNSCC, our data neither confirm nor infirm that HPV-related HNSCC can be treated with a less stringent therapy and do not necessarily represent evidence for a difference in natural history between HPV-negative and HPV-positive cancers in the absence of treatment. A combination of tumour HPV status, pack-years of tobacco smoking, and cancer stage could be used to classify patients' risk of death [26].

In this cohort, treatment with 3-week high-dose chemotherapy proved to be more advantageous. This regimen is the most widely used chemotherapy regimen in combination with radiotherapy [40, 41]. Previous studies on daily low-doses (i.e., conventional doses) have led to mitigated outcomes, with results less conclusive than those using the cisplatin 100 mg/m^2 regimen (for a cumulative dose of 300 mg/m^2) [41, 42]. Treatment regimen was modified from low-dose chemotherapy to high-dose chemotherapy in our centre in 2001; our results also show that OS, DFS, and LRC are statistically significantly different according to treatment period, that is, before and after 2001 (data not shown).

This large study, with a cohort from one centre, confirms that HPV status is strongly associated with improved prognosis among H&N cancer patients receiving CRT and should be a stratification factor for all clinical trials including HNSCC cases. Separate trials in HPV-positive and HPV-negative oropharyngeal cancers will be needed to device the optimal treatment for each of these distinct entities, with the focus in HPV-positive cancers being to determine whether a decrease in treatment intensity and consequential toxicity can be achieved without compromising currently achieved outcomes. The comparison for a new therapy could consist of a concomitant boost-accelerated-fractionation regimen of radiotherapy or a standard-fractionation regimen, combined with concurrent, high-dose cisplatin, as both methods lead to similar results in terms of overall survival [26].

Conflict of Interests

There is no conflict of interests to declare. None of the coauthors have direct financial relations with any of the trademarks mentioned in this paper.

References

[1] W. H. Westra, J. M. Taube, M. L. Poeta, S. Begum, D. Sidransky, and W. M. Koch, "Inverse relationship between human papillomavirus-16 infection and disruptive p53 gene mutations in squamous cell carcinoma of the head and neck," *Clinical Cancer Research*, vol. 14, no. 2, pp. 366–369, 2008.

[2] T. Wiest, E. Schwarz, C. Enders, C. Flechtenmacher, and F. X. Bosch, "Involvement of intact HPV16 E6/E7 gene expression in head and neck cancers with unaltered p53 status and perturbed pRB cell cycle control," *Oncogene*, vol. 21, no. 10, pp. 1510–1517, 2002.

[3] H. C. Hafkamp, J. J. Manni, A. Haesevoets et al., "Marked differences in survival rate between smokers and nonsmokers with HPV 16-associated tonsillar carcinomas," *International Journal of Cancer*, vol. 122, no. 12, pp. 2656–2664, 2008.

[4] B. Kumar, K. G. Cordell, J. S. Lee et al., "EGFR, p16, HPV titer, Bcl-xL and p53, sex, and smoking as indicators of response to therapy and survival in oropharyngeal cancer," *Journal of Clinical Oncology*, vol. 26, no. 19, pp. 3128–3137, 2008.

[5] M. L. Gillison, W. M. Koch, R. B. Capone et al., "Evidence for a causal association between human papillomavirus and a subset of head and neck cancers," *Journal of the National Cancer Institute*, vol. 92, no. 9, pp. 709–720, 2000.

[6] C. T. Allen, J. S. Lewis Jr., S. K. El-Mofty, B. H. Haughey, and B. Nussenbaum, "Human papillomavirus and oropharynx cancer: biology, detection and clinical implications," *Laryngoscope*, vol. 120, no. 9, pp. 1756–1772, 2010.

[7] A. K. Chaturvedi, E. A. Engels, W. F. Anderson, and M. L. Gillison, "Incidence trends for human papillomavirus-related and -unrelated oral squamous cell carcinomas in the United States," *Journal of Clinical Oncology*, vol. 26, no. 4, pp. 612–619, 2008.

[8] A. R. Kreimer, G. M. Clifford, P. Boyle, and S. Franceschi, "Human papillomavirus types in head and neck squamous cell carcinomas worldwide: a systemic review," *Cancer Epidemiology Biomarkers and Prevention*, vol. 14, no. 2, pp. 467–475, 2005.

[9] L. Hammarstedt, D. Lindquist, H. Dahlstrand et al., "Human papillomavirus as a risk factor for the increase in incidence of tonsillar cancer," *International Journal of Cancer*, vol. 119, no. 11, pp. 2620–2623, 2006.

[10] A. Näsman, P. Attner, L. Hammarstedt et al., "Incidence of human papillomavirus (HPV) positive tonsillar carcinoma in Stockholm, Sweden: an epidemic of viral-induced carcinoma?" *International Journal of Cancer*, vol. 125, no. 2, pp. 362–366, 2009.

[11] T. Ramqvist and T. Dalianis, "Oropharyngeal cancer epidemic and human papillomavirus," *Emerging Infectious Diseases*, vol. 16, no. 11, pp. 1671–1677, 2010.

[12] M. L. Gillison, G. D'Souza, W. Westra et al., "Distinct risk factor profiles for human papillomavirus type 16-positive and human papillomavirus type 16-negative head and neck cancers," *Journal of the National Cancer Institute*, vol. 100, no. 6, pp. 407–420, 2008.

[13] G. D'Souza, A. R. Kreimer, R. Viscidi et al., "Case-control study of human papillomavirus and oropharyngeal cancer," *The New England Journal of Medicine*, vol. 356, no. 19, pp. 1944–1956, 2007.

[14] R. Chen, L. M. Aaltonen, and A. Vaheri, "Human papillomavirus type 16 in head and neck carcinogenesis," *Reviews in Medical Virology*, vol. 15, no. 6, pp. 351–363, 2005.

[15] C. C. R. Ragin and E. Taioli, "Survival of squamous cell carcinoma of the head and neck in relation to human papillomavirus infection: review and meta-analysis," *International Journal of Cancer*, vol. 121, no. 8, pp. 1813–1820, 2007.

[16] C. Fakhry, W. H. Westra, S. Li et al., "Improved survival of patients with human papillomavirus-positive head and neck squamous cell carcinoma in a prospective clinical trial," *Journal of the National Cancer Institute*, vol. 100, no. 4, pp. 261–269, 2008.

[17] C. Fakhry and M. L. Gillison, "Clinical implications of human papillomavirus in head and neck cancers," *Journal of Clinical Oncology*, vol. 24, no. 17, pp. 2606–2611, 2006.

[18] P. M. Weinberger, Z. Yu, B. G. Haffty et al., "Molecular classification identifies a subset of human papillomavirus- associated oropharyngeal cancers with favorable prognosis," *Journal of Clinical Oncology*, vol. 24, no. 5, pp. 736–747, 2006.

[19] N. F. Schlecht, "Prognostic value of human papillomavirus in the survival of head and neck cancer patients: an overview of the evidence," *Oncology Reports*, vol. 14, no. 5, pp. 1239–1247, 2005.

[20] K. Lindel, K. T. Beer, J. Laissue, R. H. Greiner, and D. M. Aebersold, "Human papillomavirus positive squamous cell carcinoma of the oropharynx: a radiosensitive subgroup of head and neck carcinoma," *Cancer*, vol. 92, pp. 805–813, 2001.

[21] S. R. Schwartz, B. Yueh, J. K. McDougall, J. R. Daling, and S. M. Schwartz, "Human papillomavirus infection and survival in oral squamous cell cancer: a population-based study," *Otolaryngology*, vol. 125, no. 1, pp. 1–9, 2001.

[22] J. M. Ritchie, E. M. Smith, K. F. Summersgill et al., "Human papillomavirus infection as a prognostic factor in carcinomas of the oral cavity and oropharynx," *International Journal of Cancer*, vol. 104, no. 3, pp. 336–344, 2003.

[23] L. Dahlgren, H. Dahlstrand, D. Lindquist et al., "Human papillomavirus is more common in base of tongue than in mobile tongue cancer and is a favorable prognostic factor in base of tongue cancer patients," *International Journal of Cancer*, vol. 112, no. 6, pp. 1015–1019, 2004.

[24] M. L. Gillison, "Human papillomavirus and prognosis of oropharyngeal squamous cell carcinoma: implications for clinical research in head and neck cancers," *Journal of Clinical Oncology*, vol. 24, no. 36, pp. 5623–5625, 2006.

[25] D. Rischin, R. J. Young, R. Fisher et al., "Prognostic significance of p16INK4Aand human papillomavirus in patients with oropharyngeal cancer treated on TROG 02.02 phase III trial," *Journal of Clinical Oncology*, vol. 28, no. 27, pp. 4142–4148, 2010.

[26] K. K. Ang, J. Harris, R. Wheeler et al., "Human papillomavirus and survival of patients with oropharyngeal cancer," *The New England Journal of Medicine*, vol. 363, no. 1, pp. 24–35, 2010.

[27] F. Coutlée, C. Hankins, and N. Lapointe, "Comparison between vaginal tampon and cervicovaginal lavage specimen collection for detection of human papillomavirus DNA by the polymerase chain reaction," *Journal of Medical Virology*, vol. 51, no. 1, pp. 42–47, 1997.

[28] F. Coutlée, D. Rouleau, P. Petignat et al., "Enhanced detection and typing of human papillomavirus (HPV) DNA in anogenital samples with PGMY primers and the linear array HPV genotyping test," *Journal of Clinical Microbiology*, vol. 44, no. 6, pp. 1998–2006, 2006.

[29] M. V. Jacobs, A. M. de Roda Husman, A. J. C. van den Brule, P. J. F. Snijders, C. J. L. M. Meijer, and J. M. M. Walboomers, "Group-specific differentiation between high- and low-risk human papillomavirus genotypes by general primer-mediated PCR and two cocktails of oligonucleotide probes," *Journal of Clinical Microbiology*, vol. 33, no. 4, pp. 901–905, 1995.

[30] N. Reimers, H. U. Kasper, S. J. Weissenborn et al., "Combined analysis of HPV-DNA, p16 and EGFR expression to predict prognosis in oropharyngeal cancer," *International Journal of Cancer*, vol. 120, no. 8, pp. 1731–1738, 2007.

[31] C. S. Kong, B. Narasimhan, H. Cao et al., "The relationship between human papillomavirus status and other molecular prognostic markers in head and neck squamous cell carcinomas," *International Journal of Radiation Oncology Biology Physics*, vol. 74, no. 2, pp. 553–561, 2009.

[32] S. J. Smeets, A. T. Hesselink, E. J. M. Speel et al., "A novel algorithm for reliable detection of human papillomavirus in paraffin embedded head and neck cancer specimen," *International Journal of Cancer*, vol. 121, no. 11, pp. 2465–2472, 2007.

[33] C. A. Fischer, I. Zlobec, E. Green et al., "Is the improved prognosis of p16 positive oropharyngeal squamous cell carcinoma dependent of the treatment modality?" *International Journal of Cancer*, vol. 126, no. 5, pp. 1256–1262, 2010.

[34] N. F. Schlecht, R. D. Burk, L. Adrien et al., "Gene expression profiles in HPV-infected head and neck cancer," *Journal of Pathology*, vol. 213, no. 3, pp. 283–293, 2007.

[35] K. Specht, T. Richter, U. Müller, A. Walch, M. Werner, and H. Höfler, "Quantitative gene expression analysis in microdissected archival formalin-fixed and paraffin-embedded tumor tissue," *The American Journal of Pathology*, vol. 158, no. 2, pp. 419–429, 2001.

[36] R. L. Cantley, E. Gabrielli, F. Montebelli, D. Cimbaluk, P. Gattuso, and G. Petruzzelli, "Ancillary studies in determining human papillomavirus status of squamous cell carcinoma of the oropharynx: a review," *Pathology Research International*, vol. 2011, Article ID 138469, 7 pages, 2011.

[37] W. Shi, H. Kato, B. Perez-Ordonez et al., "Comparative prognostic value of HPV16 E6 mRNA compared with in situ hybridization for human oropharyngeal squamous carcinoma," *Journal of Clinical Oncology*, vol. 27, no. 36, pp. 6213–6221, 2009.

[38] J. H. Maxwell, B. Kumar, F. Y. Feng et al., "Tobacco use in human papillomavirus-positive advanced oropharynx cancer patients related to increased risk of distant metastases and tumor recurrence," *Clinical Cancer Research*, vol. 16, no. 4, pp. 1226–1235, 2010.

[39] M. L. Gillison, Q. Zhang, R. Jordan et al., "Tobacco smoking and increased risk of death and progression for patients with p16-positive and p16-negative oropharyngeal cancer," *Journal of Clinical Oncology*, vol. 30, no. 17, pp. 2102–2111, 2012.

[40] D. J. Adelstein, Y. Li, G. L. Adams et al., "An intergroup phase III comparison of standard radiation therapy and two schedules of concurrent chemoradiotherapy in patients with unresectable squamous cell head and neck cancer," *Journal of Clinical Oncology*, vol. 21, no. 1, pp. 92–98, 2003.

[41] J. P. Pignon, A. L. Maître, E. Maillard, and J. Bourhis, "Meta-analysis of chemotherapy in head and neck cancer (MACH-NC): an update on 93 randomised trials and 17,346 patients," *Radiotherapy and Oncology*, vol. 92, no. 1, pp. 4–14, 2009.

[42] A. A. Forastiere, H. Goepfert, and M. Maor, "Concurrent chemotherapy and radiotherapy for organ preservation in advanced laryngeal cancer," *The New England Journal of Medicine*, vol. 349, pp. 2091–2098, 2003.

8

Evidence of Bacterial Biofilms among Infected and Hypertrophied Tonsils in Correlation with the Microbiology, Histopathology, and Clinical Symptoms of Tonsillar Diseases

Saad Musbah Alasil,[1] Rahmat Omar,[2] Salmah Ismail,[3] Mohd Yasim Yusof,[4] Ghulam N. Dhabaan,[4] and Mahmood Ameen Abdulla[5]

[1] Department of Microbiology, Faculty of Medicine, MAHSA University, 59100 Kuala Lumpur, Malaysia
[2] Pantai Hospital Cheras, 56100 Kuala Lumpur, Malaysia
[3] Institute of Biological Science, Faculty of Science, University of Malaya, 50603 Kuala Lumpur, Malaysia
[4] Department of Medical Microbiology, Faculty of Medicine, University of Malaya, 50603 Kuala Lumpur, Malaysia
[5] Department of Biomedical Science, Faculty of Medicine, University of Malaya, 50603 Kuala Lumpur, Malaysia

Correspondence should be addressed to Salmah Ismail; salmah_r@um.edu.my

Academic Editor: Peter S. Roland

Diseases of the tonsils are becoming more resistant to antibiotics due to the persistence of bacteria through the formation of biofilms. Therefore, understanding the microbiology and pathophysiology of such diseases represent an important step in the management of biofilm-related infections. We have isolated the microorganisms, evaluated their antimicrobial susceptibility, and detected the presence of bacterial biofilms in tonsillar specimens in correlation with the clinical manifestations of tonsillar diseases. Therefore, a total of 140 palatine tonsils were collected from 70 patients undergoing tonsillectomy at University Malaya Medical Centre. The most recovered isolate was *Staphylococcus aureus* (39.65%) followed by *Haemophilus influenzae* (18.53%). There was high susceptibility against all selected antibiotics except for cotrimoxazole. Bacterial biofilms were detected in 60% of patients and a significant percentage of patients demonstrated infection manifestation rather than obstruction. In addition, an association between clinical symptoms like snore, apnea, nasal obstruction, and tonsillar hypertrophy was found to be related to the microbiology of tonsils particularly to the presence of biofilms. In conclusion, evidence of biofilms in tonsils in correlation with the demonstrated clinical symptoms explains the recalcitrant nature of tonsillar diseases and highlights the importance of biofilm's early detection and prevention towards better therapeutic management of biofilm-related infections.

1. Introduction

The ear, nose, and throat (ENT) represent a natural habitat for a broad range of microorganisms such as commensal bacteria as well as potential pathogens [1]. However, these bacteria can sometimes find their way to overcome the defense barriers of such locations and establish chronic infections that poses a challenge to both medical practice and healthcare system [2]. Infections of the ENT such as tonsillitis are diseases that occur with high frequency [3]. During the past decades, efforts have been made to manage the infectious diseases of

tonsils [4]. It has been reported that the impact of tonsillar diseases may not only affect the tonsils alone but it can reach other related anatomic structures like the paranasal sinus, upper aerodigestive tract, and Eustachian tube-middle ear complex [4]. Thus understanding the microbiology and pathophysiology of such diseases represents an important step in the management of biofilm-related infections.

Chronic infections of the ear, nose, and throat are becoming more resistant to common antimicrobial therapies [5] due to the ability of bacteria to persist through the formation of biofilms [6] which are bacterial cells attached to a surface and embedded in a matrix of exopolysaccharide [7]. The most important step in biofilm formation is the secretion of a matrix comprising of proteins and sugars outside the individual bacterial cells [8]. In addition, the biofilm structure provides mechanical stability to the bacteria and it represents a site where genetic elements are exchanged [9]. It has been estimated that more than 65% of all human bacterial infections are associated with biofilms [10]. Moreover, bacteria in the biofilm are 1000 times more resistant to antibiotics than their free-living counterparts [11, 12] which may lead to discrepancies between the *in vitro* and *in vivo* antimicrobial susceptibility results [13]. Therefore, shifting the mode of antibiotic regimens to include bacteria in a biofilm mode will improve the methods of treatment especially against biofilm-associated infections [14]. Biofilms play a major role in chronic tonsillitis which is considered one of the most common pathologies in childhood [15–17]. Despite the widespread use of antibiotics, tonsillitis is often recalcitrant and tonsillectomy is mainly performed only when antibiotic therapy fails to relieve the symptoms of infection [18] or when the enlarged tonsils cause functional obstruction to the air passage [19]. Moreover, the increasing incidence of β-lactamase-producing bacteria recovered from tonsils may protect the causing pathogens from being eliminated by host defense and antibiotics [20] which may lead to the recurrence of tonsillar infections that are caused by microorganisms shown to be susceptible *in vitro* [21]. These observations have led to the hypothesis that bacteria in a biofilm can resist eradication causing chronic inflammation and permanent changes in the tonsillar lymphoid tissue [21].

A biofilm is considered a marker of virulence which can be detected phenotypically [22]. However, proper visualization of biofilms within tissue sections is challenging due to the difficulty in staining both bacteria and glycocalyx [6]. Most of the early investigations on biofilms relied heavily on scanning electron microscopy (SEM) [23]. It has been reported that the most effective and nondestructive approach for examining biofilms within tissue sections is via confocal laser scanning microscopy (CLSM) [24]. In our study, we have identified the bacterial isolates recovered from tonsillar specimens and evaluate their antimicrobial susceptibility in addition to examining the histopathology and presence of bacterial biofilms in tonsillar tissue sections in correlation with the clinical manifestations of tonsillar diseases that are due to infection and obstruction.

2. Materials and Methods

2.1. Selection of Patients. A total of 70 patients undergoing elective tonsillectomy were enrolled in this study. Patients were diagnosed with three main clinical cases including recurrent tonsillitis, chronic tonsillitis, and obstructive sleep apnea. The duration of the study was 10 months from October 2009 to July 2010. Prior to surgery, an approval letter was obtained from the medical ethics committee at University Malaya Medical Centre (UMMC) PPUM/UPP/300/02/02 Ref. number 744.11 and written consents were recorded from each patient separately. Inclusion criteria included 3

attacks/year of chronic and recurrent tonsillitis or 5 attacks in 2 years with symptoms like fever, snoring, sore throat, and inability to take normal diet [25]. Other inclusion criteria included patients diagnosed with obstructive sleep apnea with symptoms like nocturnal snoring with partial upper airway obstruction, complete cessation of airflow with gas exchange abnormalities, and severe disturbance of sleep [26]. Exclusion criteria included patients with a history of infection who received antimicrobial therapy within one month prior to surgery, patients with grossly asymmetrical tonsillar size as noted on preoperative clinical assessment, patients undergoing tonsillectomy for emergency conditions such as peritonsillar abscess or other deep neck space infections, and patients suspected for benign or malignant tonsillar tumors [27]. Other exclusion criteria included immunocompromised and diabetic patients [28] and patients with obstructive sleep apnea that are not due to adenotonsillar hypertrophy but to other causes such as craniofacial anomalies and neurologic abnormalities [29].

2.2. Indications of Tonsillar Diseases. The clinical indications for tonsillectomy were used as a guideline to determine the assignments of tonsillar diseases among the selected patients [27]. The size of tonsils was estimated on a 1+ to 4+ scale as outlined in the group classification [30] and the grading of tonsillar hypertrophy [31]. Patients were classified into two main groups based on their clinical diagnosis and history of infection; the first group was designed the name tonsillar infection group represented by 49 patients with recurrent tonsillitis having minimally visible tonsils occupying less than 25% of the oropharyngeal airway (1+) and 9 patients with chronic tonsillitis having moderately enlarged tonsils occupying less than 50% of the oropharyngeal airway (2+). The second group was designed the name tonsillar obstruction group represented by 12 patients with obstruction sleep apnea having moderately to massively enlarged tonsils (3+ or 4+) occupying greater than 50–75% of the oropharyngeal airway.

2.3. Collection of Tonsillar Specimens. Upon surgery, the surface of palatine tonsils was swabbed with a sterile cotton applicator followed by the surgical removal [28]. Tonsillar biopsies were aseptically dissected into four parts [32]; the first part was unfixed and was referred to the Clinical Diagnostic Laboratory (CDL) at UMMC along with the tonsillar swabs to identify the type of microorganisms. The second part was fixed with 4% glutaraldehyde to detect the presence of biofilms via SEM. The third and fourth parts were fixed with 10% neutral buffered formalin to detect the presence of biofilms via CLSM and examine the histopathology of tonsils respectively.

2.4. Isolation of Tonsillar Microorganisms. Tonsillar biopsies were aseptically weighted and placed in thioglycollate broth with a volume equivalent to 1 : 10 dilution followed by tissue homogenization. Serial dilutions of 1 : 10 and 1 : 100 were performed and each dilution was poured into Columbia agar supplemented with 5% sheep blood. After incubation for 24 hours, the microbial load was assessed by colony counting as described previously [33] and bacterial identification was accomplished by routine culturing on selective and differential media. Moreover, biochemical tests were performed such as DNase test for *S. aureus*; optochin test, bile solubility test, and bacitracin test for Streptococci spp.; indole, citrate test, malonate utilization test, urease test, oxidase test, and methyl red test for *Enterobacteriacea*; and the XV factor test for *Haemophilus* spp.

2.5. Antimicrobial Susceptibility of Tonsillar Isolates. The Clinical Diagnostic Laboratory in consultation with the infectious disease practitioners at UMMC has decided which antimicrobial agent to report routinely or selectively. Therefore, susceptibility test for selected antibiotics was carried out via disk diffusion as descripted previously [34]. Briefly, a fixed volume of nutrient broth containing a standard concentration for each bacterial isolate was smeared evenly onto the surface of Mueller-Hinton agar plate and filter paper disks impregnated with antibiotic concentrations were applied to the plate surface followed by aerobic incubation. The zone of inhibition for each antibiotic was measured and the edge of these zones correlated with the antibiotic concentration that inhibits the growth of bacteria were compared to a standard table of predetermined zone widths [35].

2.6. Histopathology Examination of Tonsils. Tonsillar biopsy specimens were examined by routine staining with hematoxylin & eosin (H&E) as described previously [36]. Briefly, biopsies were embedded in paraffin wax then cut using a manual rotary microtome (Leica RM2235, Leica Microsystems. Germany) into thin sections that were later fixed onto a glass slide. Slides were then deparaffinized in xylene for 10 minutes and then rehydrated for 1 minute in a grade series of ethanol. Sections were then stained with hematoxylin for 2 minutes, rinsed, and then stained with eosin for 1 minute. Slides were then dehydrated with ethanol followed by xylene for 10 minutes and mounted to be inspected under light microscope.

2.7. Microscopic Examination of Biofilms. To visualize the biofilm presence covering the surface of tonsils, SEM was used as described previously [6]. Briefly, specimens were fixed in 4% glutaraldehyde for 24 hours followed by dehydration through a graded series of acetone solutions and then critical point drying was performed for which they were mounted on metal stubs and coated with gold prior to imaging. Specimens were examined by SEM (INCA x-sight, Oxford instruments. UK). Images were collected at an acceleration voltage of approximately 5.0 kV, a filament current of approximately 10^{-10} A, and a working distance of approximately 39 mm; images were digitized as high resolution TIFF files and were then converted to high-quality TIF files using commercially available software. To visualize the biofilm's 3D architecture, CLSM was used in combination with immunohistochemistry staining for which a fluorescent-labeled lectin named concanavalin A (Con A) will specifically bind to the biofilm's matrix as described previously [6]. Briefly, specimens were embedded in an optimal cutting temperature (OCT) media

and were frozen in a mixture of cold isopentane and liquid nitrogen forming blocks that were cut into a thickness of 5–10 μm using a cryostat (Leica CM1850, Leica Microsystems. Germany), then fixed onto a glass slide. Staining was achieved with Propidium iodide followed by Con A and sections were then embedded in an antiquenching mounting medium of phosphate-buffered saline and glycerol. Specimens were examined by CLSM (LSM 700. Carl Zeiss. Germany) and various colocalization parameters were determined with the aid of ZEN 2010 software for a more comparative analysis of biofilms. Specimens were considered having a biofilm if more than one biofilm structure was observed at the surface or within the crypts of tonsils. However, when only bacteria were visualized without any matrix surrounding them they were not considered having a biofilm [9].

3. Results

3.1. Prevalence of Clinical Cases. The prevalence of clinical cases in tonsillar infection group was 20 (28.57%) cases of recurrent tonsillitis among paediatric patients and 29 (41.42%) cases among adult patients, whereas 4 (5.71%) cases of chronic tonsillitis among paediatric patients and 5 (7.14%) cases among adult patients. Moreover, the prevalence of clinical cases in tonsillar obstructive group was 9 (12.85%) cases of obstructive sleep apnea among paediatric patients and 3 (4.28%) cases among adult patients. In recurrent tonsillitis, the age group of 1.0–10 years old was the highest with 18 (25.71%) patients followed by the 11–20 years with 16 (22.85%) patients and the 21–30 years with 14 (20%), whereas 31–40 years and 41–50 years were among the lowest with 3 (4.28%) and 1 (1.42%) patients, respectively. In chronic tonsillitis cases, the age group of 11–20 years old was the highest with 5 (7.14%) patients followed by the 1–10 years with 3 (4.28%) patients and the 21–30 years with 1 (1.42%) patient. Moreover, the highest number of age group in obstructive sleep apnea cases was the 1.0–10 years old with 7 (10%) patients followed by 11.0–20 years with 2 (2.85%) patients. The frequency and type of operative procedures performed on selected patients showed that, among all clinical cases, 44 (62.85%) patients underwent tonsillectomy alone while 26 (37.14%) patients underwent tonsillectomy and adenoidectomy (T&A). Our results showed that the clinical symptoms were correlated with the presence of biofilms in the tonsils (Table 1). A significantly higher percentage of patients presented chronic or recurrent infections rather than obstruction manifestation (P < 0.05). However, an association between the clinical symptoms like snore, apnea, nasal obstruction, and tonsillar hypertrophy were found to be related to the presence of bacterial biofilms in the tonsils.

3.2. Microbiology of Tonsillar Diseases. The weight of excised tonsils varied from 2.2 to 8.1 grams. There was no correlation between the tonsillar weight and the number and type of bacterial isolates. In addition, there was no significant difference in the recovery rate of isolates among the clinical cases. Recurrent tonsillitis cases showed a recovery average of 10.85 isolates/gram tonsil and chronic tonsillitis cases showed

TABLE 1: Association between the clinical symptoms of tonsillar diseases and the presence of biofilms in tonsils.

Clinical symptom	Patients with clinical symptom	Patients with evidence of biofilm
(1) Tonsillar hypertrophy	49 (70%)*	42 (60%)*
(2) Sore throat	40 (57%)*	40 (57%)*
(3) Adenoid hypertrophy	26 (37.14%)*	13 (18%)*
(4) Apnea	12 (17.14%)*	10 (14%)*
(5) Nasal obstruction	12 (17.14%)*	10 (14%)*

*Percentage was calculated based on the total number of patients which was 70.

3.75 isolates/gram tonsil whereas obstructive sleep apnea cases showed 3 isolates/gram tonsil. The total number of bacterial isolates recovered from tonsillar specimens was 464 isolates with 184 (39.65%) isolates of *Staphylococcus aureus* as the most common followed by 86 (18.53%) isolates of *Haemophilus influenzae* and 56 (12.06%) isolates of *Streptococcus agalactiae*. There was no significant difference between the number of isolates recovered from both tonsillar swab and biopsy specimens. However, isolates of *Haemophilus parainfluenzae* were more frequently recovered in the core of tonsils 10 (2.15%) rather than the surface 21 (4.52%). Distribution of bacterial isolates among tonsillar specimens is shown in (Table 2). Moreover, a special group of pathogens designated the name ESKAPE was isolated from tonsillar specimens; these were including *Enterococcus faecium*, *Staphylococcus aureus*, *Klebsiella pneumoniae*, *Acinetobacter baumannii*, *Pseudomonas aeruginosa*, and *Enterobacter* species. The total number of recovered ESKAPE pathogens was 225 isolates (48.46%) with 184 isolates (39.65%) of *Staphylococcus aureus*, 30 isolates (6.46%) of *Klebsiella pneumoniae*, 9 isolates (1.93%) of *Pseudomonas aeruginosa*, and 1 (0.21%) isolate for each of *Acinetobacter baumannii* and *Enterobacter cloacae* with no *Enterococcus faecium* isolates.

3.3. Antimicrobial Susceptibility of Tonsillar Diseases. The results of antimicrobial susceptibility of *S. aureus* isolates showed that 169 (91.48%) isolates were susceptible to all the selected antibiotics whereas 20 (10.87%) isolates were resistant to fusidic acid and only 1 (0.5%) isolate was resistant to both methicillin and fusidic acid [37]. The antibiotic cotrimoxazole showed the highest rate of resistance against majority of the bacterial isolates including Group A beta haemolytic streptococci (GABHS) with 11 (2.37%) resistant and 3 (0.64%) susceptible; Group B *streptococcus* with 55 (11.85%) resistant and 1 (0.21%) susceptible; Group G Streptococci with 14 (3.01%) resistant and 11 (2.37%) susceptible; *Streptococcus pneumoniae* with 3 (0.64%) resistant; *Haemophilus influenzae* with 27 (5.81%) resistant and 59 (12.71%) susceptible, and *Haemophilus parainfluenzae* with 10 (2.15%) resistant and 21 (4.52%) susceptible. The number of *Haemophilus influenzae* isolates that were β-lactamase negative ampicillin-resistant (BLNAR) was 12 (2.58%) isolates. Resistance to antimicrobial agents belonging to the penicillins class was detected including 3 (0.64%) isolates of

Streptococcus pneumoniae resistant to penicillin, 12 (2.58%) isolates of *Haemophilus influenzae* resistant to ampicillin, 30 (6.46%) isolates of *Klebsiella pneumoniae* resistant to ampicillin, 7 (1.50%) isolates of *Pseudomonas aeruginosa* resistant to ampicillin, 4 (0.86%) isolates of *Citrobacter* sp. resistant to ampicillin, and 1 (0.21%) isolate of each of *Acinetobacter baumannii*, and *Enterobacter cloacae* resistant to ampicillin. A total of 10 (2.15%) isolates recovered from infected tonsils were multidrug resistant (MDR) whereas 7 (1.50%) isolates recovered from hypertrophied tonsils were MDR including 7 isolates of *Pseudomonas aeruginosa*, 3 isolates of *Streptococcus pneumoniae* and 1 isolate of *Enterobacter cloacae*. There were an increased number of *H. influenzae* isolates in association with GABHS which may be due to a synergistic relationship between these organisms. The antimicrobial susceptibility of tonsillar bacterial isolates against selected β-lactam and non-β-lactam agents is shown in (Figures 1 and 2) respectively.

3.4. Histopathology of Tonsillar Diseases. The gross pathology examination of tonsillar specimens showed the excised palatine tonsils as a nodular to tubular irregular brownish and soft surface tissue with an average measuring size of 2 × 2 × 1 cm. However, the microscopy examination revealed that the tonsillar tissue is covered with benign stratified squamous epithelium with the stroma consisting of variably sized reactive lymphoid follicles. No malignancies were found and a rate of crypt keratination was observed in majority of the tissue sections. The overall pathological interpretation was described as reactive (benign) lymphoid hyperplasia. Moreover, there was evidence of infection with *Actinomyces* spp. in 11 (15.71%) tonsillar biopsies. These infections caused an inflammatory lesion of the tonsillar crypts and led to tonsillar hypertrophy. The most frequent rate of tonsillar grading was grade III (3+) with 39 (55.71%) patients followed by grade II (2+) with 20 (28.57%) patients and grade I (1+) with 6 (8.57%) and patients then grade IV (4+) with 5 (7.15%) patients. Tonsillar biopsies from patients with chronic and recurrent tonsillitis showed increased number of lymphatic follicles in comparison to patients with obstructive sleep apnea. Moreover, an association with adenoids hypertrophy was detected in 22 (32.85%) patients.

3.5. Evidence of Bacterial Biofilms. Microscopic examination of biofilms in the tonsils via SEM showed abnormal tonsillar mucosal surrounded by red blood cells along with small depressions between the epithelium harboring bacterial microcolonies and some inflammatory cells at the periphery. Attached bacteria were present on the surface and were clearly distinguished from smaller irregularities nearby. Bacterial cells seemed to be organized in a scaffolding network and were connected by an extracellular matrix (Figure 3). Examination of the biofilm's 3D structure via CLSM showed evidence of accumulated bacteria embedded in an amorphous polysaccharide matrix that underlines the tonsillar crypts (Figure 4). Evidence of biofilms were present in 30 out of 49 patients with recurrent tonsillitis, 5 out of 9 patients with chronic tonsillitis, and 7 out of 12 patients with obstructive sleep apnea. Double staining showed that

TABLE 2: Distribution of bacterial isolates among tonsillar specimens.

Gram-positive isolates	Tonsillar biopsy (core) no. (%)	Tonsillar swab (surface) no. (%)	Total no. (%)
Staphylococcus aureus	85 (18.31%)	99 (21.33%)	184 (39.65%)
Streptococcus agalactiae	36 (7.75%)	20 (4.31%)	56 (12.06%)
Group G streptococci	11 (2.37%)	14 (3.01%)	25 (5.38%)
Streptococcus pyogenes	6 (1.29%)	8 (1.72%)	14 (3.01%)
Group F streptococci	5 (1.07%)	6 (1.29%)	11 (2.37%)
Group C streptococci	4 (0.86%)	4 (0.86%)	8 (1.72%)
Streptococcus pneumoniae	1 (0.21%)	2 (0.43%)	3 (0.64%)
Methicillin resistant *S. aureus*	0	1 (0.21%)	1 (0.21%)
Subtotal	**148 (31.89%)**	**154 (33.18%)**	**302 (65.08%)**
Gram-negative isolates	Tonsillar biopsy (core) no. (%)	Tonsillar swab (surface) no. (%)	Total no. (%)
Haemophilus influenzae	44 (9.48%)	42 (9.05%)	86 (18.53%)
Haemophilus parainfluenzae	10 (2.15%)	21 (4.52%)	31 (6.68%)
Klebsiella pneumoniae	15 (3.23%)	15 (3.23%)	30 (6.46%)
Pseudomonas aeruginosa	5 (1.07%)	4 (0.86%)	9 (1.93%)
Citrobacter sp.	2 (0.43%)	2 (0.43%)	4 (0.86%)
Acinetobacter baumannii	1 (0.21%)	0	1 (0.21%)
Enterobacter cloacae	0	1 (0.21%)	1 (0.21%)
Subtotal	**77 (16.59%)**	**85 (18.31%)**	**162 (34.91%)**
Total	**225 (48.49%)**	**239 (51.50%)**	**464 (100%)**

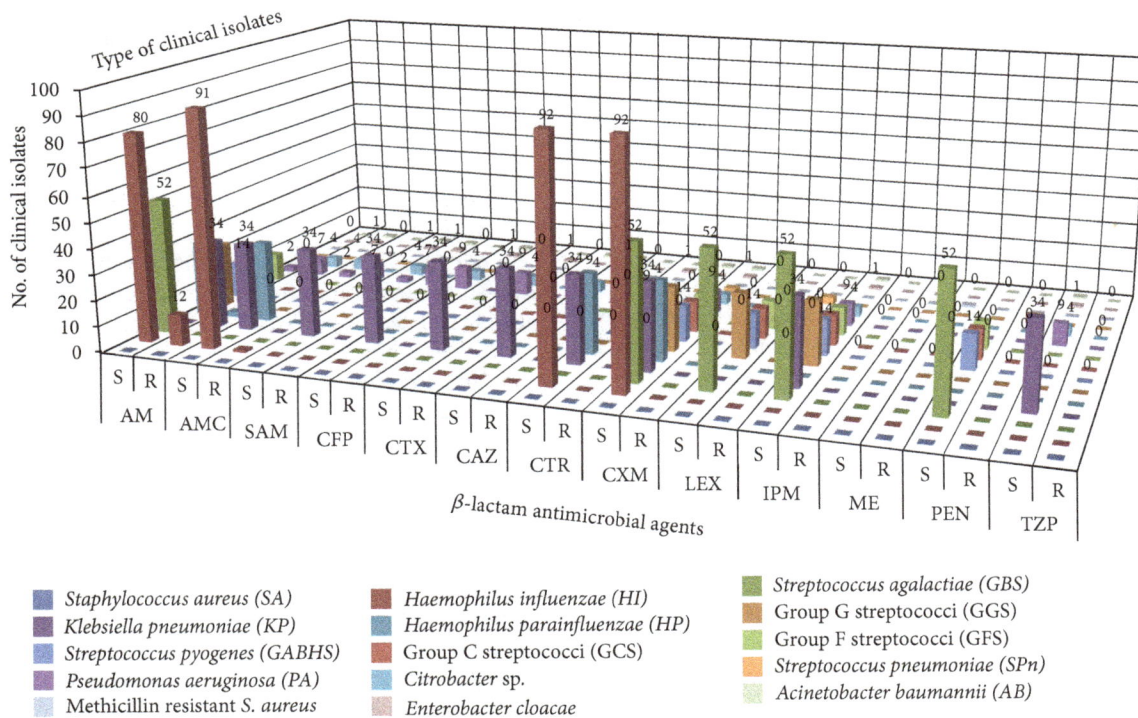

FIGURE 1: Antimicrobial susceptibility of tonsillar isolates against selected β-lactam agents. AM: ampicillin, AMC: amoxicillin-Clavulanic acid, SAM: ampicillin-Sulbactam, CFP: cefoperazone, CTX: cefotaxime, CAZ: ceftazidime, CTR: ceftriaxone, CXM: cefuroxime, LEX: cephalexin, IPM: imipenem, ME: methicillin, PEN: penicillin, TZP: piperacillin-Tazobactam. (S) indicates susceptible isolates and (R) indicates resistant isolates.

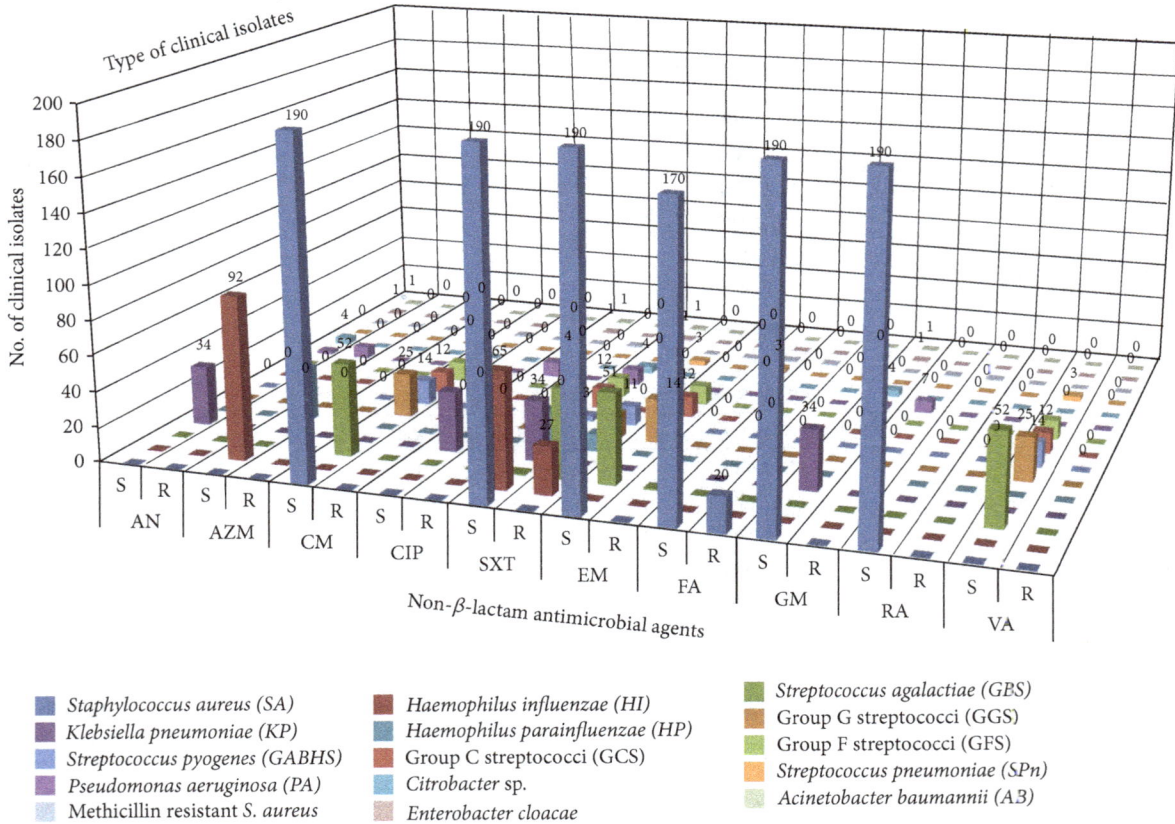

FIGURE 2: Antimicrobial susceptibility of tonsillar isolates against selected non-β-lactam agents. AN: amikacin, AZM: azithromycin, CM: clindamycin, CIP: ciprofloxacin, SXT: co-trimoxazole, EM: erythromycin, FA: fusidic Acid, GM: gentamicin, RA: rifampin, VA: vancomycin. (S) indicates susceptible isolates and (R) indicates resistant isolates.

bacterial cells and tonsillar cells were stained red whereas the biofilm's glycocalyx was stained fluorescent green. Majority of the visualized bacteria were cocci shaped with some bacilli indicating a polymicrobial biofilm community. However, the type of bacteria could not be identified based on the microscopic examination. Colocalization analysis showed red tonsillar nuclei tagged with propidium iodide and green glycocalyx tagged with Con A.

4. Discussion

Our assessment for the microbiology of tonsillar diseases showed that *Staphylococcus aureus* was the most common bacterial isolate followed by *Haemophilus influenzae* which indicates that those two pathogens might be the etiological factors for chronic and recurrent tonsillitis. This was similar to Kielmovitch et al. in which they have reported *S. aureus* and *H. influenzae* as the main causative agents of tonsillitis [38]. There was low number of recovery among *Streptococcus pneumoniae* and GABHS isolates from both infected and hypertrophied tonsils which indicates their less possible role in the development of chronic and recurrent tonsillitis in addition to obstructive sleep apnea. This was in contrast with Kielmovitch et al. where they have reported GABHS,

Streptococcus pneumonia, and *Neisseria gonorrhoeae* as the main causes of tonsillitis [38].

In our study, there was no significant difference between the tonsillar surface and core. In fact, the same type of bacteria that were isolated from the core was isolated from the surface as well. These findings were similar to those of Almadori et al. where they have reported no qualitative difference between tonsillar surface and core cultures [39]. However, this was in contrast with Brook et al. and Rosen et al. were they have reported that the isolated microorganisms from tonsillar surface may not always represent the real cause of recurrent tonsillitis [40, 41]. The only microorganism that was found to have significant difference in the recovery was *Haemophilus influenzae* for which 10 isolates where recovered from the core whereas 21 were recovered from the surface. This was similar to Gul et al. where they have reported a difference in recovery between surface and core tissue among *H. influenzae* and *S. aureus* isolates [42]. *H. influenzae* was rarely recovered from the tonsillar surface which indicates that the surface cultures commonly show normal flora whereas the tonsil core cultures show pathogenic microorganisms. Despite the contrast with previous studies in the role of swabbing, the use of swabs can still be reliable to recognize the presence of possible pathogens especially for patients who are not

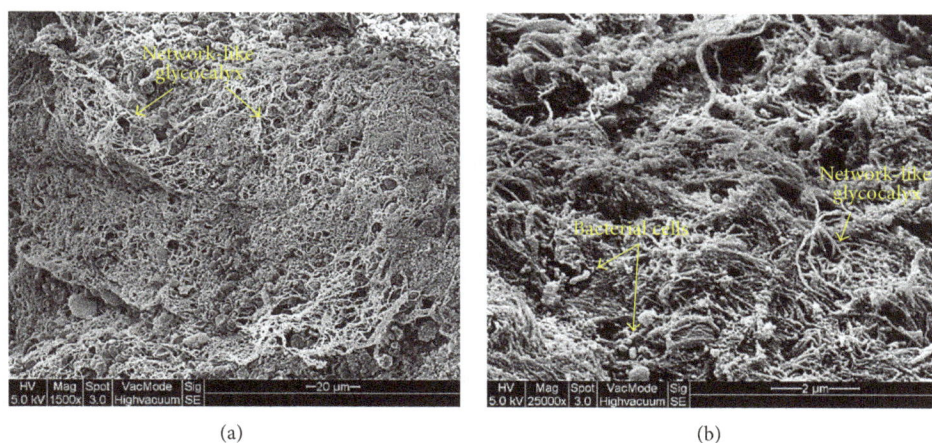

(a)   (b)

FIGURE 3: Microscopic evidence of bacterial biofilms on the tonsillar surface via SEM. (a) Overall image of biofilm from a patient with recurrent tonsillitis showing the layers of network-like glycocalyx (low magnification 1500x). (b) Representative image of biofilm from a patient with chronic tonsillitis showing bacterial cells attached to the surface of tonsillar cells and embedded in a network-like glycocalyx (high magnification 25000x). Arrows indicate the biofilm structures.

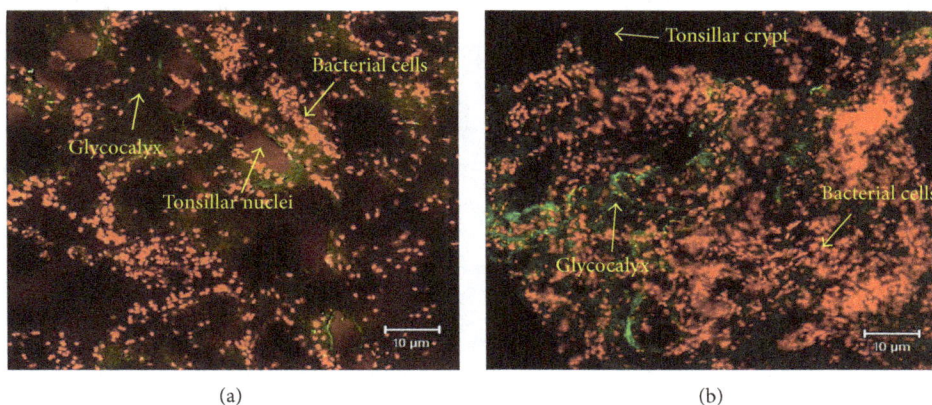

(a)   (b)

FIGURE 4: Microscopic evidence of bacterial biofilms within the tonsillar crypts via CLSM. (a) Representative image of biofilm from a patient with obstructive sleep apnea showing bacterial cells (red) embedded with glycocalyx (green) surrounding the tonsillar nuclei (red). (b) Three-dimensional image of a biofilm showing bacterial aggregates (cells) embedded in a glycocalyx matrix (100x). Arrows indicate the biofilm structures and tissue sections were stained with propidium iodide and concanavalin A.

willing to undergo surgical management despite of not being responding to antimicrobial treatment.

In the case of tonsillar infection, bacteria that inhabit the crypts can spread into the tissue and secret their toxins leading to infiltration of leukocyte and surface ulceration that can cause the bacteria to inoculate the tonsillar core [43, 44]. However, the mechanism of activating such infections is still poorly understood [28]. Therefore, knowing the microbiology of tonsils does not help in the treatment of disease however; it establishes an understanding whether the bacteria play a role in reactivating recurrent infections by using virulence factors such as forming a biofilm.

Our antimicrobial susceptibility results showed a high rate of sensitivity among majority of tonsillar isolates. This was similar to Sadoh et al. in which they have reported a 100% sensitivity to cefuroxime, azithromycin, and ceftazidime among *S. aureus* and β-haemolytic streptococci [45]. It is worthy of note that ampicillin exhibited more

resistance against pathogens such as *P. aeruginosa* and *H. influenzae*. Although the reason for this difference is not clear, we suspect it may be related to possible abuse of the easily accessible and relatively cheap ampicillin that will eventually develop resistance. Moreover, a noticeable percentage of resistance to the antibiotic cotrimoxazole was detected; these include 21.43% resistance by GABHS isolates, 68.60% by *H. influenzae* isolates, and 67.75% by *H. parainfluenzae* isolates. This was similar to Sadoh et al. where they have reported no sensitivity to ampicillin and cotrimoxazole [45]. Although our susceptibility results cannot estimate the current status of antimicrobial resistance in Malaysia, it highlights a number of important issues regarding the susceptibility and epidemiology of important respiratory tract pathogens such as *S. aureus, H. influenza,* and GABHS [37]. Our results indicates a significant resistance (10.87%) to fusidic acid among *S. aureus* isolates which was similar to Brown and Thomas where they have reported a 10.6% resistance to fusidic acid among methicillin-susceptible *S. aureus* isolates making it a less potential drug of choice for patients with chronic and recurrent tonsillitis [46]. This was also similar to another study by Norazah et al. in which they reported an increased resistant to fusidic acid between 3 and 5% among Malaysian hospitals [47]. We have found that 12 (2.58%) isolates of *H. influenzae* were β-lactamase negative ampicillin-resistant (BLNAR). This is of clinical significance, since *H. influenzae* isolates that are BLNAR are typically coresistant to other commonly prescribed β-lactams including cephalosporins, amoxicillin-clavulanate, and ampicillin-sulbactam [35].

The recovered ESKAPE pathogens showed high susceptibility against the selected antibiotics except for *P. aeruginosa* where it exhibited 22% resistance to amikacin, ampicillin-sulbactam, amoxicillin-clavulanic acid and ampicillin. This was in contrast with Rice where they reported high levels of resistance by ESKAPE isolates [48]. Bacterial interference has been shown to exist between isolates of α-haemolytic and β-haemolytic streptococci and between Gram-negative bacilli and α-haemolytic streptococci [49]. The lack of interference strains may explain the increased susceptibility of certain individuals to β-haemolytic streptococci. Since the administration of antimicrobial agents can affect the composition of the nasopharyngeal flora, a proper use of antibiotics is important in the preservation of the normal interfering flora [50].

The lack of a rapid and reproducible assay to provide a measurable antimicrobial activity against sessile bacteria represents a problem in the selection of alternative antibiotic regiments [51, 52]. Therefore, it is believed that clinical microbiology laboratories can adapt alternative diagnostic techniques to assess the susceptibility of bacteria in the biofilm. This will assist clinicians in the selection of more powerful antibiotics for their activity and efficacy.

The mean age of patients with tonsillitis where streptococci was mainly recovered, that is, streptococcal tonsillitis (ST), was 10 years old while in Nonstreptococcal tonsillitis (NST) it was 13.34 years old. The prevalence of patients with ST was significantly less than that in patients with NST which emphasizes the role of group B, C, G, and F in the clinical presentation and pathogenesis of tonsillitis infections. Our results indicate that the prevalence of bacterial biofilms among ST cases was 100% while among NST cases it was 53% indicating a role of both GABHS and non-GABHS isolates in the pathogenesis of biofilm-associated tonsillar diseases. This was similar to Diaz et al. [9] in which they have reported the correlation between chronic inflammation of the tonsils, clinical features, and the presence of biofilms among 36 patients undergoing tonsillectomy for obstructive sleep apnea and recurrent upper airway infection.

The gross pathology of tonsillar specimens showed that the highest rate of tonsillar grading was grade III (55.71%) followed by grade II (28.57%), grade I (8.57%) and grade IV (7.15%). This was similar to Dell'Aringa et al. (2005) in which they have reported grade III to be the highest with 160 (64%) patients followed by grade II with 45 (18%) patients, grade IV with 26 (10.4%) patients, and grade I with 9 (3.6%) patients [53]. In our study, there was no malignant neoplasia among our tonsillar specimens which can be attributed to the

low prevalence of adult patients submitted to tonsillectomy. Moreover, there was no evaluation of the influence of tonsillar size on patients with obstructive sleep apnea and the influence of oropharyngeal anatomy and body mass index on the actual volume of tonsils; this was mainly because we have emphasized more on the microbiology, histopathology, and clinical aspects of tonsillar diseases rather than the physiological and anatomic aspects; therefore, no such correlation was assessed.

Based on the histopathology examination, only 11 (15.71%) patients presented infections by *Actinomyces* spp. in their tonsils leading to tonsillar hypertrophy and an inflammatory lesion of the crypts. This was similar to Pransky et al. where they have reported the presence actinomycosis in 8.5% of patients with obstructive tonsillar hypertrophy and recurrent tonsillitis [54]. However, it was in contrast to Dell'Aringa et al. where they have reported only 2 patients (0.8%) with *Actinomyces* spp. infections [53]. Despite the presence of *Actinomyces* in our examined tonsils, the rate of these infections was significantly low ($P < 0.05$) suggesting no relation between the presence of *Actinomyces* and the hypertrophy of tonsils. This was mainly due to the fact that tonsillar surface is contaminated with oropharyngeal secretions which generally shows normal flora of the oropharynx such as α-hemolytic and nonhemolytic streptococci, coagulase negative staphylococci, *Neisseria*, *Corynebacterium*, *Actinomyces*, *Leptotrichia*, and *Fusobacterium* spp. [55].

In our study, bacterial biofilms were present in 60% of tonsils. This was similar to previous findings were biofilms were present in 61% and 70% of examined tonsils, respectively [6, 18]. The high prevalence of biofilm among our tonsils suggests that chronic and recurrent tonsillitis and obstructive sleep apnea are caused by biofilm-forming pathogens. This was similar to previous investigators where they have confirmed the hypothesis that chronic and recurrent tonsillitis are biofilm-related [56, 57]. Although we were able to capture images from different tonsillar specimens to minimize any potential error, these might not completely prevent the chance for false positive biofilm-like artifacts. Therefore, detecting the bacteria and its glycocalyx is crucial for a fundamental understanding of the presence of biofilms in clinical specimens. The use of concanavalin A that binds to mannose residues specific to the bacteria's glycocalyx coupled with CLSM has enabled us to visualize the biofilm's structure more clearly which was similar to a previous study [58]. However, despite the importance of CLSM as a versatile tool it has the limitation of identifying the type of microorganism(s) causing that biofilm in addition of being costly. Furthermore, we could not assess the role of fungi and viruses among our samples due to the technical difficulties in collecting, transporting, and culturing them. Therefore, further studies are needed to tackle the role of nonbacterial biofilms among larger sample size for a better and more insightful understanding of biofilm-associated infections. It has been reported that hypertrophied tonsils even without a history of infection cannot be considered as control samples which is considered as a limitation to our study due to difficulties in obtaining tonsillar specimens from age-matched individuals who never had infection or obstruction in their upper airways. This is similar to the study by Stewart and Costerton where they reported [59]. The evidence of biofilms in the tonsils of patients without a clinical history of infection does raise the possibility that biofilm formation within the tonsillar crypt is part of an immunological surveillance process which leads us to conclude that bacterial biofilms are part of the tonsillar microbial flora among clinically diseased tonsils [18]. Another explanation is that tonsils of healthy individuals are colonized with the same biofilm-forming strains found in tonsillitis patients. However, these strains might not induce a disease. Future studies can be addressed to identify a control group that comprises of volunteers scheduled for laryngeal microsurgery with no history of tonsillitis over the previous 2 years [60].

Our results investigated the correlation between tonsillar inflammations, clinical features, and the presence of biofilms among patients with recurrent infections and obstructive hypertrophy suggesting that biofilm acts a reservoir to establish a persistent infection that leads to the enlargement of tonsils. This was similar to Diaz et al. [9] in which they have demonstrated the symptoms like harsh raucous sound, tonsillar and adenoids hypertrophy, apnea, and cervical adenopathies to be related to the presence of biofilm in the tonsils. Despite the low prevalence of symptoms like apnea and nasal obstruction in comparison with tonsillar and adenoid hypertrophy due to small sample size, a direct correlation between apnea and nasal obstruction was found with the presence of biofilms in 7 out of 12 tonsils within the obstructive group. Moreover, biofilms were found in all hypertrophic tonsils which confirms that tonsillar hypertrophy is one of the important symptoms associated with the presence of biofilms. The increased number of tonsillar lymphatic follicles was related to the presence of biofilms in infected more than hypertrophied tonsils; this finding was similar to a finding in a previous study [61, 62]. The biofilm as a structure is too big to be engulfed by the host's macrophages; therefore their presence in the tonsils will interfere with the normal functions of tonsillar lymphatic tissue which eventually leads to establish a chronic or recurrent infection [62, 63]. This process explains the poor outcome of most therapeutic strategies to minimize the enlarged size of tonsils and avoid the choice of surgery [64]. Failure to respond to antimicrobial therapy leaves the tonsillitis patients with no choice but surgery. However, despite the role of tonsillectomy in relieving the symptoms of tonsillar diseases, the more likely explanation for its effectiveness is the elimination of a possible biofilm infection.

In conclusion, evidence of bacterial biofilms in the tonsils in correlation with the demonstrated clinical symptoms explains the recalcitrant nature of chronic and recurrent tonsillitis and highlights the importance of investigating the microbiology and histopathology of tonsillar diseases towards better therapeutic management of biofilm-related infections.

Conflict of Interests

The authors declare that they have no conflict of interests.

Acknowledgments

This study was supported by University of Malaya through the Fundamental Research Grant Scheme (FP026-2010B) and the Postgraduate Research Grant (PS184/2009C). The authors would like to thank all participating clinicians, nurses them and technical staff at University Malaya Medical Center who assisted in the diagnosis of clinical cases and the collection of specimens. The authors are thankful to the staff of electron microscopy unit at the Faculty of Medicine, University Malaya, and the microscopy unit at the Institute of Bioscience, Universiti Putra Malaysia (UPM), for providing all the facilities to process and examine the specimens. The principal investigator had access to all the data in the study and takes full responsibility for the integrity and accuracy of the data analysis.

References

[1] J. Á. García-Rodríguez and M. J. Fresnadillo Martínez, "Dynamics of nasopharyngeal colonization by potential respiratory pathogens," *Journal of Antimicrobial Chemotherapy*, vol. 50, supplement S2, pp. 59–73, 2002.

[2] D. P. Morris, "Bacterial biofilm in upper respiratory tract infections," *Current Infectious Disease Reports*, vol. 9, no. 3, pp. 186–192, 2007.

[3] N. Yamanaka, "Moving towards a new Era in the research of tonsils and mucosal barriers," *Advances in Oto-Rhino-Laryngology*, vol. 72, pp. 6–19, 2011.

[4] M. Bista, R. C. M. Amatya, and P. Basnet, "Tonsillar microbial flora: a comparison of infected and noninfected tonsils," *Kathmandu University Medical Journal*, vol. 4, no. 13, pp. 18–21, 2006.

[5] P. V. Vlastarakos, T. P. Nikolopoulos, P. Maragoudakis, A. Tzagaroulakis, and E. Ferekidis, "Biofilms in ear, nose, and throat infections: how important are they?" *The Laryngoscope*, vol. 117, no. 4, pp. 668–673, 2007.

[6] R. E. Kania, G. E. M. Lamers, M. J. Vonk et al., "Demonstration of bacterial cells and glycocalyx in biofilms on human tonsils," *Archives of Otolaryngology*, vol. 133, no. 2, pp. 115–121, 2007.

[7] K. W. Bayles, "The biological role of death and lysis in biofilm development," *Nature Reviews Microbiology*, vol. 5, no. 9, pp. 721–726, 2007.

[8] A. Seminara, T. E. Angelini, J. N. Wilking et al., "Osmotic spreading of *Bacillus subtilis* biofilms driven by an extracellular matrix," *Proceedings of the National Academy of Sciences of the United States of America*, vol. 109, no. 4, pp. 1116–1121, 2012.

[9] R. R. Diaz, S. Picciafuoco, M. G. Paraje et al., "Relevance of biofilms in pediatric tonsillar disease," *European Journal of Clinical Microbiology and Infectious Diseases*, vol. 30, no. 12, pp. 1503–1509, 2011.

[10] C. Potera, "Forging a link between biofilms and disease," *Science*, vol. 283, no. 5409, pp. 1837–1839, 1999.

[11] C. A. Fux, J. W. Costerton, P. S. Stewart, and P. Stoodley, "Survival strategies of infectious biofilms," *Trends in Microbiology*, vol. 13, no. 1, pp. 34–40, 2005.

[12] J. C. Nickel, I. Ruseska, J. B. Wright, and J. W. Costerton, "Tobramycin resistance of *Pseudomonas aeruginosa* cells growing as a biofilm on urinary catheter material," *Antimicrobial Agents and Chemotherapy*, vol. 27, no. 4, pp. 619–624, 1985.

[13] M. El-Azizi, S. Rao, T. Kanchanapoom, and N. Khardori, "*In vitro* activity of vancomycin, quinupristin/dalfopristin, and

linezolid against intact and disrupted biofilms of staphylococci," *Annals of Clinical Microbiology and Antimicrobials*, vol. 4, article 2, 2005.

[14] R. D. Wolcott and G. D. Ehrlich, "Biofilms and chronic infections," *Journal of the American Medical Association*, vol. 299, no. 22, pp. 2682–2684, 2008.

[15] J. N. Palmer, "Bacterial biofilms: do they play a role in chronic sinusitis?" *Otolaryngologic Clinics of North America*, vol. 38, no. 6, pp. 1193–1201, 2005.

[16] I. J. Nixon and B. J. G. Bingham, "The impact of methicillin-resistant *Staphylococcus aureus* on ENT practice," *The Journal of Laryngology and Otology*, vol. 120, no. 9, pp. 713–717, 2006.

[17] I. Brook, "Antibiotic resistance of oral anaerobic bacteria and their effect on the management of upper respiratory tract and head and neck infections," *Seminars in Respiratory Infections*, vol. 17, no. 3, pp. 195–203, 2002.

[18] R. A. Chole and B. T. Faddis, "Anatomical evidence of microbial biofilms in tonsillar tissues: a possible mechanism to explain chronicity," *Archives of Otolaryngology*, vol. 129, no. 6, pp. 634–636, 2003.

[19] A. H. Messner and R. Pelayo, "Pediatric sleep-related breathing disorders," *The American Journal of Otolaryngology*, vol. 21, no. 2, pp. 98–107, 2000.

[20] I. Brook, P. Yocum, and P. A. Foote Jr., "Changes in the core tonsillar bacteriology of recurrent tonsillitis: 1977- 1993," *Clinical Infectious Diseases*, vol. 21, no. 1, pp. 171–176, 1995.

[21] I. Brook, "Failure of penicillin to eradicate group A beta-hemolytic streptococci tonsillitis: causes and management," *Journal of Otolaryngology*, vol. 30, no. 6, pp. 324–329, 2001.

[22] A. Jain and A. Agarwal, "Biofilm production, a marker of pathogenic potential of colonizing and commensal staphylococci," *Journal of Microbiological Methods*, vol. 76, no. 1, pp. 88–92, 2009.

[23] R. M. Donlan and J. W. Costerton, "Biofilms: survival mechanisms of clinically relevant microorganisms," *Clinical Microbiology Reviews*, vol. 15, no. 2, pp. 167–193, 2002.

[24] A. Oliveira and M. D. L. R. S. Cunha, "Comparison of methods for the detection of biofilm production in coagulase-negative staphylococci," *BMC Research Notes*, vol. 3, article 260, 2010.

[25] D. H. Darrow and C. Siemens, "Indications for tonsillectomy and adenoidectomy," *The Laryngoscope*, vol. 112, supplement S100, pp. 6–10, 2002.

[26] D. Gozal, "Obstructive sleep apnea in children," *Minerva Pediatrica*, vol. 52, no. 11, pp. 629–639, 2000.

[27] J. J. Kuhn, I. Brook, C. L. Waters, L. W. P. Church, D. A. Bianchi, and D. H. Thompson, "Quantitative bacteriology of tonsils removed from children with tonsillitis hypertrophy and recurrent tonsillitis with and without hypertrophy," *Annals of Otology, Rhinology and Laryngology*, vol. 104, no. 8, pp. 646–652, 1995.

[28] A. Loganathan, U. D. Arumainathan, and R. Raman, "Comparative study of bacteriology in recurrent tonsillitis among children and adults," *Singapore Medical Journal*, vol. 47, no. 4, pp. 271–275, 2006.

[29] M. Greenfeld, R. Tauman, A. DeRowe, and Y. Sivan, "Obstructive sleep apnea syndrome due to adenotonsillar hypertrophy in infants," *International Journal of Pediatric Otorhinolaryngology*, vol. 67, no. 10, pp. 1055–1060, 2003.

[30] N. F. Weir, "Clinical interpretation of tonsillar size," *The Journal of Laryngology and Otology*, vol. 86, no. 11, pp. 1137–1144, 1972.

[31] L. Brodsky, "Modern assessment of tonsils and adenoids," *Pediatric Clinics of North America*, vol. 36, no. 6, pp. 1551–1569, 1989.

[32] M. Al Ahmary, A. Al Mastour, and W. Ghnnam, "The microbiology of tonsils in Khamis civil hospital, Saudi Arabia," *ISRN Otolaryngology*, vol. 2012, Article ID 813581, 3 pages, 2012.

[33] C. T. Sasaki and N. Koss, "Chronic bacterial tonsillitis: fact or fiction," *Otolaryngology*, vol. 86, no. 6, part 1, pp. 858–864, 1978.

[34] CLSI, *Analysis and Presentation of Cumulative Antimicrobial Susceptibility Test Data, Approved Guideline*, Clinical Laboratory and Standards Institute (CLSI), Wayne, Pa, USA, 3rd edition, 2009.

[35] CLSI, *Methods for Dilution Antimicrobial Susceptibility Tests for Bacteria That Grow Aerobically, Approved Standard*, Clinical and Laboratory Standards Institute (CLSI), Wayne, Pa, USA, 2009.

[36] C. J. Hochstim, J. Y. Choi, D. Lowe, R. Masood, and D. H. Rice, "Biofilm detection with hematoxylin-eosin staining," *Archives of Otolaryngology*, vol. 136, no. 5, pp. 453–456, 2010.

[37] S. Alasil, R. Omar, S. Ismail, M. Y. Yusof, and M. Ameen, "Bacterial identification and antibiotic susceptibility patterns of *Staphyloccocus aureus* isolates from patients undergoing tonsillectomy in Malaysian University Hospital," *African Journal of Microbiology Research*, vol. 5, no. 27, pp. 4748–4752, 2011.

[38] I. H. Kielmovitch, G. Keleti, C. D. Bluestone, E. R. Wald, and C. Gonzalez, "Microbiology of obstructive tonsillar hypertrophy and recurrent tonsillitis," *Archives of Otolaryngology*, vol. 115, no. 6, pp. 721–724, 1989.

[39] G. Almadori, L. Bastianini, F. Bistoni, G. Paludetti, and M. Rosignoli, "Microbial flora of surface versus core tonsillar cultures in recurrent tonsillitis in children," *International Journal of Pediatric Otorhinolaryngology*, vol. 15, no. 2, pp. 157–162, 1988.

[40] I. Brook, P. Yocum, and K. Shah, "Surface vs core-tonsillar aerobic and anaerobic flora in recurrent tonsillitis," *Journal of the American Medical Association*, vol. 244, no. 15, pp. 1696–1698, 1980.

[41] G. Rosen, J. Samuel, and I. Vered, "Surface tonsillar microflora versus deep tonsillar microflora in recurrent acute tonsillitis," *The Journal of Laryngology and Otology*, vol. 91, no. 10, pp. 911–913, 1977.

[42] M. Gul, E. Okur, P. Ciragil, I. Yildirim, M. Aral, and M. Akif Kilic, "The comparison of tonsillar surface and core cultures in recurrent tonsillitis," *The American Journal of Otolaryngology*, vol. 28, no. 3, pp. 173–176, 2007.

[43] L. Brodsky, L. Moore, J. F. Stanievich, and P. L. Ogra, "The immunology of tonsils in children: The effect of bacterial load on the presence of B- and T-cell subsets," *The Laryngoscope*, vol. 98, no. 1, pp. 93–98, 1988.

[44] C. W. Gross and S. E. Harrison, "Tonsils and adenoids," *Pediatrics Reviews*, vol. 21, no. 3, pp. 75–78, 2000.

[45] W. E. Sadoh, A. E. Sadoh, A. O. Oladipo, and O. O. Okunola, "Bacterial isolates of tonsillitis and pharyngitis in a paediatric casualty setting," *Journal of Medicine and Biomedical Research*, vol. 7, no. 1, pp. 37–44, 2008.

[46] E. M. Brown and P. Thomas, "Fusidic acid resistance in *Staphylococcus aureus* isolates," *The Lancet*, vol. 359, no. 9308, p. 803, 2002.

[47] A. Norazah, V. K. E. Lim, Y. T. Koh et al., "Molecular fingerprinting of fusidic acid- and rifampicin-resistant strains of methicillin-resistant *Staphylococcus aureus* (MRSA) from Malaysian hospitals," *Journal of Medical Microbiology*, vol. 51, no. 12, pp. 1113–1116, 2002.

[48] L. B. Rice, "Progress and challenges in implementing the research on ESKAPE pathogens," *Infection Control and Hospital Epidemiology*, vol. 31, supplement 1, pp. S7–S10, 2010.

[49] S. E. Holm and E. Grahn, "Bacterial interference in streptococal tonsillitis," *Scandinavian Journal of Infectious Diseases*, vol. 39, pp. 73–78, 1983.

[50] I. Brook and A. E. Gober, "Long-term effects on the nasopharyngeal flora of children following antimicrobial therapy of acute otitis media with cefdinir or amoxycillin-clavulanate," *Journal of Medical Microbiology*, vol. 54, part 6, pp. 553–556, 2005.

[51] H. Ceri, M. E. Olson, C. Stremick, R. R. Read, D. Morck, and A. Buret, "The Calgary Biofilm Device: New technology for rapid determination of antibiotic susceptibilities of bacterial biofilms," *Journal of Clinical Microbiology*, vol. 37, no. 6, pp. 1771–1776, 1999.

[52] M. E. Olson, H. Ceri, D. W. Morck, A. G. Buret, and R. R. Read, "Biofilm bacteria: formation and comparative susceptibility to antibiotics," *Canadian Journal of Veterinary Research*, vol. 66, no. 2, pp. 86–92, 2002.

[53] A. R. Dell'Aringa, A. J. C. Juares, C. de Melo, J. C. Nardi, K. Kobari, and R. M. Perches Filbo, "Histopathologic analysis of the adenotonsilectomy specimens from January 2001 to May 2003," *Revista Brasileira de Otorrinolaringologia*, vol. 71, no. 1, pp. 18–22, 2005.

[54] S. M. Pransky, J. I. Feldman, D. B. Kearns, A. B. Seid, and G. F. Billman, "Actinomycosis in obstructive tonsillar hypertrophy and recurrent tonsillitis," *Archives of Otolaryngology*, vol. 117, no. 8, pp. 883–885, 1991.

[55] J. B. Surow, S. D. Handler, S. A. Telian, G. R. Fleisher, and C. C. Baranak, "Bacteriology of tonsil surface and core in children," *The Laryngoscope*, vol. 99, no. 3, pp. 261–266, 1989.

[56] M. A. Richardson, "Sore throat, tonsillitis and adenoiditis," *Medical Clinics of North America*, vol. 83, no. 1, pp. 75–83, 1999.

[57] A. Stjernquist-Desatnik and E. Holst, "Tonsillar microbial flora: comparison of recurrent tonsillitis and normal tonsils," *Acta Oto-Laryngologica*, vol. 119, no. 1, pp. 102–106, 1999.

[58] H. Akiyama, T. Hamada, W.-K. Huh, O. Yamasaki, T. Oono, and K. Iwatsuki, "Confocal laser scanning microscopic observation of glycocalyx production by *Staphylococcus aureus* in mouse skin: does *S. aureus* generally produce a biofilm on damaged skin?" *British Journal of Dermatology*, vol. 147, no. 5, pp. 879–885, 2002.

[59] P. S. Stewart and J. W. Costerton, "Antibiotic resistance of bacteria in biofilms," *The Lancet*, vol. 358, no. 9276, pp. 135–138, 2001.

[60] J. H. Woo, S. T. Kim, I. G. Kang, J. H. Lee, H. E. Cha, and D. Y. Kim, "Comparison of tonsillar biofilms between patients with recurrent tonsillitis and a control group," *Acta Otolaryngologica*, vol. 132, no. 10, pp. 1115–1120, 2012.

[61] K. A. Al-Mazrou and A. S. Al-Khattaf, "Adherent biofilms in adenotonsillar diseases in children," *Archives of Otolaryngology*, vol. 134, no. 1, pp. 20–23, 2008.

[62] P. Ogra and R. Welliver Sr., "Effects of early environment on mucosal immunologic homeostasis, subsequent immune responses and disease outcome," *Nestle Nutrition Workshop Series: Pediatric Program*, vol. 61, pp. 145–181, 2008.

[63] Y. H. Lai and M. D'Souza, "Microparticle transport in the human intestinal M cell model," *Journal of Drug Targeting*, vol. 16, no. 1, pp. 36–42, 2008.

[64] M. E. Zernotti, N. A. Villegas, M. R. Revol et al., "Evidence of bacterial biofilms in nasal polyposis," *Journal of Investigational Allergology and Clinical Immunology*, vol. 20, no. 5, pp. 380–385, 2010.

9

Goiter and Laryngeal Sensory Neuropathy

Abdul Latif Hamdan,[1] Jad Jabour,[1] and Sami T. Azar[1,2]

[1] *Department of Otolaryngology-Head & Neck Surgery, American University of Beirut Medical Center,
P.O. Box 110-236, Beirut, Lebanon*
[2] *Department of Internal Medicine, Division of Endocrinology and Metabolism, American University of Beirut Medical Center,
P.O. Box 110-236, Beirut, Lebanon*

Correspondence should be addressed to Sami T. Azar; sazar@aub.edu.lb

Academic Editor: Bill Yates

Objective. Examining the prevalence of laryngeal sensory neuropathy (LSN) in goiter patients versus a control group. *Study Design.* Cross-sectional study. *Methods.* 33 Goiter patients were enrolled versus 25 age-matched controls. TSH levels, size of thyroid gland, and presence or absence of thyroid nodules were reported. Subjects were asked about the presence or absence of any of the following symptoms: cough, globus pharyngeus, and/or throat clearing that persistented for more than 6 weeks. The presence of one or more of these symptoms for at least six weeks in the absence of LPRD, allergy, asthma, ACE inhibitor intake, and psychogenic disorder was defined as LSN. *Results.* For goitrous patients mean age (years) was (41.73 ± 9.47) versus (37.44 ± 10.89) for controls. 82% goitrous patients had known nodules and 27% carried a simultaneous diagnosis of hypothyroidism. Among those with documented size (61%), mean total thyroid volume was 26.996 ± 14.852 cm^3, with a range from 9.430 to 67.022 cm^3. The overall prevalence of LSN among goitrous patients was 42% versus 12% among controls (P = 0.0187). There was no correlation between LSN, size of thyroid gland, and TSH level. *Conclusion.* The prevalence of LSN in goitrous patients is significantly higher than that in a nongoitrous population.

1. Introduction

Goiter is the most prevalent endocrine condition in the world affecting over 500 million with prevalence rates reaching up to 30% [1, 2]. It is believed to result from an interaction between genetics and environmental factors, namely, iodine deficiency. It has long been established that adequate iodine uptake is crucial, as low iodine levels lead to hypothyroidism which in turn increases blood levels of thyroid stimulating hormone (TSH) resulting in glandular hypertrophy [3]. Thus, certain conditions that exacerbate iodine deficiency, such as smoking or increased parity, can be considered risk factors for goiter [4]. While the exact contribution of each factor remains unclear, genetic predisposition to goiter also plays a crucial role in goitrogenesis [5].

Patients with goiter may complain of cosmetic disfigurement attributed to the visibly enlarged thyroid gland, of symptoms of hyper or hypothyroidism secondary to the altered levels of thyroid hormones, and last but not the least

of compressive neck symptoms. These include respiratory discomfort, stridor, and change in voice quality, globus pharyngeus, dysphagia, and others. The neck and throat symptoms in patients with goiter have been invariably attributed to the glandular hypertrophy of the thyroid and its mass effect on the laryngotracheal framework. The enlarged gland may impede the movement of the larynx and trachea and thus interfere with the basic functions of the larynx, namely, phonation and swallowing. Compression and invasion of the laryngotracheal complex may also result in airway symptoms with narrowing of the lumen and or impaired mobility of the vocal fold with or without recurrent laryngeal nerve neuropathy [1].

No previous study has examined the possible presence of laryngeal sensory neuropathy (LSN) in patients with goiter despite the fact that LSN is a confounding etiology for many of the throat and pharyngeal symptoms in goitrous patients. The presence of globus pharyngeus, cough, throat discomfort, and change in voice quality in patients with goiter might be the clinical manifestation of other diseases beside goiter. [6, 7]. Laryngeal sensory neuropathy is usually suspected when other etiologies have been ruled out and/or when positive response to a neuromodulator is displayed. It is considered in the differential diagnosis of chronic cough (longer than 6 weeks), when conditions such as asthma, pneumonia, bronchitis, LPR, or ACE inhibitor adverse reactions have been ruled out [7]. The presence of throat discomfort of acute onset in addition to cough should allude more to the etiological role of laryngeal sensory neuropathy [8]. What helps to confirm the diagnosis of LSN is the response to neuromodulating agents such as pregabalin and gabapentin [7]. In a retrospective chart review of 12 patients prescribed pregabalin for symptoms of LSN, the mean treatment chief complaint symptom decreased from 3.9 to 1.2 after a one-month treatment with pregabalin.

The purpose of this study is to examine the prevalence of LSN in a cross-section of goiter patients compared to a control group. Improved knowledge of the prevalence of LSN status in patients with goiter may lead to better management of symptoms previously attributed to the mass effect of thyroid gland alone. Patients with goiter and laryngopharyngeal symptoms due to LSN may be treated with neuromdulators. The resolution of these symptoms may spare goitrous patients the need for surgical intervention.

The hypothesis of the study is that the prevalence of LSN is significantly higher in a population of goitrous patients compared to that in nongoitrous controls.

2. Methods

Thirty-Three consecutive patients with goiter were recruited over a two-month period at a private endocrinology clinic at the American University of Beirut Medical Center. All goitrous patients between the ages of 18–65 were informed of a study taking place in the adjacent "Hamdan Voice Unit" regarding the possible association of goiter with laryngeal sensory neuropathy. None of the patients with goiter refused to participate in the study. The diagnosis of goiter was based on clinical and/or radiological examination using ultrasound. Thirty-three patients enrolled in the study and signed a consent form approved by the Institutional Review Board at the American University of Beirut. During the same period, twenty-five age-matched controls were recruited by word of mouth. Exclusion criteria included history of laryngeal manipulation or current upper respiratory infection symptoms.

Demographic data included age, gender, smoking status, laryngopharyngeal reflux disease, and allergy. The presence of laryngopharyngeal reflux disease was based on a reflux symptom Index above 9 using the reflux symptom index designed by Belafsky et al. [9]. The presence of allergy was confirmed using a validated questionnaire developed by Bauchau et al. [10].

For goiter patients, the following parameters were also reported: thyroid hormonal level, size of the thyroid gland, and presence or absence of thyroid nodules. The thyroid hormonal level was determined using their last Thyroid Stimulating Hormone test (TSH). A range between 0.27 and 4.20 microunit/mL was considered as normal. Findings from the most recent ultrasound were used to establish the size of the thyroid. The presence of thyroid nodule was determined on either clinical or radiological examination.

Subjects were asked about the presence or absence of any of the following symptoms: cough, globus pharyngeus, and or throat clearing that was persistent for more than 6 weeks. The presence of one or more of these symptoms for at least six weeks in the absence of laryngopharyngeal reflux disease, allergy, asthma, ACE inhibitor intake, and psychogenic disorder was defined as laryngeal sensory neuropathy based on the definition by Halum et al. [7]. Patients were considered to have no laryngopharyngeal disease when the reflux symptom index was less than nine.

Simple descriptive analysis was used to determine the prevalence of vocal symptoms suggestive of LSN in this cross-sectional sample of goiter patients. The Fisher exact test was used to make comparisons between goiter patients and controls and between goitrous patients with and without hypothyroidism. The Pearson correlation coefficient was calculated to test for associations between the presence of LSN and goiter size.

3. Results

3.1. Demographic Data. A total of 33 patients with goiter and 25 controls with no diagnosis of goiter were enrolled in the study. The mean age was 41.73 ± 9.47 for goitrous patients and 37.44 ± 10.89 for controls. The prevalence of smoking was 27% (9/33) among goitrous patients and 20% (5/25) among controls ($P = 0.5551$). The prevalence of allergies was 12% (4/33) among cases and 32% (8/25) among controls.

Among goitrous patients, 82% (27/33) had known nodules. Twenty-seven percent (9/27) carried a simultaneous diagnosis of hypothyroidism; none had hyperthyroidism. For 61% (20/33), a documented thyroid size based on ultrasound performed within the last year was available. Among those with documented size, mean total thyroid volume was $26.996 \pm 14.852 \, \text{cm}^3$, with a range from 9.430 to $67.022 \, \text{cm}^3$ (Table 1).

3.2. Prevalence of LSN in Patients with Goiter and Controls. The overall prevalence of LSN determined by the aforementioned criteria among goitrous patients was 42% (14/33). The prevalence among controls was 12% (3/25). The difference in proportions was statistically significant ($P = 0.0187$) (Table 2).

3.3. Correlation between Laryngeal Sensory Neuropathy, Size of Thyroid Gland, and Thyroid Hormonal Level. Only twenty patients with goiter had documented ultrasound measurements of their thyroid gland. Only eight of these twenty subjects had LSN. Those with LSN had a mean thyroid volume of $24.126 \pm 19.834 \, \text{cm}^3$, while those without LSN had a mean thyroid volume of $27.629 \pm 11.209 \, \text{cm}^3$ ($P = 0.5062$). The calculated Pearson correlation coefficient was $r = -0.118$, giving a two-sided P value of 0.6188 (Table 3).

The prevalence of LSN among cases with simultaneous diagnosis of hypothyroidism was 44% (4/9), compared to

TABLE 1: Demographic data for cases and controls, including prevalence of smoking, reflux, allergies, and concurrent endocrine conditions.

	Cases	Controls
Total number (n)	33	25
Mean Age ± SD	41.73 ± 9.47	37.44 ± 10.89
Gender (% males)	6	40
Smoking (%)	27	20
Reflux (%)	12	12
Allergy (%)	12	32
Mean thyroid size (cm^3)	26.996 ± 14.852	
(Range)	9.430–67.022	
Thyroid stimulating hormonal level		
Hypothyroidism (%)	27	0
Hyperthyroidism (%)	3	0
Euthyroid (%)	70	0
Thyroid nodules (%)	82	—

TABLE 2: Prevalence of Laryngeal Sensory Neuropathy (LSN) in cases and controls.

	Cases	Controls	P-value
LSN (%)	42	12	0.0187

TABLE 3: Results of Fisher exact test and Pearson correlation test for association between thyroid size and LSN prevalence, no significant P values.

Mean thyroid size (cm^3)	Goitrous pts with LSN	Goitrous patients without LSN	P value
	24.126 ± 19.834	27.629 ± 11.209	0.5062
Pearson correlation coeff. (r)	−0.118		
2-side P value	0.6118		

42% (10/24) among those without hypothyroidism (P = 1.000). There was no correlation between LSN, size of the gland, and hypothyroidism.

4. Discussion

Chronic refractory cough is present in roughly 31% of the general population [10], attributed to a wide variety of conditions. Though relatively rare, laryngeal sensory neuropathy has fairly recently gained attention as a potential cause of not only chronic cough, but also throat discomfort and possibly dysphagia and dysphonia [7, 11]. It is thought to be the result of a decrease in the laryngeal sensory threshold leading to a variety of abnormal laryngeal behavior. These include abnormal glottic closure reflexes, intractable cough, throat clearing, impaired mobility of the vocal folds and vocal fold paralysis [8, 12, 13]. The diagnosis of laryngeal sensory neuropathy is that of exclusion after having excluded the aforementioned confounding diseases, namely; reflux, allergy, asthma, ACE inhibitor intake, and psychogenic disorders. Other diagnostic tests include fiberoptic laryngeal sensory testing through the repeated application of air puffs to elicit glottic closure reflex and using surface evoked laryngeal sensory action potential evaluation [11, 14].

In view of the overlap in the laryngopharyngeal symptoms of patients with LSN and patients with goiter, the authors of this paper have been intrigued to examine the prevalence of LSN in patients with goiter. The hypothesis is that LSN is more prevalent in patients with goiter compared to controls. Fiorentino et al. had made a similar argument in relation to LPR pointing out other potential explanations for the local neck symptoms often experienced by goitrous patients and normally attributed solely to the goiter [6]. The hypothesis for the increased prevalence of LSN in the population of this study can largely be based on one or many of the suggested mechanisms for LSN previously described in the literature. Though the exact pathogenesis of LSN in general has not been elucidated, several theories have been suggested. These include viral infections, metabolic changes, and insult to either the recurrent laryngeal nerve or superior laryngeal nerve with subsequent change in the firing threshold [7]. Because LSN is thought to occur secondary to mechanical damage to nerves [7] and such damage can be associated with glandular hypertrophy [1], it is reasonable to expect a higher prevalence of LSN in patients with goiter. In view of the proximity of the thyroid gland to the laryngeal framework, hypertrophy of the thyroid gland may induce stretching of the recurrent laryngeal nerve, compression, reduction in its blood supply, perineural inflammation and fibrosis, and or simply direct invasion of the nerve [15]. All of the suggested mechanisms may result in damage to the laryngeal innervations with subsequent increase in laryngopharyngeal symptoms.

Indeed, the results of our study supported the hypothesis that the prevalence of LSN in a population of goitrous patients is significantly higher than that in a population of nongoitrous controls. Nearly half (42%) of goitrous patients in this study had LSN compared to only 12% in the control group. The prevalence of smoking in both subgroups, goitrous patients with LSN and controls with LSN, was similar (35.7% versus 33.3%, resp.). What is surprising on the other hand is the lack of correlation between the size of the gland and LSN in our study. The results of the Pearson correlation analysis suggest that there is no significant association between thyroid volume and prevalence of LSN ($r = −0.118$; $P = 0.6118$). The lack of correlation in our study might be attributed to the small size sample and the relatively moderate size of the gland in our subject population (mean of 26.996 ± 14.852 cm^3). While a correlation with thyroid size might be expected based on the proposed mechanism of association between goiter and LSN previously mentioned, further studies would be needed to elucidate this relationship.

Another possible explanation for the LSN is metabolic damage. Common example is sensory neuropathy in patients with diabetes mellitus. Poor glycemic control is known to result in nerve degeneration with resultant demyelination and poor nerve conduction [16]. Subsequently patients with diabetic neuropathy experience symptoms of numbness, paresthesia, and pain. Similarly, thyroid diseases have been reported to cause signs and symptoms of neuromuscular dysfunction [17–20]. Most often reported clinical features are proximal muscle weakness, mononeuropathy, and sensorimotor polyneuropathy. In a large case-control cross-sectional study on 40 patients with hypothyroidism, the majority had carpel tunnel syndrome [18]. In another prospective study by El-Salem and Ammari on twenty-three neurologically asymptomatic patients with primary hypothyroidism, nerve conduction studies revealed that almost half of the subjects had some abnormality predominantly of the motor demylinating pattern, and nondisfigurative myopathic changes were seen in 74% of the patients most commonly affecting the deltoid [19]. In corroboration with these results, Duyff et al., in his evaluation of patients newly diagnosed with hypo- and hyperthyroidism, indicated that neuromuscular symptoms and signs were commonly present and that 40% and 20% of hypothyroid and hyperthyroid patients had sensory signs of a sensorimotor axonal neuropathy [20].

In this study, it did not appear that hypothyroidism had an independent effect on LSN, as subgroup analysis between goitrous patients with and without hypothyroidism revealed no significant difference in prevalence of LSN ($P = 1.000$). This lack of correlation between hypothyroidism and LSN is not commensurate with the previous reports on the neuromuscular and sensory motor status in patients with hypothyroidism. This can be attributed to the small sample size and the lack of any objective measures to detect subclinical neuromuscular manifestations.

There are two main limitations to this study. The first is the relatively small sample size and the second is the lack of objective diagnostic tests for LSN employed. For instance, LSN can be associated with alterations in surface evoked laryngeal sensory action potential (SELSAP) waveforms [15]. Alternatively, fiberoptic endoscopy can be used to evaluate laryngeal sensation [17]. Nonetheless, LSN remains primarily a clinical diagnosis, and thus clinical criteria were used in this study.

To the authors' knowledge, this is the first paper to explicitly examine the prevalence of LSN in goitrous patients. A more extensive study, with similar methodologies, could be done to corroborate the findings presented here. The highly significant P value (0.0187) strongly suggests that a true difference in LSN prevalence exists between goitrous and nongoitrous patients. Consequently, it may be worthwhile to consider a neuromodulating agent to relieve the patient's symptoms, before concluding that they are a direct result of the goiter and would be relieved by surgery. Further research would need to be undertaken on this question before proposing any official recommendations.

5. Conclusion

The prevalence of laryngeal sensory neuropathy (LSN) in a population of goitrous patients is significantly higher than that in a nongoitrous population. Symptoms of persistent cough, throat clearing, dysphonia, or globus pharyngeus in those with goiter may be attributable to LSN, rather than the goiter itself. Physicians should be aware of how this possible etiology could alter the optimal management approach.

Conflict of Interests

There is no conflict of interests or financial interest relevant to this paper.

References

[1] T. A. Day, A. Chu, and K. G. Hoang, "Multinodular goiter," *Otolaryngologic Clinics of North America*, vol. 36, no. 1, pp. 35–54, 2003.

[2] C. Reiners, K. Wegscheider, H. Schicha et al., "Prevalence of thyroid disorders in the working population of Germany: ultrasonography screening in 96,278 unselected employees," *Thyroid*, vol. 14, no. 11, pp. 926–932, 2004.

[3] R. Paschke, "Nodulogenesis and goitrogenesis," *Annales d'Endocrinologie*, vol. 72, no. 2, pp. 117–119, 2011.

[4] N. Knudsen, P. Laurberg, H. Perrild, I. Bülow, L. Ovesen, and T. Jørgensen, "Risk factors for goiter and thyroid nodules," *Thyroid*, vol. 12, no. 10, pp. 879–888, 2002.

[5] J. Singer, M. Eszlinger, J. Wicht, and R. Paschke, "Evidence for a more pronounced effect of genetic predisposition than environmental factors on goitrogenesis by a case control study in an area with low normal iodine supply," *Hormone and Metabolic Research*, vol. 43, no. 5, pp. 349–354, 2011.

[6] E. Fiorentino, C. Cipolla, G. Graceffa et al., "Local neck symptoms before and after thyroidectomy: a possible correlation with reflux laryngopharyngitis," *European Archives of Oto-Rhino-Laryngology*, vol. 268, no. 5, pp. 715–720, 2011.

[7] S. L. Halum, D. L. Sycamore, and B. R. McRae, "A new treatment option for laryngeal sensory neuropathy," *Laryngoscope*, vol. 119, no. 9, pp. 1844–1847, 2009.

[8] B. Lee and P. Woo, "Chronic cough as a sign of laryngeal sensory neuropathy: diagnosis and treatment," *Annals of Otology, Rhinology and Laryngology*, vol. 114, no. 4, pp. 253–257, 2005.

[9] P. C. Belafsky, G. N. Postma, and J. A. Koufman, "Validity and reliability of the reflux symptom index (RSI)," *Journal of Voice*, vol. 16, no. 2, pp. 274–277, 2002.

[10] V. Bauchau, D. Philippart, and S. Durham, "A simple and efficient screening tool for allergic rhinitis," in *Proceedings of the 23rd Congress of the European Academy of Allergology and Clinical Immunology*, Amsterdam, The Netherlands, June 2004.

[11] J. M. Bock, J. H. Blumin, R. J. Toohill, A. L. Merati, T. E. Prieto, and S. S. Jaradeh, "A new noninvasive method for determination of laryngeal sensory function," *Laryngoscope*, vol. 121, no. 1, pp. 158–163, 2011.

[12] R. W. Bastian, A. M. Vaidya, and K. G. Delsupehe, "Sensory neuropathic cough: a common and treatable cause of chronic cough," *Otolaryngology*, vol. 135, no. 1, pp. 17–21, 2006.

[13] M. R. Amin and J. A. Koufman, "Vagal neuropathy after upper respiratory infection: a viral etiology?" *American Journal of Otolaryngology*, vol. 22, no. 4, pp. 251–256, 2001.

[14] J. E. Aviv, T. Kim, J. E. Thomson, S. Sunshine, S. Kaplan, and L. G. Close, "Fiberoptic endoscopic evaluation of swallowing with sensory testing (FEESST) in healthy controls," *Dysphagia*, vol. 13, no. 2, pp. 87–92, 1998.

[15] R. T. J. Holl-Allen, "Benign thyroid disease and vocal cord palsy," *Annals of the Royal College of Surgeons of England*, vol. 75, no. 6, p. 450, 1993.

[16] R. Jamali and S. Mohseni, "Hypoglycaemia causes degeneration of large myelinated nerve fibres in the vagus nerve of insulin-treated diabetic BB/Wor rats," *Acta Neuropathologica*, vol. 109, no. 2, pp. 198–206, 2005.

[17] S. N. Rao, B. C. Katiyar, K. R. P. Nair, and S. Misra, "Neuromuscular status in hypothyroidism," *Acta Neurologica Scandinavica*, vol. 61, no. 3, pp. 167–177, 1980.

[18] F. Eslamian, A. Bahrami, N. Aghamohammadzadeh, M. Niafar, Y. Salekzamani, and K. Behkamrad, "Electrophysiologic changes in patients with untreated primary hypothyroidism," *Journal of Clinical Neurophysiology*, vol. 28, no. 3, pp. 323–328, 2011.

[19] K. El-Salem and F. Ammari, "Neurophysiological changes in neurologically asymptomatic hypothyroid patients: a prospective cohort study," *Journal of Clinical Neurophysiology*, vol. 23, no. 6, pp. 568–572, 2006.

[20] R. F. Duyff, J. Van Den Bosch, D. M. Laman, B. J. Potter Van Loon, and W. H. J. P. Linssen, "Neuromuscular findings in thyroid dysfunction: a prospective clinical and electrodiagnostic study," *Journal of Neurology Neurosurgery and Psychiatry*, vol. 68, no. 6, pp. 750–755, 2000.

10

Radiological Assessment of the Indian Children with Congenital Sensorineural Hearing Loss

Sangeet Kumar Agarwal,[1] Satinder Singh,[1] Samarjit Singh Ghuman,[2] Shalabh Sharma,[1] and Asish Kr. Lahiri[1]

[1] *Department of Otorhinolaryngology and Head, Neck Surgery, Sir Ganga Ram Hospital, New Delhi 110049, India*
[2] *Department of Radiology, Sir Ganga Ram Hospital, New Delhi 110049, India*

Correspondence should be addressed to Sangeet Kumar Agarwal; drsangeetagarwal@gmail.com

Academic Editor: Myer III Myer

Introduction. Congenital sensorineural hearing loss is one of the most common birth defects with incidence of approximately 1 : 1000 live births. Imaging of cases of congenital sensorineural hearing loss is frequently performed in an attempt to determine the underlying pathology. There is a paucity of literature from India and for this reason we decided to conduct this study in Indian context to evaluate the various cochleovestibular bony and nerve anomalies by HRCT scan of temporal bone and MRI with 3D scan of inner ear in a tertiary care centre. *Material and Methods.* A total of 280 children with congenital deafness (158 males and 122 females), between January 2002 to June 2013 were included in the study and they were assessed radiologically by HRCT scan of temporal bone and MRI with 3D scan of inner ear. *Results.* In the present study we found various congenital anomalies of bony labyrinth and vestibulocochlear nerve. Out of 560 inner ears we found 78 anomalous inner ears. Out of these 78 inner ears 57 (73%) had cochlear anomaly, 68 (87.1%) had anomalous vestibule, 44 (56.4%) had abnormal vestibular aqueduct, 24 (30.7%) had anomalous IAC, and 23 (29.4%) had abnormal cochleovestibular nerves. *Conclusion.* In present study, we found lower incidences of congenital anomalies comparative to existing literature.

1. Introduction

Congenital sensorineural hearing loss is one of the most common birth defects with incidence of approximately 1 : 1000 live births [1]. Imaging of cases of congenital sensorineural hearing loss is frequently performed in an attempt to determine an underlying pathology. Both high resolution computed tomography scan (HRCT) of the temporal bone and magnetic resonance imaging scan (MRI) of the inner ear have been used in this set of patients with certain advantages and disadvantages of each. The HRCT scan reveals many types of bony inner ear malformations and MRI scan provides better visualization of the membranous labyrinth and the status of vestibulocochlear nerves. In such cases the most common CT scan abnormality is a dilated vestibular aqueduct (LVA) defined as measuring greater than 1.5 mm in diameter. This disorder may be unilateral or bilateral [1].

Bony inner ear malformations are fairly uncommon anomalies, representing approximately 20% of the cases of congenital sensorineural hearing loss. The remaining 80% of the cases of congenital malformations are membranous malformations in which bony architecture of the inner ear is normal and the pathology is at the cellular level. In the latter patient group, the result of radiological investigations of the inner ear falls within the normal limits [2].

Before the cochlear implant era, radiology of the temporal bone was not routinely done in prelingually deaf children. It was observed that a few cases of Michel deformity had been inadvertently fitted with hearing aids and rehabilitation was initiated. In order to avoid misfortunes like this, it is now common practice to obtain radiological evaluation of the temporal bone as soon as patient is diagnosed with severe to profound sensorineural hearing loss. Vestibulocochlear congenital anomalies may be classified as follows.

(1) Michel deformity: there is complete absence of all cochlear and vestibular structures.

(2) Cochlear aplasia: the cochlea is completely absent.

(3) Common cavity deformity: there is a cystic cavity representing the cochlea and vestibule but without showing any differentiation into cochlea and vestibule.

(4) Cochlear hypoplasia: the cochlea and vestibule are separate from each other but their dimensions are smaller than normal.

(5) Incomplete partition type I: the cochlea is lacking the entire modiolus and cribriform area resulting in a cystic appearance. This is accompanied by a large cystic vestibule.

(6) Incomplete partition type II (Mondini deformity): the cochlea consists of 1.5 turns in which the middle and apical turns coalesce to form a cystic apex, accompanied by a dilated vestibule and enlarged VA.

(7) Vestibular malformations: They include Michel deformity, common cavity, absent vestibule, and dilated vestibule.

(8) Semicircular canal malformations: They are absent, hypoplastic, or enlarged.

(9) Internal auditory canal malformations: They are absent, narrow, or enlarged.

Radiology gives information regarding the type of malformation, additional pathologies in the middle ear and mastoid, and the presence or absence of the vestibulocochlear nerve. There has been a debate about which of the two modalities, HRCT or MRI, should be used in the preoperative evaluation of candidates undergoing cochlear implantation. HRCT scan of the temporal bone should be obtained in axial and coronal sections. This gives very good details of the temporal bone. Facial nerve abnormalities and the size of any defect between the internal auditory canal (IAC) and inner ear can be better evaluated on HRCT. MRI is important to diagnose the presence of nerves in the IAC and cochlear fluids [3].

Cochlear implants in patients with severe to profound sensorineural hearing loss have proved to be the method of choice for auditory rehabilitation. Accurate preoperative imaging is necessary for selection of candidates, identification of the more suitable ear for implantation, and selection of the appropriate device. The fluid filled cochlea and the cochlear nerve are the structures of highest interest for a successful surgery [4]. Radiological imaging plays a major role in cochlear implantation with regard to preoperative candidacy evaluation, intraoperative monitoring, and postoperative evaluation as well as research and experimental techniques. Imaging the auditory pathway of the implant candidate is necessary to screen for morphological conditions that will preclude or complicate the implantation process.

The selection of candidates for cochlear implantation requires consideration of a variety of clinical and radiographic factors. With the rising use of increasingly complex multichannel implant devices, the preoperative radiographic assessment of the cochlear architecture has become more critical.

The modalities of imaging that are most pertinent to evaluation of auditory pathway are high resolution computed tomography (HRCT) and magnetic resonance imaging (MRI) scans.

Preoperative imaging often provides valuable information that would not preclude implantation but rather helps assessing in which ear it would be technically easier or better to implant a device [5].

The preoperative sectional imaging may derive additional useful information that can optimize safety and facilitate surgery, as well as influencing subsequent patient management. Proper surgical planning must involve careful review of sectional images, so that potential complications may be anticipated and properly managed [6].

There is a paucity of literature from India and for this reason we decided to conduct this study in Indian context.

Aim of the Study. To find out various congenital inner ear malformations by radiological assessment in a tertiary care centre.

2. Material and Methods

This prospective analytical study was undertaken in the Department of Otorhinolaryngology and Head and Neck Surgery at Sir Ganga Ram Hospital (SGRH), New Delhi, from January 2003 to June 2013. We evaluated a total of 280 children (males: 158, females: 122) of age of 01–14 years with standard deviation (SD) of 2.8171 and mean age 2.76 years, with bilateral congenital severe to profound sensorineural hearing loss. All patients had congenital deafness and showed bilateral severe to profound sensorineural hearing loss in observational audiometric tests, otoacoustic emissions, and auditory brain stem responses. All patients were candidates for possible cochlear implantation; the patients underwent HRCT and MRI examination of the temporal bone and inner ear. To reduce motion artifacts, the children were studied in sedation. The patients included in the study were selected on the basis of following inclusion and exclusion criteria.

> Inclusion criteria: children who were congenitally deaf.
>
> Exclusion criteria: children who were not congenitally deaf and developed hearing loss after some acquired cause.

Work-up of the patient includes the brief history of the patient which includes history of hearing loss, prenatal, natal, and postnatal history, drug intake and radiation exposure to mother during pregnancy, developmental history, hearing aid trial, any other associated diseases, and family history.

Examination of patient includes the general examination, ear, nose, and throat examination, and any syndromic signs.

Investigations includes the audiological assessment of patient which includes pure tone audiogram (PTA), free field audiometry (FFA), brain evoked response audiometry (BERA), auditory steady state response (ASSR), and otoacoustic emissions (OAE).

Radiological assessment by HRCT temporal bone and MRI head with 3D reconstruction of cochleovestibular complex to see the status of

(i) morphology of cochlea with modiolus,

(ii) vestibule,

(iii) vestibular aqueduct,

(iv) semicircular canals,

(v) internal auditory canal,

(vi) status of vestibulocochlear nerve.

2.1. Imaging Protocol

2.1.1. HRCT Scan. All HRCT investigations were performed in the axial orientation using multislice light speed with a slice thickness of 0.625 mm and ultrahigh algorithm. These were documented in a bone window. Coronal and sagittal reconstructions were performed with volume rendered images if required. All images were evaluated as advantage windows work stations.

2.1.2. MRI Scan with 3D Reconstruction of Cochlea. All MRI scans were performed on a 3T MRI scanner (Siemens Verio) using an 8-channel head coil and the SPACE (heavily T2 weighted) sequence. Images were viewed on a Siemens work station in multiple planes with MIP and 3D reconstruction.

2.1.3. Sedation. In some of the children up to age of 4 years, Triclofos (5 mL = 750 mg) was given in the dose of 50–70 mg/kg of body weight. For elderly children of age group >4 years, midazolam (0.05–0.1 mg/kg of body weight) was given intravenous.

2.1.4. Image Analysis. All printed CT and MRI were evaluated independently by a senior ENT surgeon, a senior radiologist, and ENT resident. Different parts of inner ear were studied for malformations. The morphology of the cochlea, vestibule, semicircular canals, vestibular aqueduct, and internal auditory canal along with vestibulocochlear and facial nerve is described. The malformations were classified using new classification of inner ear malformations based on CT and MRI given by Sennaroglu and Saatci [6]. The evaluation of nerves within the internal auditory canal was performed with the reconstructed axial and parasagittal MR images. The complete course, from the brain stem into the labyrinth, of the nerves was studied. A present facial nerve and vestibulocochlear nerve branching into the cochlear, inferior, and superior vestibular nerve were identified as normal.

Data was collected and entered in a predesigned proforma which includes patient's demography, patient's clinical workup, audiological findings, and radiological findings, and the results were analyzed.

Radiological findings were arranged as per classification given by Sennaroglu and Saatci [6].

3. Results and Analysis

HRCT and MRI depicted numerous congenital malformations of the inner ear. There was no difference in describing anomalies of the inner ear between both modalities. CT allowed appreciation of the bony borders of the malformations, and MRI showed the fluid filled cavities.

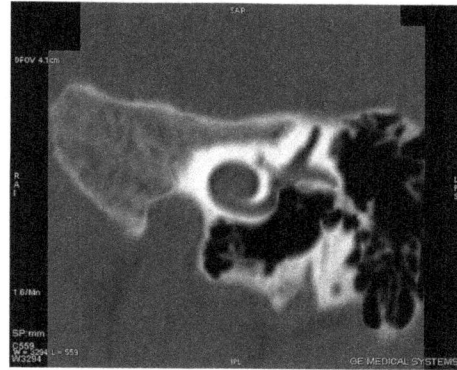

FIGURE 1: HRCT scan of temporal bone with coronal section showing cochlear anomaly in which cochlea shows 1 and 1/2 turns.

A total of 280 children (560 ears) with the age group of 01 to 14 years with bilateral congenital severe to profound sensorineural hearing loss were radiologically evaluated with HRCT of temporal bone and MRI of inner ear. Out of 280 children, 240 children were normal and 40 children (78 inner ears) were found to be congenital abnormal. All the 40 children had bilaterally abnormal inner ear except for 2 children who had unilateral abnormal ear.

4. Evaluation of the Anomalies

4.1. Cochlear Anomalies. Out of 78 abnormal inner ears, in 57 (73%) cochlea was found to be abnormal. Abnormalities of cochlea includes the incomplete partition type-I (IP-I), incomplete partition type-II (IP-II), and common cavity deformity.

In 9 (11.5%) inner ears, cochlea had no turn or only a bony mass without any turn was visualized so it was classified as incomplete partition type-I (IP-I).

In 32 (41%) inner ears, cochlea was of incomplete partition type-II (IP-II), means Mondini deformity, in this type the cochlea consists of 1.5 turns in which the middle and apical turns coalesce to form a cystic apex, accompanied by a dilated vestibule and enlarged vestibular aqueduct.

In 16 (20.5%) of cases cochlea was classified under the common cavity as there was cystic cavity representing the cochlea and vestibule, without showing any differentiation into cochlea and vestibule.

Modiolus was absent in 25 (32%) inner ears and in the rest of the cases it was normal (Figures 1, 2, and 3).

4.1.1. Vestibular Anomalies. Vestibular anomalies were the most common anomalies found. Out of 78 abnormal inner ears in 68 (87.1%) inner ears vestibule was found abnormal. In 62 (79.4%) inner ears vestibule was dilated and in the rest 6 (7.6%) it was aplastic or hypoplastic.

4.1.2. Semicircular Canal Anomalies. In 21 (26.9%) out of 78 malformed inner ears, lateral semicircular canals were found to be aplastic or hypoplastic and in 10 (12.8%) inner ears lateral semicircular canal was dilated. Superior semicircular

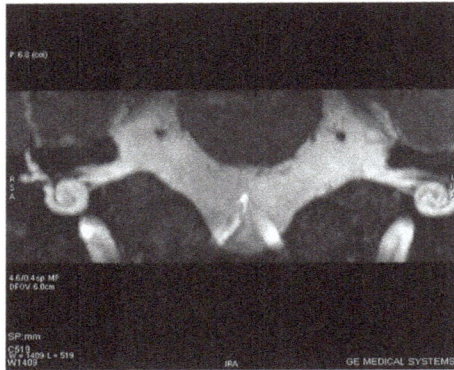

FIGURE 2: MRI scan of inner ear with axial section showing cochlear anomaly in which cochlea shows 1 and 1/2 turns.

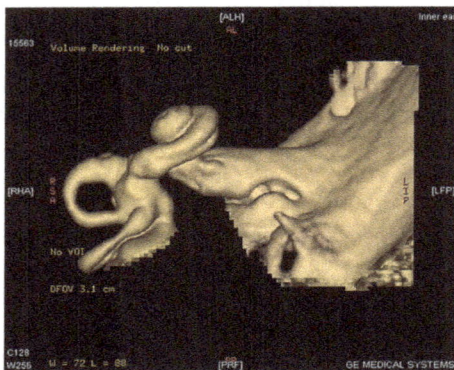

FIGURE 3: MRI scan with 3D reconstruction of inner ear showing cochlear anomaly in which cochlea shows 1 and 1/2 turns.

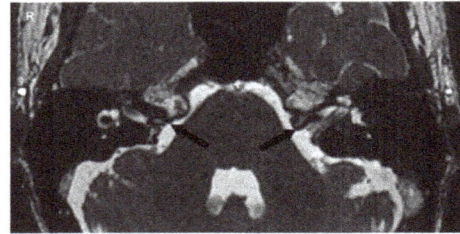

FIGURE 4: MRI scan of inner ear with axial section showing bilateral hypoplastic internal auditory canals.

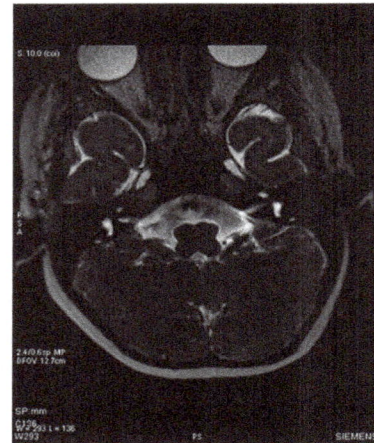

FIGURE 5: MRI scan of inner ear with axial section showing bilateral hypoplastic vestibulocochlear nerves.

canal was aplastic or hypoplastic in 11 (14.1%) cases and dilated in 3 (3.8%) cases. Posterior semicircular canal was found to aplastic or hypoplastic in 14 (17.9%) inner ears and was dilated in 3 (3.8%) cases. In 7 (8.9%) cases all the three canals were absent and in 3 (3.8%) cases all the three canals were dilated.

4.1.3. Vestibular Aqueduct Anomalies. In 44 out of 78 (56.4%) of abnormal inner ears the vestibular aqueduct was found to be abnormal. Vestibular aqueduct was found to be dilated in 41 (52.5%) of cases and in the rest 3 (3.8%) of cases it was aplastic or hypoplastic.

4.1.4. Internal Auditory Canal (IAC) Anomalies. In 24 out of 78 (30.7%) of abnormal inner ears the internal auditory canal was found to be abnormal.

In 19 (24.3%) inner ears IAC was found to be narrow in lumen and short in length. In most of the cases its diameter was <2 mm and short in length also. In 2 (2.5%) cases it was absent and only a solid bony structure which was not patent was seen. In 3 (3.8%) cases IAC was dilated with the diameter of >4 mm (Figure 4).

4.1.5. Status of Vestibulocochlear Nerves. In all cases where IAC was malformed, vestibulocochlear nerves were also malformed except for 1 case where IAC was dilated but nerves were visualized. Out of 78 inner ears, 23 (29.4%) inner ears had nerve anomalies. In 11 (14.1%) of cases nerves were thin in diameter but well visualized; in 12 (15.3%) cases nerves were absent or not visualized (Figures 5 and 6).

5. Overall Evaluation of the Malformations

A total of 313 malformations were detected in 78 abnormal inner ears in a total of 40 patients. 57 of 313 (18.2%) inner ear malformations showed malformations of cochlea and in 25 of 313 (7.9%) inner ear malformations modiolus was found to be malformed. In 44 of 313 (14%) inner ear malformations vestibular aqueduct was abnormal. In 68 of 313 (21.7%) inner ear malformations vestibule was abnormal. In 72 of 313 (23%) semicircular canals were found to be malformed. In 24 of 313 (7.6%) inner ear malformations internal auditory canal was found to be malformed. In 23 of 313 (7.3%) vestibulocochlear nerves anomalies were present.

Summary is shown in Table 1.

Maximum malformations found in a single ear were 7 structural malformations which included malformation of cochlea, modiolus, vestibule, vestibular aqueduct, semicircular canals, internal auditory canal, and vestibulocochlear nerve. Five out of 78 (6.4%) malformed inner ears showed

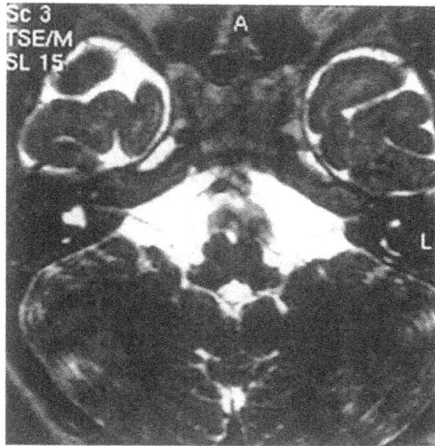

FIGURE 6: MRI scan of inner ear with axial section showing bilateral hypoplastic vestibulocochlear nerves.

TABLE 1: Overall evaluation of malformations.

Type	Number	Percent (%)
Cochlear	57/313	18.2%
Modiolus-	25/313	7.9%
Vestibular aqueduct	44/313	14%
Vestibule	68/313	21.7%
Semicircular canal	72/313	23%
Internal auditory canal	24/313	7.6%
Vestibulocochlear nerve-	23/313	7.3%

TABLE 2: Distribution of malformations.

Number of malformations	Number. of inner Ears	Percent (%)
Seven	5/78	6.4%
Six	6/78	7.6%
Five	7/78	8.9%
Four	15/78	19.2%
Three	19/78	24.3%
Two	23/78	29.4%
One	3/78	3.8%

all 7 structural malformations, 6 ears (7.6%) had 6 malformations, 7 ears (8.9%) had 5 malformations, 15 ears (19.2%) showed 4 malformations, 19 ears (24.3%) had 3 malformations, 23 ears (29.4%) had 2 malformations, and only 3 ears (3.8%) had single isolated malformation.

Summary is given in Table 2.

6. Discussion

In present study, we identified total number of 313 inner ear malformations in 78 inner ears in a total of 40 patients with HRCT scan and MRI scan. This study showed that HRCT scan and MRI scan revealed similar morphologic findings of malformed inner ears, except for vestibulocochlear nerves which were more appreciated on MRI scan. The importance of HRCT scan to study the temporal bone should not be

underestimated [7–9]. HRCT scan depicts the bony borders of malformed labyrinth. This is important because the surgeon can analyze the direction of insertion of the electrode array to minimize the risk of misplacement and by assessing the malformation preoperatively we can minimize the trauma to the vital structure. The implantation of the cochlear implant requires the knowledge about the cochleovestibular malformations. MRI scan delivers additional information that is needed in the preoperative work-up of patients with congenital sensorineural deafness. The fluid filled spaces of the normal cochlea and the malformed cochlea are necessary for the insertion of the electrode array of the cochlear implantation [10]. This can be clearly visualized with MRI scan by using a 3D T-2-weighted fast SE sequence for the surgical reasons and for proper evaluation of congenital malformations only the combined use of HRCT scan and MRI scan can be recommended to study this patient group.

One of the most important findings of our study is that MRI scan allows full appreciation of the normal anatomy and anomalies of the vestibulocochlear nerves within the internal auditory canal in children with congenital sensorineural deafness. For this we performed modified acquisitions of axial and parasagittal reformations using small field of view. In 23 inner ears MRI documented anomalies of vestibulocochlear nerves within the internal auditory canal. Clinical significance of these findings is important. A missing or ill-defined vestibulocochlear nerve is a contra indication for cochlear implantation surgery because this nerve is required to conduct the cochlear implant impulses [11–13].

In the clinical setting, evoked potentials may be used to study the presence and function of the nerve. A positive brain stem evoked potential predicts a functional nerve, but a negative test does not distinguish between a functional, damaged, or undeveloped nerve [13]. 11 inner ears were found to have bilateral ill-defined but visualized vestibulocochlear nerves and 12 inner ears had absent nerves. MRI scan detected anomaly of the vestibulocochlear nerve in 23 inner ears out of 78 (29.4%) malformed ears in this study population but in study by McClay et al. in 2008 [14] and Miyasaka et al. in 2010 [15] it found 40% and 18% of nerve anomalies, respectively. In the present study the internal auditory canal was malformed in 24 out of 78 (30.7%) abnormal inner ears; in 19 (24.3%) inner ears IAC was found to be narrow in lumen and short in length. In most of the cases its diameter was <2 mm and short in length also and this was associated with absent or thin nerves, in 2 (2.5%) cases it was absent and only a solid bony structure which was not patent was seen, and in 3 (3.8%) cases IAC was dilated with the diameter of >4 mm. Westerhof et al. in 2001 [16] found 38% of internal auditory canal anomalies in their study which is slightly higher than present study.

Anomaly of the vestibulocochlear nerve occurred along with a malformed labyrinth. Data from embryologic studies might explain this phenomenon. In the ninth embryonic week, the cochlear windings are developed and the rise of neural epithelium builds a cochlear ganglion and neural fibers (early cochlear nerve) start to develop. These fibers grow centrally to the brain stem and peripherally back into the otic epithelium. Initial afferent fibers entering the undifferentiated otic epithelium are appreciated in the 10th embryonic week [17]. A nerve growth factor like substance released by the otic vesicle which is essential for the survival of the neural cell supports this development [18]. These data explain that in case of an arrest in the developing labyrinth, the neural embryonic proceedings may be disturbed. This could result in anomaly or aplasia of the vestibulocochlear nerves, which we found in 29.4% of ears with anomaly of the bony labyrinth.

Our study illustrates that imaging studies in patients with congenitally sensorineural hearing loss should not focus just on the vestibulocochlear nerves [19] or on cochlea [20, 21]. The majority of our patients demonstrate multiple anomalies of the inner ear. We have classified the anomalies according to the latest classification of congenital inner ear malformations given by Sennaroglu and Saatci in 2002 [6].

6.1. Incomplete Partition Type-I (IP-I). Incomplete partition type-I (cystic cochleovestibular malformations) is a malformation involving the cochlea and vestibule. In a case of IP-I, a cystic dilated vestibule accompanied the cystic, empty cochlea. This pathology represents a form of common cavity that is one step more organized and differentiated than common cavity [6]. In our study 9 (11.5%) inner ears were classified under this category, in these cases the dimensions of the cochlea were normal but the internal architecture was missing, and there was no modiolus in the cochlea giving it the shape of an empty cystic structure. Vestibule was grossly enlarged and the vestibular aqueduct was also dilated. The studies conducted by Sennaroglu and Saatci in 2002 [6] and Westerhof et al. in 2001 [16] found the incidence of IP-I as 8% and 12%, respectively, and this is almost similar to our results. The arrest of development should be at the 5th week. In addition the histological presentation of the patient reported by Graham et al. [22] fits IP-I because there are two separate cavities, although they described it as common cavity. The case presented as common cavity by Swartz and Harnsberger in their radiology text book also has separate cystic cochlear and vestibular components and is, we think, another example of IP-I but we have classified these cases separately as common cavity, in which cochlea was classified under the common cavity as there was cystic cavity representing the cochlea and vestibule, without showing any differentiation into cochlea and vestibule and the incidence of these type of cases in our study was 16 (20.5%) as compared to 7% of study by the Sennaroglu and Saatci [6].

6.2. Incomplete Partition Type-2 (IP-2): Mondini Malformation. The malformation of incomplete partition type II (Mondini malformation) represents cochlea in which only the basal part of the modiolus is present. This is the type of cochlea originally described by Carlo Mondini and together with a minimally dilated vestibule and large vestibular aqueduct it constitutes the triad of the Mondini deformity. This gives the apex of the cochlea a cystic appearance due to the confluence of the middle and apical turns. In our study, out of 78, 32 (41%) inner ears were classified in incomplete partition type-II according to Sennaroglu and Saatci classification. In these 32 inner ears cochlea was malformed having 1 and 1/2

turns with normal modiolus, dilated vestibule along with dilated vestibular aqueduct. In the studies conducted by Sennaroglu and Saatci in 2002 [6] and Westerhof et al. in 2001 [16] they found the incidence of IP-II was 15% and 22%, respectively. It is thought that in these types of malformations the arrest of development is at the 7th week of gestation.

In the present study we found total 14.2% of children with vestibulocochlear anomalies which is lower incidence in comparison to the international studies, and according to them the incidence is about 20% (Sennaroglu and Saatciin 2001 [6]), 23% (Abdullah et al. in 2003 [23]), 30% (Ma et al. in 2008 [24]) and 31% (McClay et al. in 2008 [14]). All of these studies had lower sample size than our study.

7. Conclusion

The present study is the first study done in India. By this study we can find out different types of congenital inner ear malformations and their incidence in congenitally deaf children in India.

Conflict of Interests

The authors declare that there is no conflict of interests regarding the publication of this paper.

References

[1] M. B. St. Martin and B. E. Hirsch, "Imaging of hearing loss," *Otolaryngologic Clinics of North America*, vol. 41, no. 1, pp. 157–178, 2008.

[2] R. K. Jackler, W. M. Luxford, and W. F. House, "Congenital malformations of the inner ear: a classification based on embryogenesis," *Laryngoscope*, vol. 97, no. 3, pp. 2–14, 1987.

[3] L. Sennaroglu, "Cochlear implantation in inner ear malformations—a review article," *Cochlear Implants International*, vol. 11, no. 1, pp. 4–41, 2010.

[4] J. Seitz, P. Held, A. Waldeck et al., "Value of high-resolution MR in patients scheduled for cochlear implantation," *Acta Radiologica*, vol. 42, no. 6, pp. 568–573, 2001.

[5] H. R. Harnsberger, D. J. Dart, J. L. Parkin, W. R. Smoker, and A. G. Osborn, "Cochlear implant candidates: assessment with CT and MR imaging," *Radiology*, vol. 164, no. 1, pp. 53–57, 1987.

[6] L. Sennaroglu and I. Saatci, "A new classification for cochleovestibular malformations," *Laryngoscope*, vol. 112, no. 12, pp. 2230–2241, 2002.

[7] P. D. Phelps, "Cochlear implants for congenital deformities," *Journal of Laryngology and Otology*, vol. 106, no. 11, pp. 967–970, 1992.

[8] D. A. Seidman, P. M. Chute, and S. Parisier, "Temporal bone imaging for cochlear implantation," *The Laryngoscope*, vol. 104, no. 5, pp. 562–565, 1994.

[9] A. L. Woolley, A. B. Oser, R. P. Lusk, and R. S. Bahadori, "Preoperative temporal bone computed tomography scan and its use in evaluating the pediatric cochlear implant candidate," *Laryngoscope*, vol. 107, no. 8, pp. 1100–1106, 1997.

[10] W. H. Slattery III and W. M. Luxford, "Cochlear implantation in the congenital malformed cochlea," *Laryngoscope*, vol. 105, no. 11, pp. 1184–1187, 1995.

[11] T. H. Lenarz, R. Hartrampf, R. Battmer, B. Bertram, and A. Lesinski, "Cochlear implantation in very young children," *Laryngo-Rhino-Otologie*, vol. 75, no. 12, pp. 719–726, 1996.

[12] R. F. Gray, J. Ray, D. M. Baguley, Z. Vanat, J. Begg, and P. D. Phelps, "Cochlear implant failure due to unexpected absence of the eighth nerve—a cautionary tale," *Journal of Laryngology and Otology*, vol. 112, no. 7, pp. 646–649, 1998.

[13] C. J. Brown, P. J. Abbas, H. Fryauf-Bertschy, D. Kelsay, and B. J. Gantz, "Intraoperative and postoperative electrically evoked auditory brain stem responses in nucleus cochlear implant users: implications for the fitting process," *Ear and Hearing*, vol. 15, no. 2, pp. 168–176, 1994.

[14] J. E. McClay, T. N. Booth, D. A. Parry, R. Johnson, and P. Roland, "Evaluation of pediatric sensorineural hearing loss with magnetic resonance imaging," *Archives of Otolaryngology—Head and Neck Surgery*, vol. 134, no. 9, pp. 945–952, 2008.

[15] M. Miyasaka, S. Nosaka, N. Morimoto, H. Taiji, and H. Masaki, "CT and MR imaging for pediatric cochlear implantation: emphasis on the relationship between the cochlear nerve canal and the cochlear nerve," *Pediatric Radiology*, vol. 40, no. 9, pp. 1509–1516, 2010.

[16] J. P. Westerhof, J. Rademaker, B. P. Weber, and H. Becker, "Congenital malformations of the inner ear and the vestibulocochlear nerve in children with sensorineural hearing loss: evaluation with CT and MRI," *Journal of Computer Assisted Tomography*, vol. 25, no. 5, pp. 719–726, 2001.

[17] R. Pujol, M. Lavigne-Rebillard, and A. Uziel, "Development of the human cochlea," *Acta Oto-Laryngologica*, no. 482, pp. 7–13, 1991.

[18] P. P. Lefebvre, P. Leprince, T. Weber, J.-M. Rigo, P. Delree, and G. Moonen, "Neuronotrophic effect of developing otic vesicle on cochleo-vestibular neurons: evidence for nerve growth factor involvement," *Brain Research*, vol. 507, no. 2, pp. 254–260, 1990.

[19] J. W. Casselman, F. E. Offeciers, P. J. Govaerts et al., "Aplasia and hypoplasia of the vestibulocochlear nerve: diagnosis with MR imaging," *Radiology*, vol. 202, no. 3, pp. 773–781, 1997.

[20] C. R. Guirado, P. Martinez, R. Roig et al., "Three-dimensional MR of the inner ear with steady-state free precession," *The American Journal of Neuroradiology*, vol. 16, no. 9, pp. 1909–1913, 1995.

[21] J. W. Casselman, R. Kuhweide, W. Ampe et al., "Inner ear malformations in patients with sensorineural hearing loss: detection with gradient-echo (3DFT-CISS) MRI," *Neuroradiology*, vol. 38, no. 3, pp. 278–286, 1996.

[22] J. M. Graham, P. D. Phelps, and L. Michaels, "Congenital malformations of the ear and cochlear implantation in children: review and temporal bone report of common cavity," *Journal of Laryngology and Otology*, vol. 114, supplement 25, pp. 1–14, 2000.

[23] A. Abdullah, M. R. Mahmud, A. Maimunah, M. A. Zulfiqar, L. Saim, and R. Mazlan, "Preoperative high resolution CT and MR imaging in cochlear implantation," *Annals of the Academy of Medicine Singapore*, vol. 32, no. 4, pp. 442–445, 2003.

[24] H. Ma, P. Han, B. Liang et al., "Multislice spiral computed tomography imaging in congenital inner ear malformations," *Journal of Computer Assisted Tomography*, vol. 32, no. 1, pp. 146–150, 2008.

11

Risk Factors for Hearing Loss in Children following Bacterial Meningitis in a Tertiary Referral Hospital

Benson Wahome Karanja,[1] Herbert Ouma Oburra,[2] Peter Masinde,[3] and Dalton Wamalwa[4]

[1] *University of Nairobi, P.O. Box 2209-00202, KNH, Nairobi, Kenya*
[2] *Department of Surgery, University of Nairobi, P.O. Box 30197-00100, G.P.O. Nairobi, Kenya*
[3] *ENT Department, Kenyatta National Hospital (KNH), University of Nairobi, P.O. Box 20723-00202, Nairobi, Kenya*
[4] *Department of Pediatrics and Child Health, University of Nairobi, P.O. Box 19676-00202, Nairobi, Kenya*

Correspondence should be addressed to Benson Wahome Karanja; drwahome@iconnect.co.ke

Academic Editor: Michael D. Seidman

Objective. This study aimed to examine hearing function in children admitted with bacterial meningitis to determine the risk factors for sensorineural hearing loss. *Setting.* The study was conducted in the audiology unit and paediatric wards of Kenyatta National Hospital. *Subjects and Methods.* The study involved 83 children between the ages of six months and twelve years admitted with bacterial meningitis. The median age for the children examined was 14. On discharge they underwent hearing testing to evaluate for presence and degree of hearing loss. *Results.* Thirty six of the 83 children (44.4%) were found to have at least a unilateral mild sensorineural hearing loss during initial audiologic testing. Of the children with hearing loss, 22 (26.5%) had mild or moderate sensorineural hearing loss and 14 (16.9%) had severe or profound sensorineural hearing loss. Significant determinants identified for hearing loss included coma score below eight, seizures, cranial nerve neuropathy, positive CSF culture, and fever above 38.7 degrees Celsius. *Conclusions.* Sensorineural hearing loss was found to be highly prevalent in children treated for bacterial meningitis. There is need to educate healthcare providers on aggressive management of coma, fever, and seizures due to their poor prognostic value on hearing.

1. Introduction

Deafness is one of the commonest serious complications of bacterial meningitis in childhood. In developed countries, approximately 10% of survivors of bacterial meningitis are left with permanent sensorineural hearing loss [1–3]. Other children experience a transient hearing loss [3–6]. Both types of hearing impairment are thought to develop during the first few days of the illness [5–7].

Kenyatta National Hospital, KNH, is Kenya's national referral hospital. Estimates show that an average forty-five children are admitted into its pediatric wards each month with a confirmed diagnosis of bacterial meningitis.

Behavioral tests of hearing may be used when an infant reaches the developmental age (as opposed to the chronological age) of six months. Infants not at this level of development and some of those with more than one disability will need to be tested by otoacoustic emissions (OAEs) and auditory brainstem responses (ABRs). Unfortunately the equipment for these latter two sets was unavailable forcing the study to be carried out in children above 6 months of age using behavioural distraction testing.

So far, in KNH no similar study had been undertaken to determine the prevalence, burden, and risk factors for hearing loss following bacterial meningitis in children admitted to KNH.

2. Materials and Methods

2.1. Participants. The study involved 83 children (49 males and 34 females) between the ages of six months and twelve years admitted with bacterial meningitis from the pediatric wards, KNH. All cases admitted within twenty-four hours of diagnosis, who met the inclusion criteria, were recruited every weekday evening during the 3-month study period.

All participants fulfilled the following criteria: age of six months or older at the time of admission and confirmed diagnosis of bacterial meningitis. Bacterial meningitis was defined according to the World Health Organization (WHO) workbook recommendations based on laboratory findings, symptoms, or signs [8]. Those excluded from the study included all subjects with a confirmed diagnosis of tuberculosis and those on current treatment for tuberculosis; those with a prior history of hearing loss; those using ototoxic antibiotics as part of treatment; those with chronic medical conditions (diabetes, renal, cardiac diseases); those on treatment for malaria.

A full medical history was documented and factors relating to the patient and prior treatment documented by the principal investigator in the questionnaire. The history included the parents or guardians' assessment of hearing and any history of ear discharge or infection. However, there were no premeningitis audiograms, which is a potential confounding factor and weakness of the study. Otoscopy was done using a Riester hand-held otoscope and its aural speculums and the findings recorded. The children then underwent a thorough physical examination. Hematological and CSF study results were documented. The Glasgow Coma Scale, GCS, was used for the level of consciousness. All these findings were entered in the patient's data entry form.

The relevant hearing assessment was done prior to discharge from hospital and two weeks after. This identified and excluded transient hearing loss.

All participants' parents or guardians gave informed consent for the study. Five guardians declined to have their children involved in the study. The study protocol was approved by the institutional ethics and review committee of KNH.

2.2. Audiological Protocol. All patients completed age-appropriate hearing tests carried out by trained audiologists in the ENT audiology section in a sound- proofed booth. This was well lit with minimal littering to minimize the child's distraction. It was also well ventilated and large enough to accommodate the child and parent/guardian, tester, and distractor. The standard ambient noise was 35 dB.

Children between six and twenty-four months of age underwent the distraction test, those between twenty-four and thirty-six months of age had the performance tests done, while pure tone audiometry was carried out on children above thirty-six months of age. They were carried out in the following manner.

(1) *Behavioral Testing.* The behavioral testing equipment included toys that were not too bright used by the distractor to distract the child being examined. Three warblers were used: low, mid, and high frequency types. A Manchester rattle was also used to deliver high frequency sounds during behavioral testing. The G-chime was used for mid-frequency sounds and the C-chime for high frequency sound generation.

(a) *Distraction Test.* A distraction test was performed if the infant was sitting and able to turn and locate the source of a sound. It was carried out with the infant sat upon an adult's knee facing forwards where a distractor controlled the infant's attention using toys. The tester introduced the sound signals at high, mid, and moderate frequencies from 45 degrees and one meter behind, at the level of the ear. These were tested separately in order to detect hearing loss restricted to one part of the frequency range. The sounds were introduced at very quiet levels (35 dBA). Care was taken not to give clues as to the tester's position other than the test signal.

(b) *Performance Tests.* The child was shown how to wait until a sound was heard before carrying out an action. Once this could be done, the test was to be performed at a meter distance and from behind. The test was performed using "Go" for low frequencies, "S" for high frequencies, introduced at the quietest voice levels or 2 Warble tones at 500 Hz, 1, or 2 kHz, and 4 kHz introduced at a very quiet level corresponding to normal hearing. The child was said to have "passed" the screen if there were two responses at the quietest level.

(2) *Pure Tone Audiometry.* This was carried out in all children recruited for the study who were above thirty-six months of age. Pure tones (20 dD Hearing Level, HL) were introduced using headphones and testing carried out by air conduction (500 H–4000 Hz) and bone conduction (500–4000 Hz). Pure tone audiometry was performed using an Interacoustics clinical audiometer (Model AC33; serial no. SN735530, calibration date June 2009). Sound delivery and masking during pure tone audiometry was ensured using TDH-399 headphones.

The main outcome measure was presence or absence of sensorineural hearing loss in the children.

2.3. Followup. If the child had made a complete recovery from meningitis, lived far from the hospital, and had no hearing loss, followup was not done.

If the child had sequalae that required further management beyond 2 weeks, followup was continued. For those children exhibiting hearing loss, whether conductive or sensorineural, recommendations for management and followup were based on specific test findings and varied accordingly.

3. Statistical Analysis

Descriptive statistics (means for continuous variables and proportions for categorical variables) were calculated to describe the population.

The main outcome was degree of sensorineural hearing loss as measured by the age-appropriate hearing test. This had three levels of outcomes: normal, mild/moderate, and severe/profound. The population proportions and the 95% confidence interval, CI, were estimated for each category of outcome, using statistical methods to give more precise estimates. All categorical variables were cross-tabulated with the outcome and Pearson Chi Square computed.

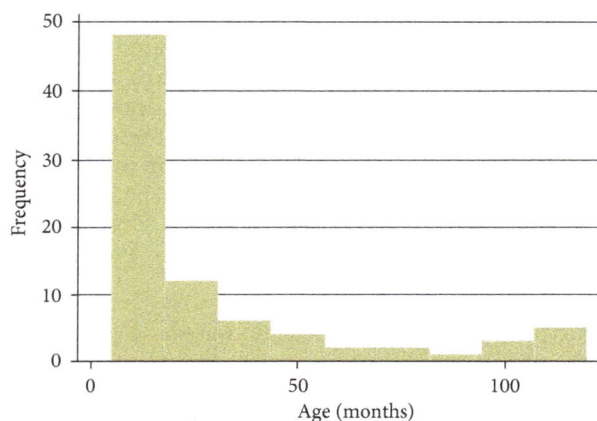

FIGURE 1: Age distribution (in months) of children evaluated.

TABLE 1: Mean and median age ranges.

Mean (SD)	Median (range)
29.09 (31.71)	14 (5–120)

4. Results

The outcomes of eighty-three children (49 males and 34 females) admitted with bacterial meningitis during the study period were analyzed. Figure 1 shows the age distribution (in months) of children evaluated. The median age for the children examined was 14 months (range from 5 to 120 months) as shown on Table 1. The characteristics of the children studied are presented in Table 2. A minority of the children were malnourished (15/83; 18.1%) and almost all caregivers (82/83; 99%) had some form of education. More than two thirds of the children presented with fever (54/83; 65%) and rarely had a cranial nerve palsy (8/83; 10%) or hydrocephalus (5/83; 6%). See Table 2 and Figure 2. Only two in ten cerebrospinal fluid culture samples yielded a growth with most being *Streptococcus pneumoniae* (10/17) (Figure 2).

On CSF microbiology, three categories were included:

(1) no cultured organism;

(2) *Streptococcus pneumoniae* (10);

(3) other (7)

    (a) *Neisseria meningitidis*—4,

    (b) *Haemophilus influenzae*—3.

Only seventeen (20.5%) of CSF specimens examined cultured any bacteria. *Streptococcus pneumoniae, Haemophilus influenza,* and *Neisseria meningitidis* were isolated in 10, 4, and 3 children, respectively. The latter two were classified as "other" microorganisms in comparison with *S. pneumoniae.* There were no distinctly different clinical presentations among children with *S. pneumoniae, H. influenza,* and *N. meningitidis* meningitis. CSF culture findings are illustrated in Figure 2.

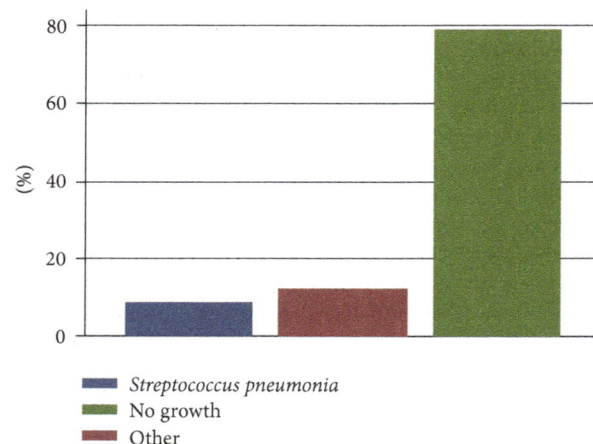

FIGURE 2: Bar chart of cerebrospinal fluid culture findings.

A significant number of patients enrolled developed sensorineural hearing loss as a sequalae (36/83). The overall prevalence of SNHL loss was estimated using bootstrap with 1000 repetitions to be 43.37% (95% CI: 33.22, 55.93). Of the children with hearing loss, 22 (26.5%) had mild or moderate sensorineural hearing loss, and 14 (16.8%) had severe or profound sensorineural hearing loss. The prevalence of specific categories of SNHL is presented in Table 3.

The results of the univariable ordinary logistic models are presented in Table 4. Comparing those who had normal hearing to those who have any SNHL, there is strong evidence to suggest that having a seizure or a positive CSF microbiological culture increased the odds of having SNHL (Model 1 on Table 5). Similarly, history of seizure or a positive culture was strongly associated with having moderate SNHL (Model 1 on Table 5). None of the predictors was significantly associated with severe SNHL. This finding may be as a result of the small numbers involved in this analysis and therefore low power to detect differences.

Table 6 shows the results of final ordinary logistic models fitted with variables significant from the univariable analysis. Overall after controlling the effect of sex and age, a positive CSF microbiological culture and history of seizure strongly predicted SNHL.

In the univariable multinomial logistic regression agitation, fever, seizure, and a positive CSF culture were associated with moderate SNHL, while only seizures were associated with severe SNHL. Estimates could not be obtained for some variables as there were too few numbers within the various categories of the variable.

From the final multivariable multinomial regression, seizures and positive CSF culture predicted both moderate and severe SNHLs, while agitation predicted moderate SNHL.

Interestingly, the ordered logistic models allowed for the inclusion of more variables which were otherwise dropped out of other models. After adjusting for age and sex, these models suggest that seizures, positive CSF culture, agitation, presence of cranial nerve palsy, and a coma score below eight strongly predicted both moderate and severe SNHL. These

TABLE 2: Characteristics and findings in children with meningitis included in this study ($n = 83$).

Variable	Overall n/N (%)	Sensorineural hearing loss (SNHL)			
		Normal ($n = 47$)	Mild/moderate ($n = 22$)	Severe/profound ($n = 14$)	Test
Biometrics					
Age in months (median, range)	14 (5–120)	15 (5–120)	10 (6–108)	14 (6–120)	$P = 0.38^*$
Males	49/83 (59%)	29/47	13/22	7/14	$P = 0.73$
Anthropometric					
Weight, mean z score (SD)^ξ	−0.89 (1.96)	−0.81 (2.10)	−1.24 (1.76)	−0.60 (1.84)	$P = 0.59^*$
Malnourished (Yes)	15/83 (18.1%)	9/47	4/22	2/14	$P = 0.91$
Clinical variables					
History					
Seizures	64/82 (78.1%)	30/46	21/22	13/14	**P = 0.006**
Examination					
Fever (Y)	54/83 (65.1%)	32/47	17/22	5/14	**P = 0.03**
Level of consciousness (GCS)					
Coma score < 8	13/83 (15.7%)	1/47	9/22	3/14	
Coma score > 8	70/83 (84.3%)	46/47	13/22	11/14	**P < 0.001**
Cranial nerve palsy (Y)†	8/83 (9.6)	0/47	4/22	4/14	**P = 0.002**
Laboratory					
CSF culture					
No growth	66/83 (79.5%)	46/47	13/22	7/14	
Other	7/83 (8.4%)	1/47	4/22	2/14	
Streptococcus pneumonia	10/83 (12.1%)	0/47	5/22	7/14	**P < 0.000**
CSF biochemistry					
CSF glucose					
Median, range (g/dL)	29.7 (21.5–90)	31.2 (21.5–90)	27.7 (22.2–90)	27.2 (21.5–90)	$P = 0.63^*$
>40 mg/dL	7/83 (8.4%)	2/47	4/22	1/14	$P = 0.150$
<40 mg/dL	76/83 (91.6%)				
CSF protein					
Median, range	225 (11–952)	231 (123–952)	222.5 (11–952)	189.5 (128–653)	$P = 0.37^*$
<100 mg/dL	0/83 (0)	0	0	0	
>100 mg/dL,	83/83 (100%)	47/47	22/22	14/14	—

† All palsies involved the Abducens (Cranial nerve VI); ^{ξ}based on CDC growth charts, US version 2000; *Levene's robust test statistic for the equality of variances between the groups.
GCS: Glasgow Coma Scale.

TABLE 3: Prevalence of SNHL.

SHNL category	Prevalence (%)	Normal based 95% CI
Normal	47/83 (56.62)	[44.79, 66.05]
Mild/moderate	22/83 (26.51)	[17.33, 35.68]
Severe/profound	14/83 (16.87)	[10.22, 25.93]
Overall SNHL	36/83 (43.37)	[33.22, 55.93]

models probably provide the most efficient and consistent results. The assumption of proportional odds was not violated by any of the ordered logistic models fitted. Thus, an assumption that there was some ordering in the severity of SNHL seems sensible and appropriate. That is to say that moderate SNHL is proportionally worse than normal, and severe SNHL is proportionally worse than moderate SNHL. Thus, the models provide, for instance, the ordered odds ratio

estimate of comparing those with positive CSF culture with those with no growth given that they had a certain severity of SNHL, when other variables are held constant. In this example, those with a positive culture are at an eightfold increased odds of having moderate SNHL compared to those with a negative culture, after controlling for other factors.

Age, nutritional status, gender, number of siblings, caregiver level of education, length of illness prior to admission, and stiff neck were not found to be significant risk factors for hearing loss.

All children with positive culture for *S. pneumoniae* and *H. influenzae* developed hearing loss, while two of three children with positive culture for *N. meningitidis* developed hearing loss.

Lowered CSF glucose and elevated CSF protein were both found to influence development of hearing loss although this did not reach statistical significance.

TABLE 4: Univariable ordinary logistic regression models.

Variable	Model 1			Model 2			Model 3		
	OR	95% CI	P value	OR	95% CI	P value	OR	95% CI	P value
Age category	0.631	0.331–1.206	0.164	0.551	0.254–1.196	0.132	0.782	0.331–1.848	0.575
Gender	1.450	0.601–3.500	0.409	1.181	0.418–3.340	0.754	1.950	0.600–6.331	0.267
Number of siblings	1.218	0.475–3.123	0.681	1.185	0.393–3.570	0.763	1.269	0.363–4.433	0.709
Caregiver level of education	0.872	0.473–1.609	0.661	0.788	0.388–1.599	0.509	1.035	0.440–2.431	0.937
Length of illness	1.141	0.464–2.806	0.773	1.298	0.457–3.688	0.624	0.938	0.273–3.217	0.918
Fever	0.642	0.259–1.592	0.338	1.487	0.458–4.833	0.509	0.219	0.0631–0.759	**0.0166**
Agitation	1.642	0.684–3.940	0.267	0.726	0.248–2.127	0.559	6.222	1.539–25.15	**0.0103**
Altered consciousness	1.659	0.632–4.357	0.304	1.143	0.387–3.376	0.809	3.467	0.695–17.30	0.130
Seizure	9.655	2.049–45.50	**0.00415**	11.59	1.423–94.32	**0.0220**	7.724	0.928–64.26	**0.0586**
Glasgow Coma score[¶]	1	1-1		1	1-1		1	1-1	
Bulging fontanel[¶]	1	1-1		1	1-1		1	1-1	
Cranial nerve palsy[¶]	1	1-1		1	1-1		1	1-1	
Hydrocephalus	1.941	0.307–12.28	0.481	2.200	0.289–16.75	0.447	1.571	0.132–18.66	0.720
Stiff neck	1.056	0.434–2.572	0.904	1.125	0.393–3.219	0.826	0.964	0.293–3.172	0.952
Protein (log base e)	0.514	0.245–1.081	**0.08**	0.412	0.127–1.328	0.138	0.564	0.257–1.237	0.153
Glucose	3.437	0.627–18.85	0.155	4.889	0.821–29.10	**0.0812**	1.571	0.132–18.66	0.720
CSF culture	34.29	4.259–276.0	**0.000895**	31.15	3.607–269.1	**0.00177**	39.37	4.250–364.8	**0.00122**

Model 1: normal versus any SNHL; Model 2: normal versus moderate SNHL; Model 3: normal versus severe SNHL. OR: odds ratio. [¶]Explanatory variable perfectly predicted outcome and estimates could not be obtained by maximum likelihood. The P values are based on Wald tests.

TABLE 5: Multivariable ordinary logistic regression.

Variable	Model 1			Model 2			Model 3		
	OR	95% CI	P value	OR	95% CI	P value	OR	95% CI	P value
Age category									
2–11 months	Ref								
12–60 months	0.807	0.239–2.733	0.731	0.324	0.0688–1.523	0.153	10.16	0.696–148.4	0.0901
>61 months	0.107	0.00955–1.201	0.0701	0.242	0.0206–2.850	0.260	8.08e − 08		0.995
Gender									
Male	Ref								
Female	2.090	0.652–6.700	0.215	0.853	0.180–4.040	0.841	6.489	0.897–46.96	0.0640
Fever									
No	Ref								
Yes							0.273	0.0321–2.332	0.236
Agitation									
No	Ref								
Yes							12.44	0.851–181.8	0.0654
Seizure									
No	Ref								
Yes	8.289	1.394–49.28	0.0201	11.79	0.994–139.7	**0.0506**	3.363	0.237–47.78	0.370
Glucose									
Normal	Ref								
Elevated				7.973	0.785–80.97	0.0792			
CSF culture							1.487e + 09		0.994
No growth	Ref								
Growth	56.83	4.058–795.9	0.00270	62.75	3.623–1,087	**0.00444**			
Protein (log base e)	0.499	0.182–1.367	0.176						

Model 1: normal versus any SNHL; Model 2: normal versus moderate SNHL; Model 3: normal versus severe SNHL. OR: odds ratio. The P values are based on Wald tests. Only variables significant at P value 0.1 level from the univariable models included for each model. Ref is the reference group. Estimates obtained from maximum likelihood.

TABLE 6: Multivariable multinomial and ordered logistic regression.

Variables	Multinomial				Ordered logistic			
	Normal versus moderate		Normal versus severe		Normal versus moderate		Normal versus severe	
	RRR	95% CI	RRR	95% CI	OR	95% CI	OR	95% CI
Age category								
2–11 months	Ref							
12–60 months	4.519	0.622–32.85	0.435	0.108–1.756	0.746	0.223–2.490	0.746	0.223–2.490
>61 months	0.310	0.00790–12.13	0.114*	0.00983–1.326	0.299	0.0437–2.046	0.299	0.0437–2.046
Gender								
Male	Ref							
Female	3.363	0.682–16.59	1.662	0.437–6.318	1.773	0.564–5.571	1.773	0.564–5.571
Fever								
No	Ref							
Yes	0.206*	0.0351–1.209	2.907	0.629–13.44	1.359	0.348–5.311	14.22***	2.304–87.77
CSF culture								
No growth	Ref							
Growth	225.8***	5.987–8.518	51.35***	3.189–826.6	12.45***	2.720–56.99	12.45***	2.720–56.99
Seizure								
No	Ref							
Yes	2.752	0.244–31.03	13.85**	1.353–141.7	24.02**	2.107–274.0	24.02**	2.107–274.0
Agitation								
No	Ref							
Yes	8.165**	1.257–53.02	0.701	0.188–2.612	0.639	0.215–1.897	0.639	0.215–1.897
Coma score								
>8	Ref							
<8					8.108***	1.856–35.41	8.108***	1.856–35.41
Cranial nerve palsy								
No	Ref							
Yes					22.21***	2.652–186.1	22.21***	2.652–186.1

In parentheses, ***$P < 0.01$, **$P < 0.05$, and *$P < 0.1$. RRR: relative risk ratio; OR: odds ratio. The P values are based on Wald tests. Estimates obtained by maximum likelihood.

5. Discussion

In the present study, children proven by history and CSF findings to have bacterial meningitis were evaluated and found to have a sensorineural hearing loss prevalence of 43.4% (95% CI). This was greater than findings of previous studies. Kutz et al. reported an incidence of 14% [8] consistent with other reports [2, 4, 9, 10]. This is likely due to several factors. The study institution is a tertiary referral center for a major metropolitan area that understandably receives a disproportionate number of very sick children. In addition, perhaps current pathogens are more virulent owing to continued drug resistance. Finally, most children in this study had not had previous objective audiologic testing, and a negative history for hearing loss was based on history alone. Therefore, a few of them may have had a previously undiagnosed hearing loss despite attempts at identifying that by the principal investigator using the questionnaire. This could potentially inflate the prevalence of hearing loss; however, it is unlikely that this would significantly affect the overall prevalence.

Consistent with most prior studies, this work did not reveal any relationship between occurrence and severity of hearing loss to the male gender. Forty-nine (59%) of the children evaluated were males, while 34 (41%) were females. There were no differences in the prevalence of hearing loss between the two groups. Kutz et al. showed that being male was a significant independent risk factor for hearing loss [8].

Early age at illness was identified by Grimwood et al. as a significant risk factor for hearing loss, with children suffering from meningitis before twelve months of age performing more poorly than children suffering from meningitis later in infancy and childhood, as well as age-matched controls, on measures of language and reading skills [10]. However, neither age nor sex was found to affect hearing outcome. This is in agreement with most previously reported studies [8, 9, 11–13].

Only seventeen (20.5%) of cerebrospinal fluid specimens were reported as positive for microorganism culture. The isolates, *Streptococcus pneumonia*, *Haemophilus influenza*, and *Neisseria meningitides*, were 59%, 23%, and 17.9%, respectively. A study in KNH revealed that in 82% of the cases, the cerebrospinal fluid cultures were bacteriologically positive [14]. Common isolates included *S. pneumoniae* (45%), *N.*

meningitidis (14%), and *H. influenzae* (12%). Other studies describe distinctly different clinical presentations between these different causative organisms. This studies' low pick-up rate may have reduced the power to determine the same. Fortnum found no differential risk of hearing impairment by causative agent in one study from Nottingham, UK [2].

All children with *S. pneumoniae* meningitis developed hearing loss. However, a very low proportion of CSF specimens (20.5%) cultured bacteria and so this may be an overestimate. Richardson et al. showed that the incidence of sensorineural hearing loss in children with *S. pneumoniae* meningitis was 36% [15]. Patients who developed hearing loss required longer hospitalization compared with patients who retained normal hearing.

Seizures and a coma score of less than eight were found to be the most significant determinants for hearing loss. Thirteen children (15.7%) had coma scores of less than eight on admission and all but one developed hearing loss. Seizures occurred in 64 (78%) of the patients. Woolley et al. found no correlation between hearing loss and seizures or hearing loss and altered level of consciousness [16]. Seizures are a common complication of meningitis in most studies occurring in 20%–30% of patients, but the cause of hearing loss in meningitis may be a different pathogenic process than the one that results in neurologic deficits [17]. In the large retrospective study by Woolley et al., 26% had seizures. Of children with hearing loss, 32% had seizures compared with 24% of those without hearing loss. Walter et al. showed that in patients who were found to have hearing loss, 45% also developed seizures. This rate is comparable with a seizure incidence of 25% in patients without hearing loss. Of the children with seizures and hearing loss, 69% developed at least severe hearing loss. Chang et al. demonstrated an overall worse prognosis for patients who develop seizures [18]. The development of seizures is multifactorial and may be due to high fevers, metabolic disturbances, or focal cerebral irritation.

Concurrent cranial nerve neuropathy was found to be a strong predictor for the subsequent development of hearing loss, with all eight of the children (8/83; 10%) with cranial nerve neuropathy developing hearing loss. The only cranial nerve neuropathy found was Abducens nerve palsy. The presence of a cranial nerve neuropathy is certainly a sign of a severe infection and is highly correlated with the development of hearing loss. Of the patients with hearing loss and cranial nerve neuropathy, seventy-one had at least a severe sensorineural hearing loss. Kutz et al. found that 6% of the patients developed a cranial nerve neuropathy, and all but three were found to have hearing loss [8].

Decreased CSF glucose and elevated CSF protein as risk factors for hearing loss did not reach statistical significance. Decreased CSF glucose was the most consistent predictor of hearing loss, as illustrated by Woolley et al. and in previous studies [8, 16, 19]. It is unclear why a low CSF glucose level is such a strong predictor of hearing loss. It may be assumed that a low CSF glucose level correlates with high bacterial concentration of the CSF, increasing the likelihood of suppurative labyrinthitis as an etiology of subsequent hearing loss. However, other studies have demonstrated a much weaker association with elevated CSF protein and CSF pleocytosis, two factors that are elevated in patients with a high CSF bacterial concentration. In the study by Woolley et al., patients with hearing loss infected with *S. pneumococcus* were found to have a significantly higher CSF protein level. Another potential sequalae of low CSF glucose is direct damage to the cochlea neuroepithelium.

Presence on fever above 38.7 degrees was a significant risk factor for hearing loss with 22/54 children recording these high fevers developing hearing loss. Duration of illness beyond one week prior to admission and caregiver level of education were not found to be significant determinants for hearing loss following bacterial meningitis. Reports of the effect of delay in treatment on hearing outcome differ [11, 12, 18, 20–22]. If children with histories of more than seven days are excluded, as the symptoms were nonspecific and may be unrelated to the onset of meningitis, they found a nonsignificant increase in incidence of hearing loss in those with a longer history of fever (50% versus 36%, $P = 0.13$). Radetsky and Kilpi et al. found that the length of history of nonspecific signs and symptoms did not correlate with outcome [23, 24]. Kutz et al. found that length of hospitalization was a significant predictor of hearing loss [8].

Malnutrition was not found to have any significance in the development of hearing loss. Poor nutrition is associated with a poor outcome from meningitis, and a low weight for age was associated with a poor outcome in a study by Molyneux et al. [11].

6. Conclusions

Hearing loss is highly prevalent in children treated for bacterial meningitis in Kenyatta National Hospital with a prevalence of 43.4%.

Strong risk factors for hearing loss following bacterial meningitis include coma score on admission of less than eight, development of seizures, concurrent cranial nerve neuropathy, positive CSF culture, and fever above 38.7 degrees Celsius. This is similar to the findings of studies done elsewhere.

Length of illness prior to admission was found not to be a determinant of hearing loss following bacterial meningitis. This is contrary to other studies done.

Age at illness, male gender, malnutrition, and primary caregivers' level of education were found not to be significant determinants of hearing loss following bacterial meningitis. The prior three were found in other studies to be significant predictors for the development of hearing loss.

Lowered CSF glucose and elevated CSF protein are minimally correlated with development of hearing loss following bacterial meningitis. This is different from other studies that place lowered CSF glucose high on the list of most significant predictors for hearing loss following bacterial meningitis.

There exists a need for objective hearing assessment in infants and young children following bacterial meningitis. This should be mandatory in all patients treated for bacterial meningitis.

Disclosure

As a requirement of publication, authors have provided to the publisher signed confirmation of compliance with legal and ethical obligations including but not limited to the following: authorship and contribution, conflict of interests, privacy and confidentiality, and (where applicable) protection of human and animal research subjects. The authors have read and confirmed their agreement with the Hindawi authorship and conflict of interests criteria. The authors have also confirmed that this paper is unique and not under consideration or published in any other publication, and that they have permission from rights holders to reproduce any copyrighted material. Any disclosures are made in this section. The external blind peer reviewers report no conflict of interests.

Conflict of Interest

No sponsorship or conflict of interests has been disclosed for this paper.

Author's Contribution

B. W. Karanja. conceived and designed the experiments, analyzed the data, and wrote the first draft of the manuscript, H. O. Oburra and D. Wamalwa contributed to the writing of the paper, H. O. Oburra, D. Wamalwa and P. Masinde agree with paper results and conclusions, B. W. Karanja, H. O. Oburra and P. Masinde jointly developed the structure and arguments for the paper, H. O. Oburra and D. Wamalwa made critical revisions and approved final version. All authors reviewed and approved of the final paper.

Acknowledgments

I acknowledge the support of my family and entire ENT fraternity in Kenyatta National Hospital.

References

[1] J. A. Dawson and R. Wardle, "Detection and prevalence of hearing loss in a cohort of children following serogroup B, meningococcal infection 1983–1987," *Public Health*, vol. 104, no. 2, pp. 99–102, 1990.

[2] H. M. Fortnum, "Hearing impairment after bacterial meningitis: a review," *Archives of Disease in Childhood*, vol. 67, no. 9, pp. 1128–1133, 1992.

[3] L. J. Baraff, S. I. Lee, and D. L. Schriger, "Outcomes of bacterial meningitis in children: a meta-analysis," *Pediatric Infectious Disease Journal*, vol. 12, no. 5, pp. 389–394, 1993.

[4] P. R. Dodge, H. Davis, and R. D. Feigin, "Prospective evaluation of hearing impairment as a sequela of acute bacterial meningitis," *The New England Journal of Medicine*, vol. 311, no. 14, pp. 869–874, 1984.

[5] H. Guiscafré, L. Benitez-Díaz, M. C. Martínez et al., "Reversible hearing loss after meningitis: prospective assessment using auditory evoked responses," *Annals of Otology, Rhinology, and Laryngology*, vol. 93, no. 3, part 1, pp. 229–232, 1984.

[6] H. Vienny, P. A. Despland, and J. Lutschg, "Early diagnosis and evolution of deafness in childhood bacterial meningitis: a study using brainstem auditory evoked potentials," *Pediatrics*, vol. 73, no. 5, pp. 579–586, 1984.

[7] J. O. Klein, R. D. Feigin, and G. H. McCracken Jr., "Report of the task force on diagnosis and management of meningitis," *Paediatrics*, vol. 78, pp. S959–S982, 1986.

[8] J. W. Kutz, L. M. Simon, S. K. Chennupati, C. M. Giannoni, and S. Manolidis, "Clinical predictors for hearing loss in children with bacterial meningitis," *Archives of Otolaryngology*, vol. 132, no. 9, pp. 941–945, 2006.

[9] M. Zaki, A. S. Daoud, Q. ElSaleh et al., "Childhood bacterial meningitis in Kuwait," *Journal of Tropical Medicine*, vol. 93, no. 1, pp. 7–11, 1990.

[10] K. Grimwood, V. A. Anderson, L. Bond et al., "Adverse outcomes of bacterial meningitis in school-age survivors," *Pediatrics*, vol. 95, no. 5, pp. 646–656, 1995.

[11] E. Molyneux, A. Walsh, A. Phiri, and M. Molyneux, "Acute bacterial meningitis in children admitted to the Queen Elizabeth Central Hospital, Blantyre, Malawi in 1996-1997," *Tropical Medicine and International Health*, vol. 3, no. 8, pp. 610–618, 2000.

[12] J. B. Nadol, "Hearing loss as a sequela of meningitis," *Laryngoscope*, vol. 88, no. 5, pp. 739–755, 1978.

[13] P. E. Brookhouser, M. C. Auslander, and M. E. Meskan, "The pattern and stability of postmeningitic hearing loss in children," *Laryngoscope*, vol. 98, no. 9, pp. 940–948, 1988.

[14] M. N. Wanyoike, P. G. Waiyaki, S. O. McLiegeyo, and E. M. Wafula, "Bacteriology and sensitivity patterns of pyogenic meningitis at Kenyatta National Hospital, Nairobi, Kenya," *East African Medical Journal*, vol. 72, no. 10, pp. 658–660, 1995.

[15] M. P. Richardson, A. Reid, M. J. Tarlow, and P. T. Rudd, "Hearing loss during bacterial meningitis," *Archives of Disease in Childhood*, vol. 76, no. 2, pp. 134–138, 1997.

[16] A. L. Woolley, K. A. Kirk, A. M. Neumann et al., "Risk factors for hearing loss from meningitis in children: the Children's Hospital experience," *Archives of Otolaryngology*, vol. 125, no. 5, pp. 509–514, 1999.

[17] N. Rasmussen, N. J. Johnsen, and V. A. Bohr, "Otologic sequelae after pneumococcal meningitis: a survey of 164 consecutive cases with a follow-up of 94 survivors," *Laryngoscope*, vol. 101, no. 8, pp. 876–882, 1991.

[18] C. J. Chang, H. W. Chang, W. N. Chang et al., "Seizures complicating infantile and childhood bacterial meningitis," *Pediatric Neurology*, vol. 31, no. 3, pp. 165–171, 2004.

[19] P. E. Brookhouser, M. C. Auslander, and M. E. Meskan, "The pattern and stability of postmeningitic hearing loss in children," *Laryngoscope*, vol. 98, no. 9, pp. 940–948, 1988.

[20] H. M. Fortnum and A. Davis, "Hearing impairment in children after bacterial meningitis: incidence and resource Implications," *British Journal of Audiology*, vol. 27, no. 1, pp. 43–52, 1993.

[21] M. Eisenhut, T. Meehan, and S. D. G. Stephens, "Risk factors for hearing loss in bacterial meningitis: delay in treatment and clinical manifestations," *Journal of Audiological Medicine*, vol. 11, no. 2, pp. 86–97, 2002.

[22] C. M. Benjamin, R. W. Newton, and M. A. Clarke, "Risk factors for death from meningitis," *British Medical Journal*, vol. 296, no. 6614, p. 20, 1988.

[23] M. Radetsky, "Duration of symptoms and outcome in bacterial meningitis: an analysis of causation and the implications of a delay in diagnosis," *Pediatric Infectious Disease Journal*, vol. 11, no. 9, pp. 694–698, 1992.

[24] T. Kilpi, M. Anttila, M. J. T. Kallio, and H. Peltola, "Length of prediagnostic history related to the course and sequelae of childhood bacterial meningitis," *Pediatric Infectious Disease Journal*, vol. 12, no. 3, pp. 184–188, 1993.

12

How Neuroscience Relates to Hearing Aid Amplification

K. L. Tremblay and C. W. Miller

Department of Speech and Hearing Sciences, University of Washington, Seattle, WA 98105, USA

Correspondence should be addressed to C. W. Miller; christim@u.washington.edu

Academic Editor: Michael D. Seidman

Hearing aids are used to improve sound audibility for people with hearing loss, but the ability to make use of the amplified signal, especially in the presence of competing noise, can vary across people. Here we review how neuroscientists, clinicians, and engineers are using various types of physiological information to improve the design and use of hearing aids.

1. Introduction

Despite advances in hearing aid signal processing over the last few decades and careful verification using recommended clinical practices, successful use of amplification continues to vary widely. This is particularly true in background noise, where approximately 60% of hearing aid users are satisfied with their performance in noisy environments [1]. Dissatisfaction can lead to undesirable consequences, such as discontinued hearing aid use, cognitive decline, and poor quality of life [2, 3].

Many factors can contribute to aided speech understanding in noisy environments, including device centered (e.g., directional microphones, signal processing, and gain settings) and patient centered variables (e.g., age, attention, motivation, and biology). Although many contributors to hearing aid outcomes are known (e.g., audibility, age, duration of hearing loss, etc.), a large portion of the variance in outcomes remains unexplained. Even less is known about the influence interacting variables can have on performance. To help advance the field and spawn new scientific perspectives, Souza and Tremblay [4] put forth a simple framework for thinking about the possible sources in hearing aid performance variability. Their review included descriptions of emerging technology that could be used to quantify the acoustic content of the amplified signal and its relation to perception. For example, new technological advances (e.g., probe microphone recordings using real speech) were making it possible to explore the relationship between amplified speech

signals, at the level of an individual's ear, and the perception of those same signals. Electrophysiological recordings of amplified signals were also being introduced as a potential tool for assessing the neural detection of amplified sound. The emphasis of the framework was on signal audibility and the ear-to-brain upstream processes associated with speech understanding. Since that time, many new directions of research have emerged, as has an appreciation of the cognitive resources involved when listening to amplified sounds. We therefore revisit this framework when highlighting some of the advances that have taken place since the original Souza and Tremblay [4] article (e.g., SNR, listening effort, and the importance of outcome measures) and emphasize the growing contribution of neuroscience (Figure 1).

2. Upstream, Downstream, and Integrated Stages

A typical example highlighting the interaction between upstream and downstream contributions to performance outcomes is that involving the cocktail party. The cocktail party effect is the phenomenon of a listener being able to attend to a particular stimulus while filtering out a variety of competing stimuli, similar to partygoer focusing on a single conversation in a noisy room [5, 6]. The ability of a particular individual to "tune into" a single voice and "tune out" all that is coming out of their hearing aid is also an example of how variables specific to the individual can also contribute to performance outcomes.

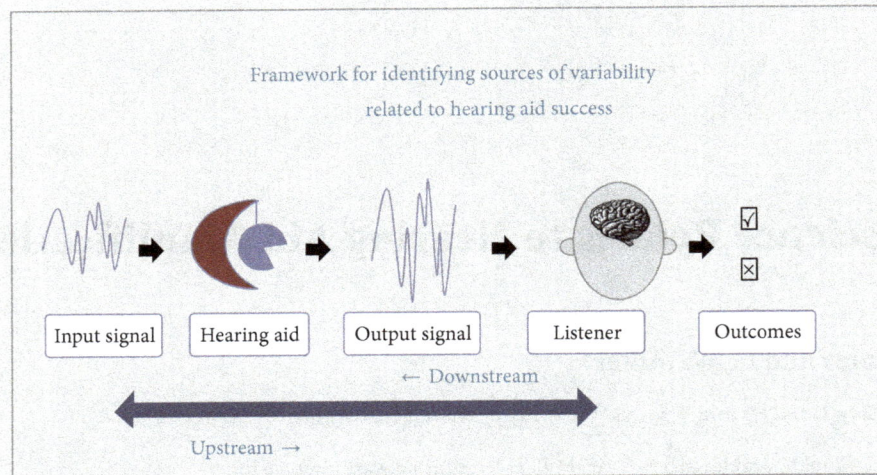

FIGURE 1: Framework for identifying sources of variability related to hearing aid success.

When described as a series of upstream events that could take place in someone's everyday life, the *input signal* refers to the acoustic properties of the incoming signal and/or the context in which the signal is presented. It could consist of a single or multiple talkers; it could be an auditory announcement projected overhead from a loudspeaker at the airport, or it could be a teacher giving homework instructions to children in a classroom. It has long been known that the ability to understand speech can vary in different types of listening environments because the signal-to-noise ratio (SNR) can vary from −2 dB, when in the presence of background noise outside the home, to +9 dB SNR, a level found inside urban homes [7]. Support for the idea that environmental SNR may influence a person's ability to make good use of their hearing aids comes from research showing that listeners are more dissatisfied and receive less benefit with their aids in noise than in quiet environments (e.g., [1, 8, 9]). From of a large-scale survey, two of the top three reasons for nonadoption of aids were that aids did not perform well in noise (48%) and/or that they picked up background sounds (45%; [10]). And of the people who did try aids, nearly half of them returned their aids due to lack of perceived benefit in noise or amplification of background noise. It is therefore not surprising that traditional hearing aid research has focused on hearing aid engineering in attempt to improve signal processing in challenging listening situations, so that optimal and audible signals can promote effective real-world hearing.

The next stage emphasizes the contribution of the *hearing aid* and how it modifies the acoustic signal (e.g., compression, gain and advanced signal processing algorithms). Examples include the study of real-world effectiveness of directional microphone and digital noise reduction features in hearing aids (e.g., [11, 12]). Amplification of background noise is one of the most significant consumer-based complaints associated with hearing aids, and directional hearing aids can improve the SNR of speech occurring in a noisy background (e.g., [13, 14]). However, these findings in the laboratory may not translate to perceived benefit in the real world. When participants were given a four-week take-home trial, omnidirectional microphones were preferred over directional microphones [15]. Over the past several decades, few advances in hearing aid technology have been shown to result in improved outcomes (e.g., [9, 16]). Thus, attempts at enhancing the quality of the signal do not guarantee improved perception. It suggests that something, in addition to signal audibility and clarity, contributes to performance variability.

What is received by the individual's auditory system is not the signal entering the hearing aid but rather a modified signal leaving the hearing aid and entering the ear canal. Therefore, quantification of the signal at the *output of the hearing aid* is an important and necessary step to understanding the biological processing of amplified sound. Although simple measures of the hearing aid output (e.g., gain for a given input level) in a coupler (i.e., simulated ear canal) have been captured for decades, current best practice guidelines highlight the importance of measuring hearing aid function in the listener's own ear canal. Individual differences in ear canal volume and resonance and how the hearing aid is coupled to an individual's ear can lead to significant differences in ear canal output levels [17]. Furthermore, as hearing aid analysis systems become more sophisticated, we are able to document the hearing aid response to more complex input signals such as speech or even speech and noise [18], which provides greater ecological validity than simple pure tone sweeps. In addition, hearing aid features can alter other acoustic properties of a speech signal. For example, several researchers have evaluated the effects of compression parameters on temporal envelope or the slow fluctuations in a speech signal [19–23], spectral contrast or consonant vowel ratio [20, 24–26], bandwidth [24], effective compression ratio [23, 24, 27], dynamic range [27], and audibility [24, 27, 28]. For example, as the number of compression channels increases, spectral differences between vowel formants decrease [26], the level of consonants compared to the level of vowels increases [29], and dynamic range decreases [27]. Similarly, as compression time constants get shorter, the temporal envelope will reduce/smear [20, 21, 23] and the effective compression ratio will increase [27]. A stronger compression ratio has been linked to greater temporal envelope changes [21, 23]. Linear amplification may also create acoustic changes, such as changes in spectral contrast if the high frequencies have much more gain than the low frequencies (e.g., [24]). The acoustic changes caused by compression processing have been linked to perceptual changes in many cases [19–22, 24, 26, 30]. In general, altering compression settings (e.g., time constants or compression ratio) modifies the acoustics of the signal and the perceptual effects can be detrimental. For this reason, an emerging area of interest is to examine how frequency compression hearing aid technology affects the neural representation and perception of sound [31].

Characteristics of the *listener* (e.g., biology) can also contribute to a person's listening experience. Starting with bottom-up processing, one approach in neuroscience has been to model the auditory-nerve discharge patterns in normal and damaged ears in response to speech sounds so that this information can be translated into new hearing aid signal processing [32, 33]. The impact of cochlear dead regions on the fitting of hearing aids is another example of how biological information can influence hearing aid fitting [34]. Further upstream, Willott [49] established how aging and peripheral hearing loss affects sound transmission, including temporal processing, at higher levels in the brain. For this reason, brainstem and cortical evoked potentials are currently being used to quantify the neural representation of sound onset, offset and even speech envelope, in children and adults wearing hearing aids, to assist clinicians with hearing aid fitting [36–39]. When evoked by different speech sounds at suprathreshold levels, patterns of cortical activity (e.g., P1-N1-P2—also called acoustic change responses (ACC)) are highly repeatable in individuals and can be used to distinguish some sounds that are different from one another [4, 37]. Despite this ability, we and others have since shown that P1-N1-P2 evoked responses do not reliably reflect hearing aid gain, even when different types of hearing aids (analog and digital) and their parameters (e.g., gain and frequency response) are manipulated [40–45]. What is more, the signal levels of phones when repeatedly presented in isolation to evoke cortical evoked potentials are not the same as hearing aid output levels when phonemes are presented in running speech context [46]. These examples are provided because they reinforce the importance of examining the output of the hearing aid. Neural activity is modulated by both endogenous and exogenous factors and, in this example, the P1-N1-P2 complex was driven by the signal-to-noise ratio (SNR) of the amplified signal. Figure 2 shows the significant effect hearing aid amplification had on SNR when Billings et al. [43] presented a 1000 Hz tone through a hearing aid. Hearing aids are not designed to process steady-state tones, but results are similar even when naturally produced speech syllables were used [37]. Acoustic waveforms, recorded in-the-canal, are shown (unaided = left; aided=right). The output of the hearing aid, as measured at the 1000 Hz centered 1/3 octave band, was approximately equivalent at 73 and 74 dB SPL for unaided and aided conditions. Noise levels in that same 1/3

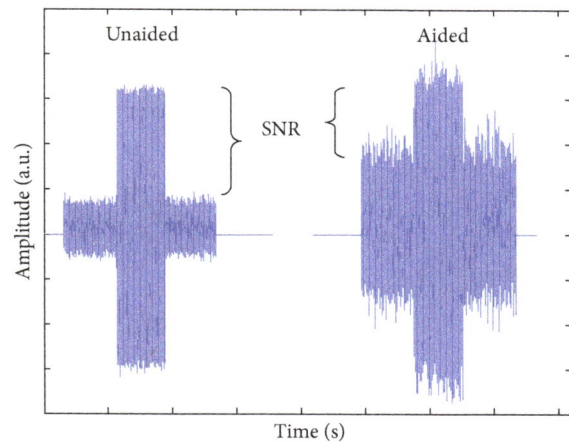

FIGURE 2: Time waveforms of in-the-canal acoustic recordings for one individual. The unaided (left) and aided (right) conditions are shown together. Signal output as measured at the 1000 Hz centered 1/3 octave band was approximately equivalent at 73 and 74 dB SPL for the unaided and aided conditions. However, noise levels in the same 1/3 octave band were approximately 26 and 54 dB SPL, demonstrating the significant change in SNR.

octave band, however, approximated 26 dB in the unaided condition and 54 dB SPL in the aided condition. Thus SNRs in the unaided and aided conditions, measured at the output of the hearing aid, were very different, and time-locked evoked brain activity shown in Figure 3 was influenced more by SNR than absolute signal level. Most of these SNR studies have been conducted in normal hearing listeners and thus the noise was audible, something unlikely to occur at some frequencies if a person has a hearing loss. Nevertheless, noise is always present in an amplified signal and contributors may range from amplified ambient noise to circuit noise generated by the hearing aid. It is therefore important to consider the effects of noise, among the many other modifications introduced by hearing aid processing (e.g., compression) on evoked brain activity. This is especially important because commercially available evoked potential systems are being used to estimate aided hearing sensitivity in young children [47].

What remains unclear is how neural networks process different SNRs, facilitate the suppression of unwanted competing signals (e.g., noise), and process simultaneous streams of information when people with hearing loss wear hearing aids. Individual listening abilities have been attributed to variability involving motivation, selective attention, stream segregation, and multimodal interactions, as well as many other cognitive contributions [48]. It can be mediated by the biological consequences of aging and duration of hearing loss, as well as the peripheral and central effects of peripheral pathology (for reviews see [44, 49]). Despite the obvious importance of this stage and the plethora of papers published each year on the topics of selective attention, auditory streaming, object formation, and spatial hearing, the inclusion of people with hearing loss and who wear hearing aids remains relatively slim.

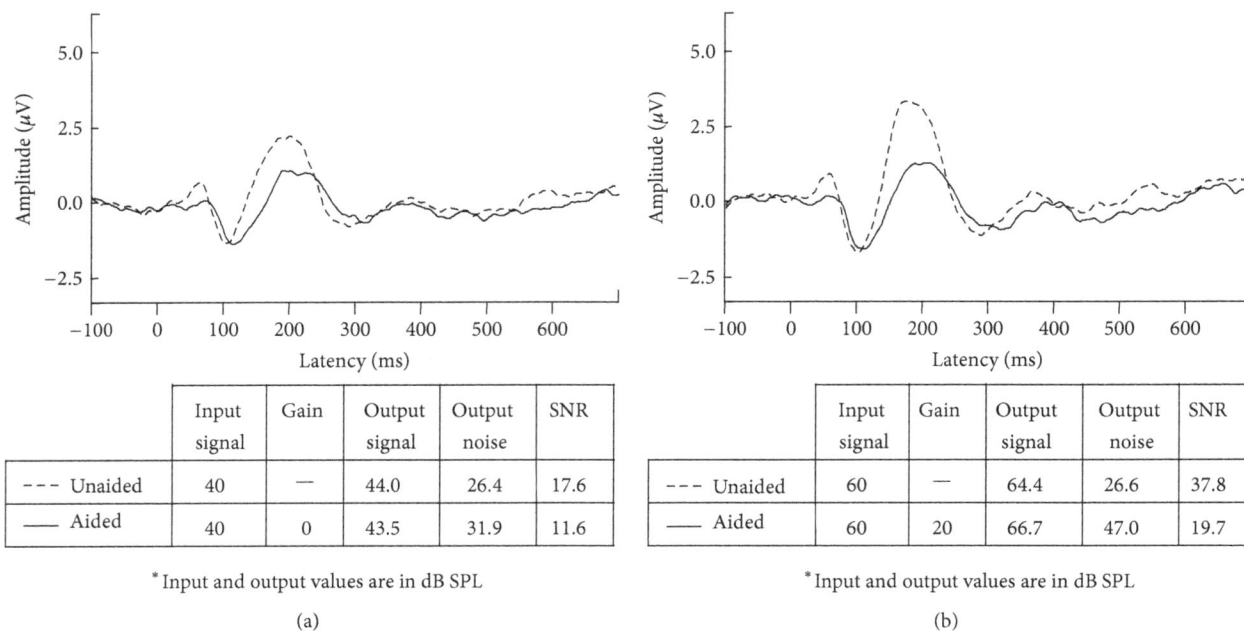

	Input signal	Gain	Output signal	Output noise	SNR
- - - Unaided	40	—	44.0	26.4	17.6
—— Aided	40	0	43.5	31.9	11.6

*Input and output values are in dB SPL

(a)

	Input signal	Gain	Output signal	Output noise	SNR
- - - Unaided	60	—	64.4	26.6	37.8
—— Aided	60	20	66.7	47.0	19.7

*Input and output values are in dB SPL

(b)

FIGURE 3: Two examples showing grand mean CAEPs recorded with similar mean output signal levels. Panels: (a) 40 dB input signals and (b) 60 dB input signals show unaided and aided grand mean waveforms evoked with corresponding in-the-canal acoustic measures. Despite similar input and output signal levels, unaided and aided brain responses are quite different. Aided responses are smaller than unaided responses, perhaps because the SNRs are poorer in the aided condition.

Over a decade ago, a working group that included scientists from academia and industry gathered and discussed the need to include central factors when considering hearing aid use [50] and since then there has been increased awareness about including measures of cognition, listening effort, and other top-down functions when discussing rehabilitation involving hearing aid fitting [51]. However, finding universally agreed upon definitions and methods to quantify cognitive function remains a challenge. Several self-report questionnaires and other subjective measures have evolved to measure listening effort, for example, but there are also concerns that self-report measures do not always correlate with objective measures [52, 53]. For this reason, new explorations involving objective measures are underway.

There have been tremendous advances in technology that permit noninvasive objective assessments of sensory and cognitive function. With this information it might become possible to harness cognitive resources in ways that have been previously unexplored. For example, it might become possible to use brain measures to guide manufacturer designs. Knowing how the auditory system responds to gain, noise reduction, and/or compression circuitry could influence future generations of biologically motivated changes in hearing aid design. The influence of brain responses is especially important with current advances in hearing aid design featuring binaural processing, which involve algorithms making decisions based on cues received from both hearing aids. Returning to the example of listening effort, pupillometry [54], an objective measure of pupil dilation, and even skin conductance (EMG activity; [55]) are being explored as an objective method for quantifying listening effort and cognitive load.

Other approaches include the use of EEG and other neuropsychological correlates of auditive processing for the purpose of setting a hearing device by detecting listening effort [56]. In fact, there already exist a number of existing patents for this purpose by hearing aid manufacturers such as Siemens, Widex, and Oticon, to name a few. These new advances in neuroscience make it clear that multidisciplinary efforts that combine neuroscience and engineering and are verified using clinical trials are innovative directions in hearing aid science. Taking this point one step further, biological codes have been used to innervate motion of artificial limbs/prostheses, and it might someday be possible to design a hearing prosthesis that includes neuromachine interface systems driven by a person's listening effort or attention [57–59]. Over the last decade, engineers and neuroscientists have worked together to translate brain-computer-interface systems from the laboratory for widespread clinical use, including hearing loss [60]. Most recently, eye gaze is being used as a means of steering directional amplification. The visually guided hearing aid (VGHA) combines an eye tracker and an acoustic beam-forming microphone array that work together to tune in the sounds your eyes are directed to while minimizing others [61]. The VGHA is a lab-based prototype whose components connect via computers and other equipment, but a goal is to turn it into a wearable device. But, once again, the successful application of future BCI/VGHA devices will likely require interdisciplinary efforts, described within our framework, given that successful use of amplification involves more than signal processing and engineering.

If a goal of hearing aid research is to enhance and empower a person's listening experience while using hearing aids, then a critical metric within this framework is the outcome measure. Quantifying a person's listening experience using a hearing aid as being positive [√] or negative [✗] might seem straight forward, but decades of research on the topic of outcome measures show this is not the case. Research aimed at modeling and predicting hearing aid outcome [9, 62] shows that there are multiple variables that influence various hearing aid outcomes. A person's age, their expectations, and the point in time in which they are queried can all influence the outcome measure. The type of outcome measure, self-report or otherwise, can also affect results. It is for this reason that a combination of measures (e.g., objective measures of speech-understanding performance; self-report measures of hearing aid usage; and self-report measures of hearing aid benefit and satisfaction) is used to characterize communication-related hearing aid outcome. Expanding our knowledge about the biological influences on speech understanding in noise can inspire the development of new outcome measures that are more sensitive to a listener's perception and to clinical interventions. For example, measuring participation in communication may assess a listener's use of their auditory reception on a deeper level than current outcomes asking how well speech is understood in various environments [63], which could be a promising new development in aided self-report outcomes.

3. Putting It All Together

Many factors can contribute to aided speech understanding in noisy environments, including device centered (e.g., directional microphones, signal processing, and gain settings) and patient centered variables (e.g., age, attention, motivation, and biology). The framework (Figure 1) proposed by Souza and Tremblay [4] provides a context for discussing the multiple stages involved in the perception of amplified sounds. What is more, it illustrates how research aimed at exploring one variable in isolation (e.g., neural mechanisms underlying auditory streaming) falls short of understanding the many interactive stages that are involved in auditory streaming in a person who wears a hearing aid. It can be argued that it is necessary to first understand how normal hearing ear-brain systems stream, but it can also be argued that interventions based on normal hearing studies are limited in their generalizability to hearing aid users.

A person's self-report or aided performance on an outcome measure can be attributed to many different variables illustrated in Figure 1. Each variable (e.g., input signal) could vary in different ways. One listener might describe themselves as performing well [√] when the input *signal* is a single speaker in moderate noise conditions, provided they are paying *attention* to the speaker while using a hearing aid that makes use of a *directional microphone*. This same listener might struggle [✗] if this single speaker is a lecturer in the front of a large classroom who paces back and forth across the stage and intermittently speaks into a microphone. In this example, changes in the quality and direction of a single source of input may be enough to negatively affect a person's use of sound upstream because of a reduced neural capacity

to follow sounds when they change in location and in space. This framework and these examples are overly simplistic, but they are used to emphasize the complexity and multiple interactions that contribute to overall performance variability. We also argue that it is overly simplistic for clinicians and scientists to assume that explanations of performance variability rest solely one stage/variable. For this reason, interdisciplinary research that considers the contribution of neuroscience as an important stage along the continuum is encouraged.

The experiments highlighted here serve as examples to show how far, and multidisciplinary, hearing aid research has come. Since the original publication of Souza and Tremblay [4], advances have been made on the clinical front as shown through the many studies aimed at using neural detection measures to assist with hearing aid fitting. And it is through neuroengineering that that next generation of hearing prostheses will likely come.

Conflict of Interests

The authors declare that there is no conflict of interests regarding the publication of this paper.

Acknowledgments

The authors wish to acknowledge funding from NIDCD R01 DC012769-02 as well as the Virginia Merrill Bloedel Hearing Research Center Traveling Scholar Program.

References

[1] S. Kochkin, "Customer satisfaction with hearing instruments in the digital age," *Hearing Journal*, vol. 58, no. 9, pp. 30–39, 2005.

[2] E. M. Chia, J. J. Wang, E. Rochtchina, R. R. Cumming, P. Newall, and P. Mitchell, "Hearing impairment and health-related quality of life: The blue mountains hearing study," *Ear and Hearing*, vol. 28, no. 2, pp. 187–195, 2007.

[3] T. H. Chisolm, C. E. Johnson, J. L. Danhauer et al., "A systematic review of health-related quality of life hearing aids: final report of the American Academy of Audiology Task Force on the Health-Related Quality of Life Benefits of Amplication in Adults," *Journal of the American Academy of Audiology*, vol. 18, no. 2, pp. 151–183, 2007.

[4] P. E. Souza and K. L. Tremblay, "New perspectives on assessing amplification effects," *Trends in Amplification*, vol. 10, no. 3, pp. 119–143, 2006.

[5] E. C. Cherry, "Some experiments on the recognition of speech, with one and with two ears," *The Journal of the Acoustical Society of America*, vol. 25, no. 5, pp. 975–979, 1953.

[6] N. Wood and N. Cowan, "The cocktail party phenomenon revisited: how frequent are attention shifts to one's name in an irrelevant auditory channel?" *Journal of Experimental Psychology: Learning, Memory, and Cognition*, vol. 21, no. 1, pp. 255–260, 1995.

[7] K. S. Pearsons, R. L. Bennett, and S. Fidell, EPA Report 600/1-77-025, 1977.

[8] R. M. Cox and G. C. Alexander, "Maturation of hearing aid benefit: objective and subjective measurements," *Ear and Hearing*, vol. 13, no. 3, pp. 131–141, 1992.

[9] L. E. Humes, J. B. Ahlstrom, G. W. Bratt, and B. F. Peek, "Studies of hearing-aid outcome measures in older adults: a comparison of technologies and an examination of individual differences," *Seminars in Hearing*, vol. 30, no. 2, pp. 112–128, 2009.

[10] S. Kochkin, "MarkeTrak VII: Obstacles to adult non-user adoption of hearing aids," *Hearing Journal*, vol. 60, no. 4, pp. 24–51, 2007.

[11] R. A. Bentler, "Effectiveness of directional microphones and noise reduction schemes in hearing aids: a systematic review of the evidence," *Journal of the American Academy of Audiology*, vol. 16, no. 7, pp. 473–484, 2005.

[12] R. Bentler, Y. H. Wu, J. Kettel, and R. Hurtig, "Digital noise reduction: Outcomes from laboratory and field studies," *International Journal of Audiology*, vol. 47, no. 8, pp. 447–460, 2008.

[13] C. V. Palmer, R. Bentler, and H. G. Mueller, "Amplification with digital noise reduction and the perception of annoying and aversive sounds," *Trends in Amplification*, vol. 10, no. 2, pp. 95–104, 2006.

[14] Y. H. Wu and R. A. Bentler, "Impact of visual cues on directional benefit and preference: Part I-laboratory tests," *Ear and Hearing*, vol. 31, no. 1, pp. 22–34, 2010.

[15] Y. H. Wu and R. A. Bentler, "Impact of visual cues on directional benefit and preference. Part II-field tests," *Ear and Hearing*, vol. 31, no. 1, pp. 35–46, 2010.

[16] R. A. Bentler and M. R. Duve, "Comparison of hearing aids over the 20th century," *Ear and Hearing*, vol. 21, no. 6, pp. 625–639, 2000.

[17] S. Fikret-Pasa and L. J. Revit, "Individualized correction factors in the preselection of hearing aids," *Journal of Speech and Hearing Research*, vol. 35, no. 2, pp. 384–400, 1992.

[18] Audioscan, *Verifit Users Guide Version 3.10*, Etymonic Design Inc, Ontario, Canada, 2012.

[19] L. Hickson and N. Thyer, "Acoustic analysis of speech-through a hearing aid: Perceptual effects of changes with two-channel compression," *Journal of the American Academy of Audiology*, vol. 14, no. 8, pp. 414–426, 2003.

[20] L. M. Jenstad and P. E. Souza, "Quantifying the effect of compression hearing aid release time on speech acoustics and intelligibility," *Journal of Speech, Language, and Hearing Research*, vol. 48, no. 3, pp. 651–667, 2005.

[21] L. M. Jenstad and P. E. Souza, "Temporal envelope changes of compression and speech rate: combined effects on recognition for older adults," *Journal of Speech, Language, and Hearing Research*, vol. 50, no. 5, pp. 1123–1138, 2007.

[22] M. A. Stone and B. C. J. Moore, "Quantifying the effects of fast-acting compression on the envelope of speech," *Journal of the Acoustical Society of America*, vol. 121, no. 3, pp. 1654–1664, 2007.

[23] P. E. Souza, L. M. Jenstad, and K. T. Boike, "Measuring the acoustic effects of compression amplification on speech in noise," *Journal of the Acoustical Society of America*, vol. 119, no. 1, pp. 41–44, 2006.

[24] P. G. Stelmachowicz, J. Kopun, A. Mace, D. E. Lewis, and S. Nittrouer, "The perception of amplified speech by listeners with hearing loss: acoustic correlates," *Journal of the Acoustical Society of America*, vol. 98, no. 3, pp. 1388–1399, 1995.

[25] L. Hickson, N. Thyer, and D. Bates, "Acoustic analysis of speech through a hearing aid: consonant-vowel ratio effects with two-channel compression amplification," *Journal of the American Academy of Audiology*, vol. 10, no. 10, pp. 549–556, 1999.

[26] S. Bor, P. Souza, and R. Wright, "Multichannel compression: effects of reduced spectral contrast on vowel identification," *Journal of Speech, Language, and Hearing Research*, vol. 51, no. 5, pp. 1315–1327, 2008.

[27] R. L. W. Henning and R. A. Bentler, "The effects of hearing aid compression parameters on the short-term dynamic range of continuous speech," *Journal of Speech, Language, and Hearing Research*, vol. 51, no. 2, pp. 471–484, 2008.

[28] P. E. Souza and C. W. Turner, "Quantifying the contribution of audibility to recognition of compression-amplified speech," *Ear and Hearing*, vol. 20, no. 1, pp. 12–20, 1999.

[29] L. Hickson, B. Dodd, and D. Byrne, "Consonant perception with linear and compression amplification," *Scandinavian Audiology*, vol. 24, no. 3, pp. 175–184, 1995.

[30] A. H. Schwartz and B. G. Shinn-Cunningham, "Effects of dynamic range compression on spatial selective auditory attention in normal-hearing listeners," *Journal of the Acoustical Society of America*, vol. 133, no. 4, pp. 2329–2339, 2013.

[31] D. Glista, V. Easwar, D. W. Purcell, and S. Scollie, "A pilot study on cortical auditory evoked potentials in children: aided caeps reflect improved high-frequency audibility with frequency compression hearing aid technology," *International Journal of Otolaryngology*, vol. 2012, Article ID 982894, 12 pages, 2012.

[32] L. H. Carney, "A model for the responses of low-frequency auditory-nerve fibers in cat," *Journal of the Acoustical Society of America*, vol. 93, no. 1, pp. 401–417, 1993.

[33] M. B. Sachs, I. C. Bruce, R. L. Miller, and E. D. Young, "Biological basis of hearing-aid design," *Annals of Biomedical Engineering*, vol. 30, no. 2, pp. 157–168, 2002.

[34] R. M. Cox, J. A. Johnson, and G. C. Alexander, "Implications of high-frequency cochlear dead regions for fitting hearing aids to adults with mild to moderately severe hearing loss," *Ear and Hearing*, vol. 33, no. 5, pp. 573–587, 2012.

[35] J. F. Willott, "Anatomic and physiologic aging: a behavioral neuroscience perspective," *Journal of the American Academy of Audiology*, vol. 7, no. 3, pp. 141–151, 1996.

[36] K. L. Tremblay, L. Kalstein, C. J. Billings, and P. E. Souza, "The neural representation of consonant-vowel transitions in adults who wear hearing aids," *Trends in Amplification*, vol. 10, no. 3, pp. 155–162, 2006.

[37] K. L. Tremblay, C. J. Billings, L. M. Friesen, and P. E. Souza, "Neural representation of amplified speech sounds," *Ear and Hearing*, vol. 27, no. 2, pp. 93–103, 2006.

[38] S. A. Small and J. F. Werker, "Does the ACC have potential as an index of early speech-discrimination ability? A preliminary study in 4-month-old infants with normal hearing," *Ear and Hearing*, vol. 33, no. 6, pp. e59–e69, 2012.

[39] S. Anderson and N. Kraus, "The potential role of the cABR in assessment and management of hearing impairment," *International Journal of Otolaryngology*, vol. 2013, Article ID 604729, 10 pages, 2013.

[40] L. M. Jenstad, S. Marynewich, and D. R. Stapells, "Slow cortical potentials and amplification. Part II: acoustic measures," *International Journal of Otolaryngology*, vol. 2012, Article ID 386542, 14 pages, 2012.

[41] S. Marynewich, L. M. Jenstad, and D. R. Stapells, "Slow cortical potentials and amplification. Part I: n1-p2 measures," *International Journal of Otolaryngology*, vol. 2012, Article ID 921513, 11 pages, 2012.

[42] C. J. Billings, K. L. Tremblay, P. E. Souza, and M. A. Binns, "Effects of hearing aid amplification and stimulus intensity on cortical auditory evoked potentials," *Audiology and Neurotology*, vol. 12, no. 4, pp. 234–246, 2007.

[43] C. J. Billings, K. L. Tremblay, and C. W. Miller, "Aided cortical auditory evoked potentials in response to changes in hearing aid gain," *International Journal of Audiology*, vol. 50, no. 7, pp. 459–467, 2011.

[44] C. J. Billings, K. L. Tremblay, and J. W. Willott, "The aging auditory system," in *Translational Perspectives in Auditory Neuroscience: Hearing Across the Lifespan. Assessment and Disorders*, K. Tremblay and R. Burkard, Eds., Plural Publishing, Inc, San Diego, Calif, USA, 2012.

[45] C. J. Billings, "Uses and limitations of electrophysiology with hearing aids," *Seminars in Hearing*, vol. 34, no. 4, pp. 257–269, 2013.

[46] V. Easwar, D. W. Purcell, and S. D. Scollie, "Electroacoustic comparison of hearing aid output of phonemes in running speech versus isolation: implications for aided cortical auditory evoked potentials testing," *International Journal of Otolaryngology*, vol. 2012, Article ID 518202, 11 pages, 2012.

[47] K. J. Munro, S. C. Purdy, S. Ahmed, R. Begum, and H. Dillon, "Obligatory cortical auditory evoked potential waveform detection and differentiation using a commercially available clinical system: HEARLab," *Ear and Hearing*, vol. 32, no. 6, pp. 782–786, 2011.

[48] M. Rudner and T. Lunner, "Cognitive spare capacity as a window on hearing aid benefit," *Seminars in Hearing*, vol. 34, no. 4, pp. 298–307, 2013.

[49] J. F. Willott, "Physiological plasticity in the auditory system and its possible relevance to hearing aid use, deprivation effects, and acclimatization," *Ear and Hearing*, vol. 17, pp. 66S–77S, 1996.

[50] J. Kiessling, M. K. Pichora-Fuller, S. Gatehouse et al., "Candidature for and delivery of audiological services: special needs of older people," *International Journal of Audiology*, vol. 42, no. 2, pp. S92–S101, 2003.

[51] P. A. Gosselin and J.-P. Gagné, "Use of a dual-task paradigm to measure listening effort," *Canadian Journal of Speech-Language Pathology and Audiology*, vol. 34, no. 1, pp. 43–51, 2010.

[52] G. H. Saunders and A. Forsline, "The Performance-Perceptual Test (PPT) and its relationship to aided reported handicap and hearing aid satisfaction," *Ear and Hearing*, vol. 27, no. 3, pp. 229–242, 2006.

[53] L. M. Shulman, I. Pretzer-Aboff, K. E. Anderson et al., "Subjective report versus objective measurement of activities of daily living in Parkinson's disease," *Movement Disorders*, vol. 21, no. 6, pp. 794–799, 2006.

[54] T. Koelewijn, A. A. Zekveld, J. M. Festen, J. Rönnberg, and S. E. Kramer, "Processing load induced by informational masking is related to linguistic abilities," *International Journal of Otolaryngology*, vol. 2012, Article ID 865731, 11 pages, 2012.

[55] C. L. Mackersie and H. Cones, "Subjective and psychophysiological indexes of listening effort in a competing-talker task," *Journal of the American Academy of Audiology*, vol. 22, no. 2, pp. 113–122, 2011.

[56] D. J. Strauss, F. I. Corona-Strauss, C. Trenado et al., "Electrophysiological correlates of listening effort: Neurodynamical modeling and measurement," *Cognitive Neurodynamics*, vol. 4, no. 2, pp. 119–131, 2010.

[57] S. Debener, F. Minow, R. Emkes, K. Gandras, and M. de Vos, "How about taking a low-cost, small, and wireless EEG for a walk?" *Psychophysiology*, vol. 49, no. 11, pp. 1617–1621, 2012.

[58] N. J. Hill and B. Schölkopf, "An online brain-computer interface based on shifting attention to concurrent streams of auditory stimuli," *Journal of Neural Engineering*, vol. 9, no. 2, Article ID 026011, 2012.

[59] M. Wronkiewicz, E. Larson, and A. K. Lee, "Towards a next-generation hearing aid through brain state classification and modeling," *Annual International Conference of the IEEE Engineering in Medicine and Biology Society*, vol. 2013, pp. 2808–2811, 2013.

[60] J. R. Wolpaw, N. Birbaumer, D. J. McFarland, G. Pfurtscheller, and T. M. Vaughan, "Brain-computer interfaces for communication and control," *Clinical Neurophysiology*, vol. 113, no. 6, pp. 767–791, 2002.

[61] G. Kidd Jr., S. Favrot, J. G. Desloge, T. M. Streeter, and C. R. Mason, "Design and preliminary testing of a visually guided hearing aid," *Journal of the Acoustical Society of America*, vol. 133, no. 3, pp. EL202–EL207, 2013.

[62] L. E. Humes and T. A. Ricketts, "Modelling and predicting hearing aid outcome," *Trends in Amplification*, vol. 7, no. 2, pp. 41–75, 2003.

[63] C. Baylor, M. Burns, T. Eadie, D. Britton, and K. Yorkston, "A Qualitative study of interference with communicative participation across communication disorders in adults," *The American Journal of Speech-Language Pathology*, vol. 20, no. 4, pp. 269–287, 2011.

13

Role of Intranasal Steroid in the Prevention of Recurrent Nasal Symptoms after Adenoidectomy

Tamer S. Sobhy

Faculty of Medicine, Ain Shams University, 15 Khalifa Maamoon, Heliopolis, Cairo, Egypt

Correspondence should be addressed to Tamer S. Sobhy; tamshok2008@hotmail.com

Academic Editor: Charles Monroe Myer

Background. Intranasal steroid provides an efficient nonsurgical alternative to adenoidectomy for theimprovement of adenoid nasal obstruction. *Objective.* To demonstrate the role of intranasal steroid in the prevention of adenoid regrowth after adenoidectomy. *Methods.* Prospective randomized controlled study. Two hundred children after adenoidectomy were divided into 2 groups. Group I received postoperative intranasal steroid and group II received postoperative intranasal saline spray. Both medications were administered for 12 weeks postoperatively. Patients were followed up for 1 year. Followup was done using the nasopharyngeal lateral X-rays, reporting the degree of the symptoms. *Results.* Significant difference between both groups after 6 months and after 1 year. The intranasal steroid group had significantly lower score after 6 months and after 1 year as regards nasal obstruction, nasal discharge, and snoring than the intranasal saline group. 2 weeks postoperatively, there was no difference between both groups as regards nasal obstruction, discharge, or snoring. As regards lateral radiographs, there was statistically significant difference between both groups 1 year but not 6 months postoperatively. *Conclusion.* Factors influencing the outcome of intranasal steroids therapy in the prevention of adenoid regrowth have not been identified. However, this treatment may obtain successful results in children to avoid readenoidectomy.

1. Introduction

Nasal obstruction is one of the main symptoms of adenoid hypertrophy; they are also presented with chronic rhinorrhea, snoring, hyponasal speech, and obstructive sleep disorder [1]. Adenoidectomy can reduce both nasal obstructions and upper respiratory infections. However, some patients display clinically significantly persistent nasal symptoms even after surgery. Symptoms, such as nasal obstruction or recurrent upper respiratory infections, persist in 19–26% of patients [2]. Adenoidectomy remains a commonly performed procedure, although it produces short-term benefits [3]. There are 2 difficulties that have been described to prevent complete adenoidal removal. Firstly, lymphoid tissue in the pharyngeal recess is considered by all authors as difficult to remove [4]. The second difficulty is the bulging adenoidal tissue into the posterior choanae, which was addressed by Pearl and Manoukian [5]; they found choanal adenoids in 9% of their study group.

Although there are few nonsurgical alternative treatment options, these may be considered in less serious cases.

Accordingly, studies about intranasal steroid applications under various protocols have been presented in the literature, but none of these studies addressed the efficacy of intranasal steroids to prevent recurrence of adenoid after adenoidectomy.

2. Patients and Methods

This study was a prospective randomized controlled parallel clinical study. As the study had no connection with any of the manufacturers of the drugs or the pharmaceutical industry at all, it was not possible to obtain a placebo, and therefore the study could not be double blinded. Simple randomization was done with every other patient consecutively.

The study was approved by the Institutional Review Board of the Otorhinolaryngology Department, Faculty of Medicine, Ain Shams University, Cairo, Egypt. Children presented to ENT outpatient clinic at Ain Shams University hospitals during the period from April 2009 to June 2011, diagnosed as adenoid hypertrophy, were included in the study. The study included 2 groups; each included 100 children. Written informed consents from the parents were taken about the participation of their children in the study.

The diagnosis was based on the following symptoms: nasal obstruction, nasal discharge, and/or snoring and lateral radiographs (enlarged convex bulge in the roof of the nasopharynx compressing the nasopharyngeal airway). Exclusion criteria included the use of intranasal or systemic steroids within the last 1 year, use of any intranasal medication within the previous 2 weeks of entering the study, acute URTI within 2 weeks of entering the study, history of epistaxis, immunodeficiency disorders, or hypersensitivity to the mometasone furoate. Also, children were excluded from the study if there is a history of craniofacial neuromuscular or genetic disorder.

Assessment of each child upon entering the study included the following: history and physical examination, parental questionnaire, and lateral nasopharyngeal radiograph. All patients under the study had complete head and neck evaluation, including flexible fiber-optic nasal endoscopy (according to the compliance of the child). Due to the difficulty of the use of the flexible endoscopy for all patients, it was not feasible to be used in the assessment of the nasopharynx pre or postoperatively.

The patients were all assessed before and after adenoidectomy as regards the nasal obstruction, discharge, and snoring. These symptoms were all graded as Grade 1: mild, Grade 2: moderate, and Grade 3: severe.

The lateral view nasopharyngeal radiograph, the size of the adenoids was graded according to the palatal airway measured from the most convex point of the adenoid tissue to the soft palate. The narrowest distance between the nasopharyngeal soft tissue and the soft palate was taken. Grading was as follows, Grade 1: >6 mm; Grade 2: 4–6 mm; Grade 3: 0–3 mm. The lateral radiographs were done before surgery and 6 months and 12 months postoperatively.

The parents were asked (using the questionnaire) about their overall satisfaction of the nasal condition of the child after adenoidectomy. They were also asked about the number of upper respiratory tract infections in the previous years and postoperatively.

Adenoidectomy was done using the classical method using the adenoid curette. After adenoidectomy, children were then simply randomized into 2 groups, group I which included (100 children) with postoperative intranasal steroids and group II (100 children) who had postoperative intranasal saline spray. Patients in group I received 12-week course of single intranasal spray administration in each nostril with mome tasone furoate (40 mcg/day). After this course, all patients in group I were reassessed to evaluate the efficacy of treatment. All patients or parents were asked to report the degree of the symptom after 2 weeks, 6 months, and 1 year postoperatively with the questionnaire that is fulfilled by the parents. No other medication was allowed during the treatment. Patients who used systemic steroids for any other reason were excluded from the study. Patients in group II received intranasal saline nasal spray for the same period (12 weeks), and assessment was done in the same way as group I. All patients were followed up after adenoidectomy after 2

TABLE 1: Demographic data of the 2 groups of the study.

		Intranasal steroid group		Intranasal saline group	
		N	%	N	%
Sex	Male	54	56.3%	42	45.7%
	Female	42	43.8%	50	54.3%
Age	Mean ± SD	7.42	2.86	5.89	2.72

weeks, 6 months, and 1 year. Lateral radiographs were done after 6 months and after 1 year in the postoperative period.

Statistical Analysis. The collected data was revised, coded, tabulated, and introduced to a PC using statistical package for Social Science (SPSS 15.0.1 for windows; SPSS Inc., Chicago, IL, USA, 2001).

3. Results

In group I patients with intranasal steroids, there were 96 patients (4 patients were excluded from the study) with age range from 3 to 13 years (mean age = 7.42 years), and there were 54 males (56.3%) and 42 females (43.8%), while in group II with intranasal saline included 92 patients (8 patients were excluded) with age range from 3 to 13 years (mean age = 5.89 years); this group included 42 males (45.7%) and 50 females (54.3%). Demographic data of the patients in both groups are shown in Table 1.

As regard nasal obstruction, highly significant difference towards group I with intranasal steroids, when compared with group II with intranasal saline 6 months (P = .001) and 1 year (P = .031) postoperatively. However, 2 weeks in the postoperatively period, there was no significant difference between both groups.

Regarding nasal discharge, there was a highly significant difference (P = .0001) between both groups, towards group I with intranasal steroids after 6 months and after 1 year (P = .001), in the postoperative period. While after 2 weeks in the postoperative period, there was no significant difference (P = 1.00) between both groups.

Regarding snoring, there was a highly significant difference between both groups after 6 months (P = .0001) and after 1 year (P = .001). There was no significant difference after 2 weeks (P = .363) in the postoperative period.

In group I, comparing data after 1 year with the data of the preoperative period, there was a highly significant difference elicited in all the 3 symptoms (P = .0001). Comparing data after 1 year with the data after 2 weeks in the postoperative period, there was significant difference regarding nasal obstruction only (P = .0001) but no difference regarding nasal discharge and snoring. When comparing data after 1 year with the data after 6 months, there was significant difference as regards the 3 symptoms with P = .011 in nasal obstruction, P = .008 in nasal discharge, and P = .003 in snoring. This can be illustrated in Figure 1.

Significant difference (P = .003) was noted towards group I patients regarding nasopharyngeal radiograph after 1 year in the postoperative period. However, there was no

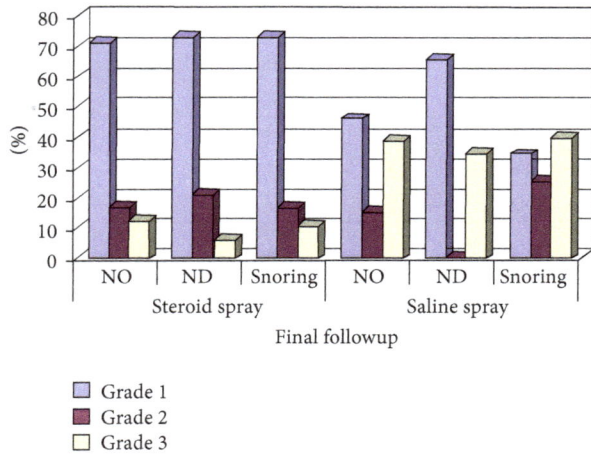

FIGURE 1: Description of nasal symptoms grades among steroid and saline patients at the last followup, 1 year postoperatively. This graph shows the differences between the nasal symptoms grades between both study groups after 1 year (NO: nasal obstruction, ND: nasal discharge, Grade 1 = mild, Grade 2 = moderate, and Grade 3 = severe).

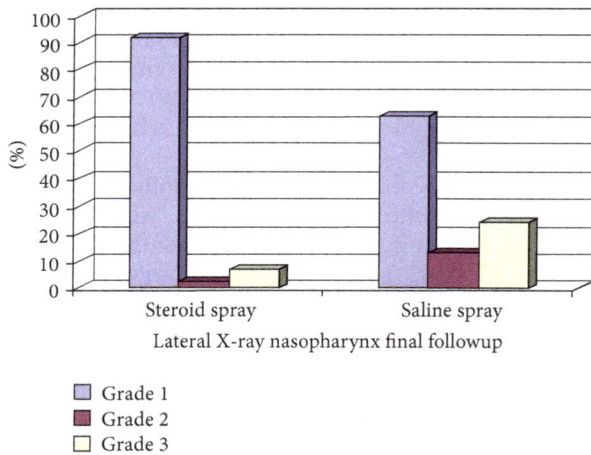

FIGURE 2: Description of X-ray findings among steroid and saline patients at the last followup, 1 year postoperatively. This graph shows the differences between patients as regards the adenoid enlargement grade between both study groups after 1 year (Grade 1 = >6 mm, Grade 2 = 4–6 mm, and Grade 3 = 0–3 mm).

significant difference between both groups (P = .191) 6 months postoperatively.

In group I patients, there was a highly significant difference (P = .0001) of the nasopharyngeal radiographs when comparing the data after 6 months with the data in the preoperative period. A highly significant difference (P = .0001) could be elucidated when comparing the data after 1 year with the data in the preoperative period despite failing to find any difference of the radiograph data after 1 year when compared with the data after 6 months which is shown in Figure 2.

In the current study, it was found that the overall satisfaction among parents of group I patients was 85.4%. Overall satisfaction among parents of group II was 76.1%. When comparing the overall satisfaction between both groups, there was no statistically significant difference. Also, there was a highly significant difference of the number of URTI when comparing data of the pre- and postoperative periods. The same data was found in group II with a significant difference (P = .0001).

There were no intraoperative or postoperative complications in group I. While in group II, post operatively, 3 patients developed secondary bleeding after 7 days.

4. Discussion

Revision adenoidectomies are not unheard of. However, a review of the literature, including some prominent textbooks, does not illuminate the issue or its frequency [4]. Buchinsky and coworkers [4] failed to find a new obstructing adenoid pad after adenoidectomy in a large series of children, while, on the contrary, Joshua and his colleagues in [2] found a new obstructing adenoid tissue in the clinical practice. They reported infrequent occurrence of adenoid re-growth after adenoidectomy that causes nasal obstruction which accounts for 3% of patients with persistent postadenoidectomy symptoms.

Successful use of intranasal steroid treatment in children with adenoid hypertrophy was introduced by Demain and Goetz [6]. Although it is not yet clear by which mechanisms the steroids reduce the nasal airway obstruction, however, there are some theories such as the anti-inflammatory effect of steroids that help to reduce adenoidal and nasopharyngeal inflammation [6].

The present study showed that the use of intra nasal steroids after adenoidectomy was beneficial to relieve nasal obstruction and prevent recurrence of adenoid after adenoidectomy after a follow-up period of 1 year. There is a difference in age across groups (7.4 in group I and 5.89 in group II) which might account for the difference across groups as the Waldeyer's ring involutes with puberty. However, Buchinsky and colleagues [4] failed to find any significant difference between children younger than 10 years and those older than 10 years as the proportions between both groups were identical.

In the current study we could not perform endoscopy for all children, although it is now the best diagnostic technique for diagnosis of adenoid-related nasal obstruction because it depends on the age and compliance of the child.

The use of postoperative intranasal steroid gives advantage to avoid the 2nd intervention. This is in contrast to Lepcha and coworkers [7], who did not find any significant efficacy of intranasal steroids in improving nasal blockage, nasal discharge, or snoring, although a fivefold reduction in adenoid size was observed in intranasal steroid group when compared with the placebo group. However, this difference did not reach a statistical significance.

Steroids are generally well tolerated in children. Studies showed only one case of episodic nasal bleeding [8]. The effect of intranasal steroids on growth was studied by Allen and his colleagues in [9], in a randomized, double-blind, placebo-controlled study. The growth rate in pre-puberty children who had used intranasal steroids for 1 year was reported to be equal to the growth rate of the placebo control group.

The mechanisms by which topical steroids improve nasal airway obstructive symptoms remain unclear. Three main trials succeeded to demonstrate the improvement of nasal obstruction with reduction of adenoid size with the use of intranasal steroids [6, 10, 11].

Nonsurgical alternatives for adenoid hypertrophy are limited to treatment of the coexisting upper airway infections. However, it was reported that treatment with intranasal steroids can decrease the size of adenoid hypertrophy, using beclomethasone [6], fluticasone [12], and mometasone [13]. Among several commercially available steroid nasal sprays, we selected mometasone furoate for this study. This drug had been reported previously not to cause any adverse effects on growth and hypothalamic pituitary adrenal axis. Also, the systemic availability of the drug after topical administration is lower than that of other steroids [14].

Ciprandi and coworkers in [15] found that the use of intranasal flunisolide was associated with a significant reduction of adenoid hypertrophy in 72.6 % of the children. On the contrary, isotonic saline solution was associated with a nonsignificant improvement of adenoid hypertrophy as reported in 30.7% of children. A recent study provided evidence that treatment with nasal steroids could represent for some children an effective means of avoiding adenoidectomy [16]. The current study also clarified similar results as Ciprandi and his colleagues [15], as there was significant reduction in the size of the adenoid in lateral radiographs after 1 year with a P value = .003.

In this study, it was found that the overall satisfaction among parents of group I patients was 85.4%. Similar results were reported by Lesinskas and Drigotas [1]; they showed that 82.7% of the parents were satisfied with the results of adenoidectomy.

The duration of treatment with intranasal steroids in previous studies varied from 8 to 24 weeks. None of these trials established the optimal duration of treatment in children. The effects are expected after 2 weeks of the initiation of the treatment as described by Criscuoli et al. [16].

The study is limited by the absence of the nasal endoscopic examination which is considered the best diagnostic technique for the diagnosis of the adenoid-related nasal manifestations. We did not include nasal endoscopy because of the noncompliance of the children. One of the limitations is the noncompliance of the children to the intranasal steroids which is observed mainly in the young children. Another limitation of the study is the method of adenoidectomy which is limited to the adenoid curette, although other methods are used, but the most feasible method of adenoidectomy was the adenoid curette. A multicenter study with longer follow-up periods on the study patients should elicit a more informative data.

5. Conclusion

Factors influencing the outcome of intranasal steroids therapy have not been identified. However, this treatment may obtain successful results in children to avoid surgery for adenoid recurrence. The most appropriate drug, the most efficient dose, and optimal treatment duration need to be investigated and determined.

Conflict of Interests

No potential conflict of interests relevant to this paper was reported.

Authors' Contribution

The author made substantial contribution for the designing of the study, acquisition of data, analysis and interpretation of data, and drafting the paper.

Acknowledgment

The author is thankful to the entire staff of the Clinic of Otorhinolaryngology at Ain Shams University hospitals for their help in performing this study. Also, the author thanks Dr. Walid Salah, M. D., lecturer of community medicine for his generous statistical help.

References

[1] E. Lesinskas and M. Drigotas, "The incidence of adenoidal regrowth after adenoidectomy and its effect on persistent nasal symptoms," *European Archives of Otorhinolaryngol*, vol. 266, no. 4, pp. 469–473, 2009.

[2] B. Joshua, G. Bahar, J. Sulkes, T. Shpitzer, and E. Raveh, "Adenoidectomy: long-term follow-up," *Otolaryngology*, vol. 135, no. 4, pp. 576–580, 2006.

[3] S. J. Vandenberg and D. G. Heatley, "Efficacy of adenoidectomy in relieving symptoms of chronic sinusitis in children," *Archives of Otolaryngology*, vol. 123, no. 7, pp. 675–678, 1997.

[4] F. J. Buchinsky, M. A. Lowry, and G. Isaacson, "Do adenoids regrow after excision?" *Otolaryngology*, vol. 123, no. 5, pp. 576–581, 2000.

[5] A. J. Pearl and J. J. Manoukian, "Adenoidectomy: indirect visualization of choanal adenoids," *Journal of Otolaryngology*, vol. 23, no. 3, pp. 221–224, 1994.

[6] J. G. Demain and D. W. Goetz, "Pediatric adenoidal hypertrophy and nasal airway obstruction: reduction with aqueous nasal beclomethasone," *Pediatrics*, vol. 95, no. 3, pp. 355–364, 1995.

[7] A. Lepcha, M. Kurien, A. Job, L. Jeyaseelan, and K. Thomas, "Chronic adenoid hypertrophy in children—is steroid nasal spray beneficial?" *Indian Journal of Otolaryngology and Head and Neck Surgery*, vol. 54, no. 4, pp. 280–284, 2002.

[8] M. Berlucchi, L. Valetti, G. Parrinello, and P. Nicolai, "Long-term follow-up of children undergoing topical intranasal steroid therapy for adenoidal hypertrophy," *International Journal of Pediatric Otorhinolaryngology*, vol. 72, no. 8, pp. 1171–1175, 2008.

[9] D. B. Allen, E. O. Meltzer, R. F. Lemanske et al., "No growth suppression in children treated with the maximum recommended dose of fluticasone propionate aqueous nasal spray for one year," *Allergy and Asthma Proceedings*, vol. 23, no. 6, pp. 407–413, 2002.

[10] M. Berlucchi, D. Salsi, L. Valetti, G. Parrinello, and P. Nicolai, "The role of mometasone furoate aqueous nasal spray in

the treatment of adenoidal hypertrophy in the pediatric age group: preliminary results of a prospective, randomized study," *Pediatrics*, vol. 119, no. 6, pp. 1392–1397, 2007.

[11] H. Demirhan, F. Aksoy, O. Ozturan, Y. S. Yildirim, and B. Veyseller, "Medical treatment of adenoid hypertrophy with "fluticasone propionate nasal drops"," *International Journal of Pediatric Otorhinolaryngology*, vol. 74, no. 7, pp. 773–776, 2010.

[12] R. T. Brouillette, J. J. Manoukian, F. M. Ducharme et al., "Efficacy of fluticasone nasal spray for pediatric obstructive sleep apnea," *Journal of Pediatrics*, vol. 138, no. 6, pp. 838–844, 2001.

[13] S. Cengel and M. U. Akyol, "The role of topical nasal steroids in the treatment of children with otitis media with effusion and/or adenoid hypertrophy," *International Journal of Pediatric Otorhinolaryngology*, vol. 70, no. 4, pp. 639–645, 2006.

[14] Y. G. Jung, H. Y. Kim, J. Y. Min, H. J. Dhong, and S. K. Chung, "Role of intranasal topical steroid in pediatric sleep disordered breathing and influence of allergy, sinusitis, and obesity on treatment outcome," *Clinical and Experimental Otorhinolaryngology*, vol. 4, no. 1, pp. 27–32, 2011.

[15] G. Ciprandi, A. Varricchio, M. Capasso et al., "Intranasal flunisolide treatment in children with adenoidal hypertrophy," *International Journal of Immunopathology and Pharmacology*, vol. 20, no. 4, pp. 833–836, 2007.

[16] G. Criscuoli, S. D'Amora, G. Ripa et al., "Frequency of surgery among children who have adenotonsillar hypertrophy and improve after treatment with nasal beclomethasone," *Pediatrics*, vol. 111, no. 3, pp. 236–238, 2003.

14

Clinical and Pathological Characteristics of Organized Hematoma

Nobuo Ohta,[1] **Tomoo Watanabe,**[1] **Tsukasa Ito,**[1] **Toshinori Kubota,**[1] **Yusuke Suzuki,**[1]
Akihiro Ishida,[1] **Masaru Aoyagi,**[1] **Atsushi Matsubara,**[2] **Kenji Izuhara,**[3] **and Seiji Kakehata**[1]

[1] *Department of Otolaryngology, Head and Neck Surgery, Faculty of Medicine, Yamagata University, 2-2-2 Iida-nishi,*
  Yamagata 990-9585, Japan
[2] *Department of Otorhinolaryngology, Hirosaki University Graduate School of Medicine,*
  Hirosaki 036-8562, Japan
[3] *Division of Medical Biochemistry, Department of Biomolecular Sciences, Faculty of Medicine,*
  Saga University, Saga 840-8502, Japan

Correspondence should be addressed to Nobuo Ohta; noohta@med.id.yamagata-u.ac.jp

Academic Editor: David W. Eisele

Objective. To study the clinical and pathological characteristics of patients with organized hematoma with malignant features in maxillary sinuses. *Subjects and Methods.* This was a retrospective study of five patients who were treated surgically for organized hematoma. The preoperative CT and MRI findings were studied clinically. The expressions of CD31, CD34, and periostin in surgical samples were investigated by immunohistochemistry. *Results.* The clinical features of organized hematoma, such as a mass expanding from the maxillary sinus with bone destruction, resembled those of maxillary carcinoma. However, CT and MRI provided sufficient and useful information to differentiate this condition from malignancy. Surgical resection was the first-line treatment because of the presence of a firm capsule. Characteristic histopathological findings were a mixture of dilated vessels, hemorrhage, fibrin exudation, fibrosis, hyalinization, and neovascularization. The expressions of periostin, CD31, and CD34 were observed in organized hematoma of the maxillary sinus. *Conclusion.* The expressions of periostin, CD31, and CD34 were observed in organized hematoma of the maxillary sinus. Organized hematoma is characterized pathologically by a mixture of bleeding, dilated vessels, hemorrhage, fibrin exudation, fibrosis, hyalinization, and neovascularization. CT and MRI show heterogeneous findings reflecting a mixture of these pathological entities.

1. Introduction

Nonneoplastic hemorrhagic lesions causing mucosal swelling and bone destruction can develop in the maxillary sinus. This type of lesion was reported in the Japanese literature in 1917 as a "blood boil of the maxillary sinus" by Tadokoro and is comparatively well known in Japan as one of the differential diagnoses of maxillary carcinoma. However, in the English literature, this type of lesion tends to be referred to as hemangioma of the maxillary sinus, organized hematoma of the maxillary sinus, or organized hematoma of the maxillary sinus mimicking tumor [1–8]. Although their clinical manifestations are very similar, the relationships between these entities have not been described.

We recently resected five such lesions and examined the associated clinical and histological features. Histologically, a combination of dilated vessels, hemorrhage, fibrin exudation, fibrosis, hyalinization, and neovascularization was characteristic. The lesion mimicked not only hematoma but also hemangioma. Therefore, either of the terms hemangioma or hematoma reflects the complete histological picture. In this paper, we report the clinicopathological characteristics of this entity and the relationship between the imaging and histopathological findings.

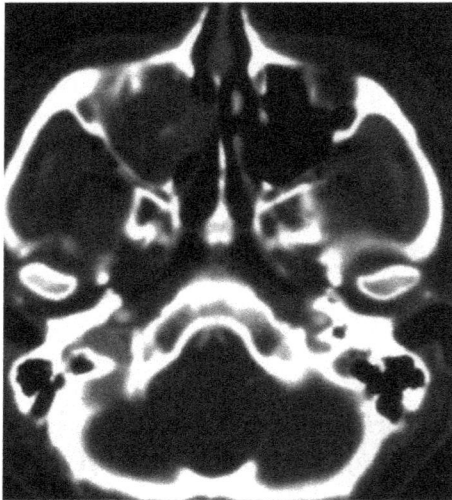

FIGURE 1: A 36-year-old female had a 2-month history of recurrent epistaxis. Initial coronal contrast-enhanced computed tomography scan of the paranasal sinuses revealed a 36 × 24 mm heterogeneous enhanced mass in the right maxillary sinus. The central region of the mass was strongly enhanced. Compression and thinning of the lateral wall of the right nasal cavity were observed (case III).

2. Subjects and Methods

2.1. Subjects. To evaluate the clinicopathological entity of the organized hematoma, we recruited subjects with lesions that met the following criteria. (1) CT demonstrated an expanding unilateral maxillary lesion, with thinning or destruction of the surrounding bony tissue; (2) MRI demonstrated a heterogeneous mass; (3) macroscopically, a mass with a hemorrhagic and heterogeneous appearance was observed; (4) histologically, nonneoplastic tissue with mucosal hemorrhage was observed.

Of all the patients referred to our department between 1996 and 2010 with suspected maxillary tumor, five met these criteria. These patients underwent clinical evaluation, followed by either transmaxillary or endonasal endoscopic sinus surgery and histopathological examination of the resected tissue.

2.2. Immunohistochemistry to Detect CD31, CD34, and Periostin. For immunohistochemical detection of CD31, CD34, and periostin, we used the labeled streptavidin-biotin-complex (SABC) method. Deparaffinized tissue sections were rehydrated in alcohols. The sections were autoclaved for 10 min at 120°C in citrate phosphate buffer (pH 6.0) for antigen retrieval. Endogenous peroxidase activity was blocked with 0.3% H_2O_2 for 30 min. The sections were then incubated with skim milk normal in phosphate-buffered saline (PBS) for 10 min to block nonspecific background staining. Monoclonal anti-CD31 and CD34 antibodies were purchased from Dako Japan (Tokyo, Japan). A polyclonal anti-Pendrin or anti-Periostin antibody was generated by immunising the rabbits with specific peptides. Polyclonal antibody against Pendrin was applied as a primary antibody

at a dilution of 1:100 and incubated at 4°C overnight. Polyclonal antibody against Periostin was applied as a primary antibody at a dilution of 1:500 and incubated at 4°C overnight. After the sections had been washed with PBS, biotinylated goat anti-rabbit IgG was applied, and they were then incubated for 1 h at room temperature. Slides were developed by using diaminobenzidine and were counterstained with hematoxylin.

2.3. Assessment of Slides. Immunostained sections were assessed at 200x magnification under an Olympus microscope with an eyepiece reticle. Cell counts are expressed as means per high-power field (0.202 mm^2). At least two sections were immunostained, and more than five areas were evaluated via the reticle. Results are expressed as number of positive cells per field, as follows: (−): negative; (+): fewer than 10 cells in each high-power field (×400); (++): 10 to 20 cells; (+++): more than 20 cells.

3. Results

Patient characteristics and the clinical features of the five cases are summarized in Table 1. The age of the patients ranged from 14 to 56 years. The clinical features resembled those of maxillary carcinoma. The most frequently observed primary sign was recurrent epistaxis, although a wide variety of clinical features were observed, including nasal obstruction, cheek pain, and nasal pain. In most cases, the clinical course before diagnosis had been a for few months; however, one patient visited an ENT clinic because of hemorrhage from right nasal cavity mass and right nasal obstruction that had gradually enlarged over the course of 11 months. No patient exhibited coagulation abnormalities or reported a history of facial trauma. CT showed unilateral maxillary masses with thinning or destruction of the surrounding bony structures (Figure 1). The expansion pattern was not invasive. On MRI, the masses were well demarcated from the surrounding structures and heterogeneous in signal density on both T1-weighted, T2-weighted, and Gd-DTPA-enhanced images (Figure 2). CT and MRI provided sufficient information to differentiate these lesions from malignancy (Table 2).

A transmaxillary surgical approach was used in two patients and endonasal endoscopic sinus surgery in three patients. None of the patients required a blood transfusion as a result of intraoperative bleeding. The masses had firm capsules and were therefore removed easily, even in all cases in which the lesion extended from the maxillary sinus. Before the surgery, three patients underwent angiography, which revealed that the maxillary artery was the feeder artery. Two of the patients had strongly enhanced lesions, which were embolized with Gelform (Table 3).

Histologically, the specimens consisted of dilated vessels, hemorrhage, fibrin exudation, fibrosis, hyalinization, and neovascularization, without tumor cells (Figure 3). CD31-positive cells (endothelial cells) were identified in separate sections from each mass. CD34-positive cells (progenitors of endothelial cells) were also observed in the specimens

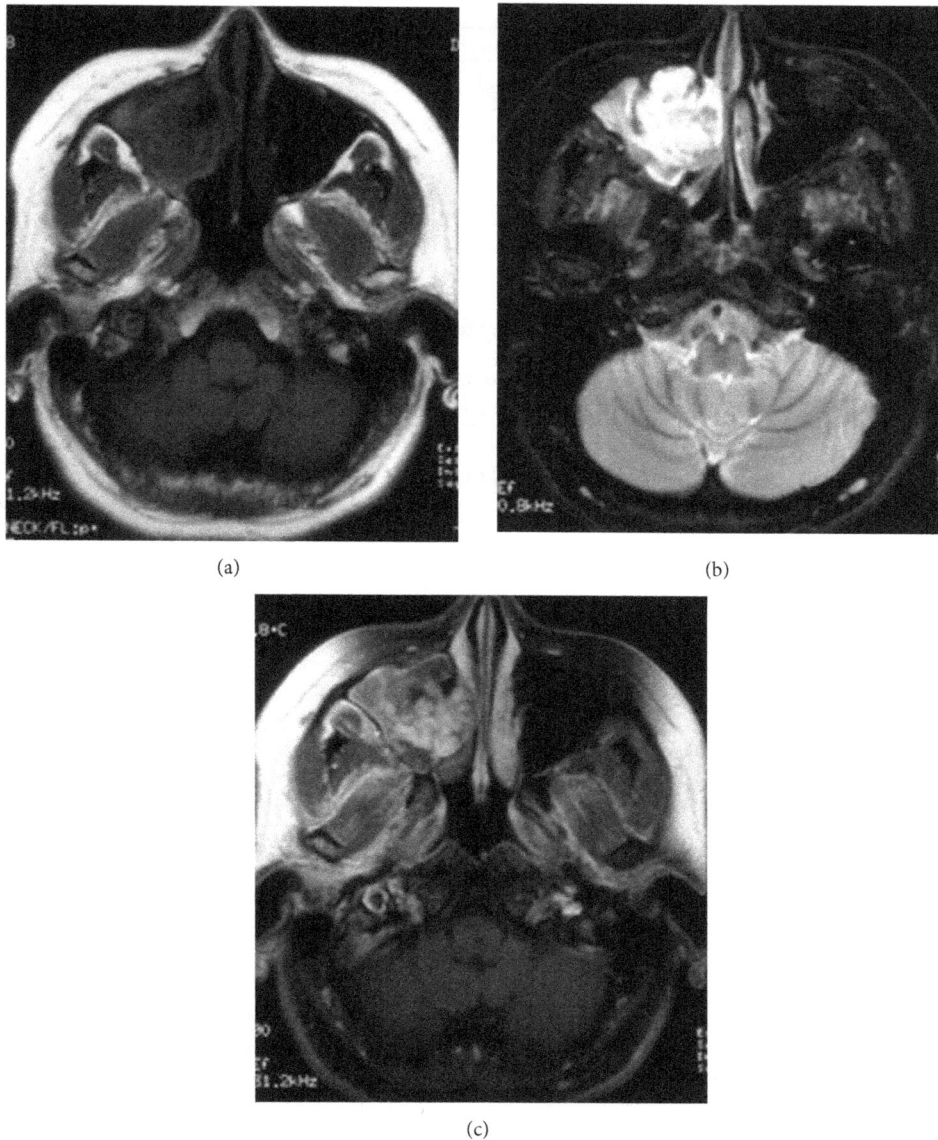

(a)

(b)

(c)

FIGURE 2: A 36-year-old female had a 2-month history of recurrent epistaxis. (a) Initial T1-weighted magnetic resonance image before treatment, showing a slightly low intensity in the central region of the mass (coronal view). (b) Initial T2-weighted magnetic resonance image before treatment, showing a heterogeneous mass. The central portion had high signal intensity, and the surrounding region had lower signal intensity than the central portion. The paranasal mucosa was thickened but kept its structure (axial view). (c) Initial Gd-DTPA magnetic resonance image before treatment, showing that the central portion was strongly enhanced. The surrounding region was less enhanced than the central portion. The thickened mucosa of the paranasal sinus was also strongly enhanced (axial view).

(Figure 4). The expression of periostin was also observed in the specimens (Figure 5). These characteristic findings were generally seen in separate sections from each mass; the pattern of the mixture of findings differed among parts of the same mass, masses from the same patient, and patients. The appearance of the findings also varied among different parts of the masses and among patients. To obtain all of these findings, we needed to examine several sections from different parts of each mass (Table 4). These characteristic findings were all subepithelial, and the lining of the epithelium was intact.

Followup to date (range from 6 to 108 months) has demonstrated all patients to be free of recurrence.

4. Discussion

Preoperative CT showed a heterogeneously enhanced mass expanding out of the maxillary sinus, with thinning or destruction of the adjacent bone. This expansion did not exhibit an invasive pattern but is commonly seen in malignancy, so the CT findings were not specific to this disease. This limitation was overcome by using MRI. MRI was able

TABLE 1: Patient demographics and clinical features.

Case	age/gender	Chief complaint	Location	Side	Intranasal findings	Duration (m)
I	38/M	Epistaxis	MS	R	Mass in the MM	1
II	14/M	Epistaxis	MS	L	Mass in the MM	3
III	36/F	Nasal obstruction	MS	R	Polyps in the MM	2
IV	31/M	Nasal obstruction	MS	R	Bulging of the LW	6
V	56/F	Epistaxis	MS	R	Mass in the MM	11

M: male; F: female; MS: maxillary sinus; R: right; L: left; MM: middle meatus; LW: lateral wall.

TABLE 2: The CT and MRI findings of the five cases.

Case	Size on CT (mm)	CT (bone destruction)	MRI (T1-weighted)		MRI (T2-weighted)		MRI (Gd-DPTA)	
			Central	Surrounding	Central	Surrounding	Central	Surrounding
I	43 × 57 × 46	+(L,P)	Low	Low	High	Iso to high	High	Low
II	37 × 28 × 30	+(L)	Low	Low to iso	High	Iso to high	High	Low
III	30 × 31 × 28	+(L)	Low	Low	High	high	Iso to high	Low to iso
IV	35 × 31 × 29	+(L)	Low	Low to iso	High	high	Iso to high	Low to iso
V	25 × 30 × 27	+(L,P)	Low	Low to iso	High	Iso to high	High	Low

L: lateral wall of nasal cavity; P: posterior wall of maxillary sinus; Low: low signal intensity; iso: iso signal intensity; high: high signal intensity; central: central portion of the mass; surrounding: surrounding portion of the mass; Gd-DPTA: Gd-DPTA enhanced.

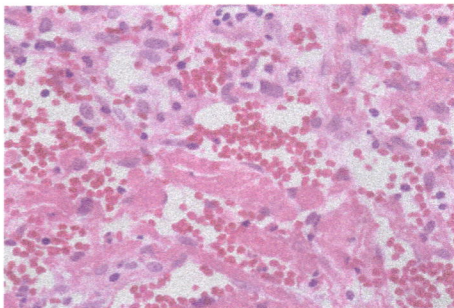

FIGURE 3: Representative pathological findings of organized hematoma. Nonneoplastic tissue with hemorrhage, fibrin exudation, and hyalinization was observed. (HE, original magnification ×100).

to demonstrate the apparent morphological heterogeneity of this disease and thus clearly differentiated it from neoplasms and mucoceles. A heterogeneous signal intensity on MRI was commonly observed. MRI showed thickening of the paranasal sinus mucosa surrounding the mass. The mucosa was well enhanced on T1-weighted images with contrast and had high signal intensity on T2-weighted images. These findings suggested the presence of inflammatory change due to obstruction by the lesion. In addition, the central part of the lesion had low signal intensity on T1-weighted imaging and high signal intensity on T2-weighted imaging and was well enhanced. These findings suggested that this central region contained blood with a low flow speed, thus matching the pathological finding of hematoma. The periphery was less well enhanced, thus matching the zone of fibrosis. This biphasic appearance is an important imaging aspect of this lesion and needs to be considered in the differential diagnosis before a decision is made on a treatment strategy. Recognizing the

location of the hematoma preoperatively could be useful for avoiding intraoperative bleeding from the mass.

Microscopic examination revealed dilated vessels, hemorrhage, fibrin exudation, fibrosis, hyalinization, and neovascularization in the subepithelium. The appearance of these findings varied among different parts of the masses, and as for the disease etiology, Omura et al. suggest the negative spiral theory during the healing process as follows [8]. First, a blood clot accumulates in the closed space owing to bleeding of various causes, including hemangioma formation, facial injury, or inflammation. Next, necrosis, fibrosis, and hyalinization occur in turn, and neovascularization develops as part of the biological healing processes. As a result, the new vessels become weak, and rebleeding might easily occur. To examine this negative spiral theory immunohistopathologically, CD31, CD34, and periostin were used for immunostaining. These results showed that the endothelial cells kept their structural integrity and dilated pattern in limited areas. CD 34 is expressed on the progenitors of endothelial cells and might play an important role in neovascularization and wound healing [9–11]. CD34 immunostaining showed that these endothelial cell progenitors were present in the lesions. Periostin is a regulator of fibrosis and collagen deposits, and although it has been recognized for the important role it plays in myocardial repair/remodeling following myocardial infarction [12], there are indicators that its overexpression in the nasal mucosa contributes to tissue repair and fibrosis. These findings may support the negative spiral theory immunohistopathologically.

Surgery is mandatory to remove the organized hematoma as first-line treatment. To differentiate the organized hematoma from a malignant tumor, the complete absence of neoplastic cells in the totally removed specimen should be confirmed [1–8]. Thus, total removal under general

(a)

(b)

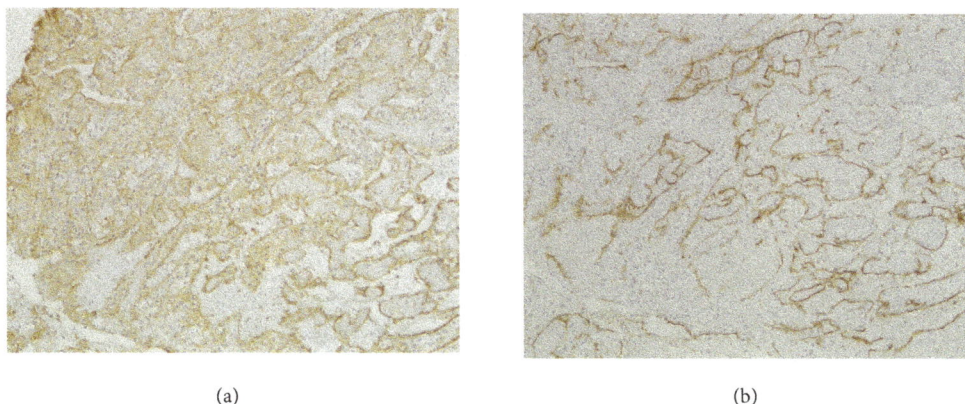

FIGURE 4: Immunohistochemical staining for CD31 and CD34 in organized hematoma (original magnification ×100). CD31-positive cells were observed in the organized hematoma, and dilated vessels were found (a). CD34-positive cells were observed in the organized hematoma (b). (Immunostaining, original magnification ×100 and ×200.)

TABLE 3: Treatment and outcomes.

Case	Angiography	Feeding artery	Embolization	Operation method	Bleeding volume (mL)	followup (m)	recurrence
I	(+)	(−)	(−)	Transmaxillary	56	108	none
II	(+)	MA	Gelform	ESS	5	48	none
III	(+)	MA	Gelform	ESS	8	6	none
IV	(−)			ESS	65	12	none
V	(−)			Transmaxillary	120	76	none

(+): performed; (−): not performed or not confirmed; MA: maxillary artery; m: months; ESS: endonasal endoscopic sinus surgery; transmaxillary: transmaxillary approach with sublabial incision.

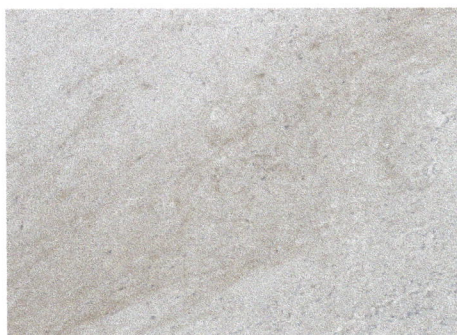

FIGURE 5: Immunohistochemical staining for periostin in organized hematoma (original magnification ×100). The expression of periostin was observed in the organized hematoma.

anesthesia is usually performed, and the surgical procedure should be chosen depending on the size of the lesion. ESS should be considered as the first line in limited lesion with adequate working space for the endoscopic operative field. In case of large lesion with thinning the bone structure of the paranasal sinuses, the transmaxillary approach should be chosen. There was little difference in the intraoperative bleeding volume between patients who received endoscopic sinus surgery (ESS) and those who underwent the transmaxillary approach. To decrease the intraoperative bleeding volume, embolization of the feeder artery is necessary if the feeder artery is identified by angiography. In our series, angiography was performed in only three patients and embolization in two. In the two patients that received embolization, the volume of intraoperative bleeding was less than that in the patients who did not receive embolization.

In summary, we have reported the distinct clinicopathological entity of organized hematoma. Organized hematoma of the maxillary sinus was characterized pathologically by a mixture of bleeding, dilated vessels, hemorrhage, fibrin exudation, fibrosis, hyalinization, and neovascularization. CT and MRI gave heterogeneous findings reflecting a mixture of these pathological conditions.

Consent

Written informed consent in Japanese was obtained from the patient for publication of this case report and accompanying images. A copy of the written consent is available for review by the Editor-in-Chief of this journal.

Conflict of Interests

The authors declare that they have no conflict of interests.

TABLE 4: Pathological findings.

Case	Bleeding	Necrosis	Fibrosis	Hyalinization	neovascularization	Vascular dilatation	CD31	CD34
I	(+)	(+)	(+)	(++)	(++)	(+)	(+++)	(++)
II	(+)	(+)	(++)	(++)	(+)	(+)	(++)	(+)
III	(+)	(−)	(+)	(+)	(+)	(−)	(+)	(+)
IV	(+)	(−)	(+)	(+)	(+)	(−)	(+)	(+)
V	(+)	(++)	(+)	(+)	(++)	(+)	(++)	(++)

Authors' Contribution

N. Ohta used all the data available and wrote the majority of this report. S. Kakehata supplied the principles of surgical information in this paper. T. Kubota, T. Watanabe, T. Ito, Y. Suzuki, A. Ishida, and M. Aoyagi saw the patient in hospital and contributed the case history notes used in this paper. A. Matsubara and K. Izuhara reported and provided us with the histopathological findings and slides. All authors read and approved the final paper.

Acknowledgments

This work was supported by a Grant-in-Aid for Scientific Research (C) from the Ministry of Education, Science, Sports, and Culture of Japan and Ministry of Health, Labour, and Welfare.

References

[1] H. M. Song, Y. J. Jang, Y. S. Chung, and B. J. Lee, "Organizing hematoma of the maxillary sinus," *Otolaryngology—Head and Neck Surgery*, vol. 136, no. 4, pp. 616–620, 2007.

[2] M. Yagisawa, J. Ishitoya, and M. Tsukuda, "Hematoma-like mass of the maxillary sinus," *Acta Oto-Laryngologica*, vol. 126, no. 3, pp. 277–281, 2006.

[3] M. Lim, S. Lew-Gor, T. Beale, A. Ramsay, and V. J. Lund, "Maxillary sinus hematoma," *Journal of Laryngology & Otology*, vol. 122, pp. 210–212, 2007.

[4] R. R. Ricalde, A. C. E. Lim, R. A. B. Lopa, and J. M. Carnate, "A benign maxillary tumour with malignant features," *Rhinology*, vol. 48, no. 2, pp. 146–149, 2010.

[5] B.-J. Lee, H.-J. Park, and S.-C. Heo, "Organized hematoma of the maxillary sinus," *Acta Oto-Laryngologica*, vol. 123, no. 7, pp. 869–872, 2003.

[6] A. Tabaee and A. Kacker, "Hematoma of the maxillary sinus presenting as a mass: a case report and review of literature," *International Journal of Pediatric Otorhinolaryngology*, vol. 65, no. 2, pp. 153–157, 2002.

[7] H. H. Unlu, C. Mutlu, S. Ayhan, and S. Tarhan, "Organized hematoma of the maxillary sinus mimicking tumor," *Auris Nasus Larynx*, vol. 28, no. 3, pp. 253–255, 2001.

[8] G. Omura, K. Watanabe, Y. Fujishiro, Y. Ebihara, K. Nakao, and T. Asakage, "Organized hematoma in the paranasal sinus and nasal cavity-Imaging diagnosis and pathological findings," *Auris Nasus Larynx*, vol. 37, no. 2, pp. 173–177, 2010.

[9] K. Oe, M. Miwa, Y. Sakai, S. Y. Lee, R. Kuroda, and M. Kurosaka, "An in vitro study demonstrating that haematomas found at the site of human fractures contain progenitor cells with multilineage capacity," *Journal of Bone and Joint Surgery B*, vol. 89, no. 1, pp. 133–138, 2007.

[10] I. E. Pleşea, A. Cameniţa, C. C. Georgescu et al., "Study of cerebral vascular structures in hypertensive intracerebral haemorrhage," *Romanian Journal of Morphology and Embryology*, vol. 46, no. 3, pp. 249–256, 2005.

[11] S. A. Dreger, P. M. Taylor, S. P. Allen, and M. H. Yacoub, "Profile and localization of matrix metalloproteinases (MMPs) and their tissue inhibitors (TIMPs) in human heart valves," *Journal of Heart Valve Disease*, vol. 11, no. 6, pp. 875–880, 2002.

[12] G. Takayama, K. Arima, T. Kanaji et al., "Periostin: a novel component of subepithelial fibrosis of bronchial asthma downstream of IL-4 and IL-13 signals," *Journal of Allergy and Clinical Immunology*, vol. 118, no. 1, pp. 98–104, 2006.

15

The Potential Role of the cABR in Assessment and Management of Hearing Impairment

Samira Anderson[1,2,3] **and Nina Kraus**[1,2,4,5]

[1] *Auditory Neuroscience Laboratory, Northwestern University, Evanston, IL 60208, USA*
[2] *Department of Communication Sciences, Northwestern University, Evanston, IL 60208, USA*
[3] *Department of Hearing and Speech Sciences, University of Maryland, 0100 Lefrak Hall, College Park, MD 20742, USA*
[4] *Department of Neurobiology and Physiology, Northwestern University, Evanston, IL 60208, USA*
[5] *Department of Otolaryngology, Northwestern University, Evanston, IL 60208, USA*

Correspondence should be addressed to Samira Anderson; sander22@umd.edu

Academic Editor: Kelly Tremblay

Hearing aid technology has improved dramatically in the last decade, especially in the ability to adaptively respond to dynamic aspects of background noise. Despite these advancements, however, hearing aid users continue to report difficulty hearing in background noise and having trouble adjusting to amplified sound quality. These difficulties may arise in part from current approaches to hearing aid fittings, which largely focus on increased audibility and management of environmental noise. These approaches do not take into account the fact that sound is processed all along the auditory system from the cochlea to the auditory cortex. Older adults represent the largest group of hearing aid wearers; yet older adults are known to have deficits in temporal resolution in the central auditory system. Here we review evidence that supports the use of the auditory brainstem response to complex sounds (cABR) in the assessment of hearing-in-noise difficulties and auditory training efficacy in older adults.

1. Introduction

In recent years, scientists and clinicians have become increasingly aware of the role of cognition in successful management of hearing loss, particularly in older adults. While it is often said that "we hear with our brain, not just with our ears," the focus of the typical hearing aid fitting continues to be one of providing audibility. Despite evidence of age-related deficits in temporal processing [1–6], abilities beyond the cochlea are seldom measured. Moreover, when auditory processing is assessed, behavioral measures may be affected by reduced cognitive abilities in the domains of attention and memory [7, 8]; for example, an individual with poor memory will struggle to repeat back long sentences in noise. The assessment and management of hearing loss in older adults would be enhanced by an objective measure of speech processing. The auditory brainstem response (ABR) provides such an objective measure of auditory function; its uses have included

evaluation of hearing thresholds in infants, children, and individuals who are difficult to test, assessment of auditory neuropathy, and screening for retrocochlear function [9]. Traditionally, the ABR has used short, simple stimuli, such as pure tones and tone bursts, but the ABR has also been recorded to complex tones, speech, and music for more than three decades, with the ABR's frequency following response (FFR) reflecting the temporal discharge of auditory neurons in the upper midbrain [10, 11]. Here, we review the role of the ABR to complex sounds (cABR) in assessment and documentation of treatment outcomes, and we suggest a potential role of the cABR in hearing aid fitting.

2. The cABR Approach

The cABR provides an objective measure of subcortical speech processing [12, 13]. It arises largely from the inferior colliculus of the upper midbrain [14], functioning as part of a circuit that interacts with cognitive, top-down influences. Unlike the click-evoked response, which bears no resemblance to the click waveform, the cABR waveform is remarkably similar to its complex stimulus waveform, whether a speech syllable or a musical chord, allowing for fine-grained evaluations of timing, pitch, and timbre representation. The click is short, nearly instantaneous, or approximately 0.1 ms, but the cABR may be elicited by complex stimuli that can persist for several seconds. The cABR's response waveform can be analyzed to determine how robustly it represents different segments of the speech stimulus. For example, in response to the syllable /da/, the onset of the cABR occurs at approximately 9 ms after stimulus onset, which would be expected when taking into account neural conduction time. The cABR onset is analogous to wave V of the brainstem's response to a click stimulus, but the cABR has potentially greater diagnostic sensitivity for certain clinical populations. For example, in a comparison between children with learning impairments versus children who are typically developing, significant differences were found for the cABR but not for responses to click stimuli [15]. The FFR comprises two regions: the transition region corresponding to the consonant-vowel (CV) formant transition and the steady-state region corresponding to the relatively unchanging vowel. The CV transition is perceptually vulnerable [16], particularly in noise, and the transition may be more degraded in noise than the steady state, especially in individuals with poorer speech-in-noise (SIN) perception [17].

The cABR is recorded to alternating polarities, and the average response to these polarities is added to minimize the cochlear microphonic and stimulus artifact [18, 19]. Phase locking to the stimulus envelope, which is noninverting, enhances representation of the envelope and biases the response towards the low frequency components of the response. On the other hand, phase locking to the spectral energy in the stimulus follows the inverting phase of the stimulus; therefore, adding responses to alternating polarities cancels out much of the spectral energy [13, 20]. Subtracting responses to alternating polarities, however, enhances the representation of spectral energy while minimizing the response to the envelope. One might choose to use added or subtracted polarities, or both, depending on the hypothetical question. For example, differences between good and poor readers are most prominent in the spectral region corresponding to the first formant of speech and are therefore more evident in subtracted polarities [21]. In contrast, the neural signature of good speech-in-noise perception is in the low frequency component of the response, which is most evident with added polarities [22]. The average response waveform of 17 normal hearing older adults (ages 60 to 67) and its evoking stimulus and stimulus and response spectra (to added and subtracted polarities) are displayed in Figure 1.

The cABR is acoustically similar to the stimulus. That is, after the cABR waveform has been converted to a .wav file, untrained listeners are able to recognize monosyllabic words from brainstem responses evoked by those words [23]. The fidelity of the response to the stimulus permits evaluation of the strength of subcortical encoding of multiple

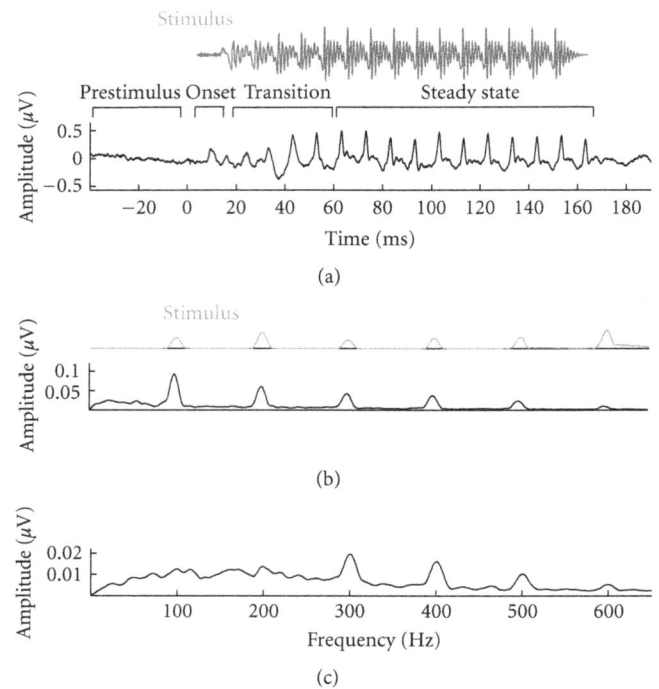

FIGURE 1: The stimulus /da/ (gray) is displayed with its response (black) in time and frequency domains. (a) Time domain. The response represents an average of 17 older adults (ages 60 to 67) all of whom have audiometrically normal hearing. The periodicity of the stimulus is reflected in the response with peaks repeating every ~10 ms (the F_0 of the vowel /a/). (b) and (c) Frequency domain. Fast Fourier transforms were calculated over the steady-state region of the response, showing frequency energy at the F_0 (100 Hz) and its integer harmonics for responses obtained by adding (b) and subtracting (c) responses to alternating polarities.

acoustic aspects of complex sounds, including timing (onsets, offsets), pitch (the fundamental frequency, F_0), and timbre (the integer harmonics of the F_0) [13]. Analyses of the cABR include measurement of latency and amplitude in the time domain and magnitude of the F_0 and individual harmonics in the frequency domain. Because of the cABR's remarkable stimulus fidelity, cross-correlation between the stimulus and the response also provides a meaningful measure [24]. In addition, responses between two conditions can be cross-correlated to determine the effects of a specific condition such as noise on a response [25].

Latency analysis has traditionally relied on picking individual peaks, a subjective task that is prone to error. Phase analysis provides an objective method for assessing temporal precision. Because the brainstem represents stimulus frequency differences occurring above 2000 Hz (the upper limits of brainstem phase locking) through timing [26] and phase representation [27, 28], the phase difference between two waveforms (in radians) can be converted to timing differences and represented in a "phaseogram." This analysis provides an objective measure of the response timing on a frequency-specific basis. For example, the brainstem's ability to encode phase differences in the formant trajectories between syllables such as /ba/ and /ga/ can be assessed and compared to a normal standard or between groups in a way that would not be feasible if the analysis was limited to peak picking (Figure 2). Although the response peaks corresponding to the F_0 are discernible, the peaks in the higher frequency formant transition region such as in Figure 2 would be difficult to identify, even for the trained eye.

In natural speech, frequency components change rapidly, and a pitch tracking analysis can be used to evaluate the ability of the brainstem to encode the changing fundamental frequency over time. From this analysis, a measure of pitch strength can be computed using short-term autocorrelation, a method which determines signal periodicity as the signal is compared to a time-shifted copy of itself. Pitch-tracking error is determined by comparing the stimulus F_0 with the response F_0 for successive periods of the response [29, 30]. These and other measures produced by the pitch-tracking analysis reveal that the FFR is malleable and experience dependent, with better pitch tracking in individuals who have heard changing vowel contours or frequency sweeps in meaningful contexts, such as in tonal languages or music [24, 31].

Other automated analyses which could potentially be incorporated into a clinical protocol include the assessment of response consistency and phase locking. Response consistency provides a way of evaluating trial-to-trial within-subject variability, perhaps representing the degree of temporal jitter or asynchronous neural firing that might be seen in an impaired or aging auditory system [6]. Auditory neuropathy spectrum disorder would be an extreme example of dyssynchronous neural firing, affecting even the response to the click [32–34]. A mild form of dyssynchrony, however, may not be evident in the results of the typical audiologic or ABR protocol but might be observed in a cABR with poor response consistency. The phase-locking factor is another measure of response consistency, providing a measure of trial-to-trial phase coherence [35, 36]. Phase locking refers to the repetitive neural response to periodic sounds. While response consistency is determined largely by the stimulus envelope, the phase-locking factor is a measure of consistency of the stimulus-evoked oscillatory activity [37].

3. The cABR and Assessment of Hearing Loss and the Ability to Hear in Noise

The cABR may potentially play an important role in assessment of hearing loss and hearing in noise. It has good test-retest reliability [39, 40], a necessity for clinical comparisons and for documentation of treatment outcomes. Just as latency differences of 0.2 ms for brainstem responses to click stimuli can be considered clinically significant when screening for vestibular schwannomas [9], similar differences on the order of fractions of milliseconds in the cABR have been found to reliably separate clinical populations [41, 42]. Banai et al. [41] found that the onset and other peaks in the cABR are delayed 0.2 to 0.3 ms in children who are good readers compared to poor readers. In older adults, the offset latency is a strong predictor of self-assessed SIN perception in older adults, with latencies ranging from 47 to 51 ms in responses to a 40 ms /da/ (formant transition only) [43]. Temporal processing deficits

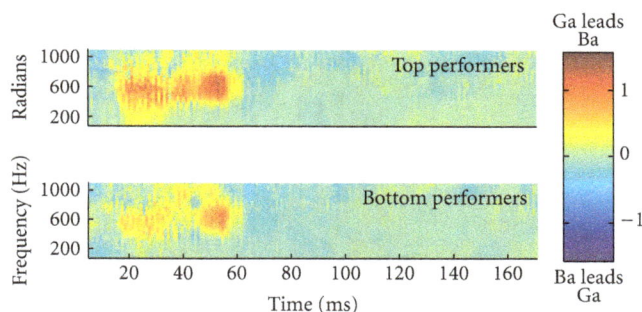

FIGURE 2: A phaseogram displaying differences in phase (radians, colorbar) in responses to /ba/ and /ga/ syllables, which have been synthesized so that they differ only in the second formant of the consonant-to-vowel transition. The top and bottom groups are children (ages 8 to 12) who differ on a speech-in-noise perception measure, the Hearing in Noise Test (HINT). The red color indicates greater phase difference, with /ga/ preceding /ba/, as expected given cochlear tonotopicity. Note that phase differences are only present in the transition, not in the steady state, during which the syllables are identical. Modified from [27].

are also seen in children with specific language impairment, who have decreased ability to track frequency changes in tonal sweeps, especially at faster rates [44].

Because of the influence of central and cognitive factors on speech-in-noise perception, the pure-tone audiogram, a largely peripheral measure, does not adequately predict the ability to hear in background noise, especially in older adults [45–47]. Due to the convergence of afferent and efferent transmission in the inferior colliculus (IC) [48, 49], we propose that the cABR is an effective method for assessing the effects of sensory processing and higher auditory function on the IC. While the cABR does not directly assess cognitive function, it is influenced by higher-level processing (e.g., selective attention, auditory training). The cABR is elicited passively without the patient's input or cooperation beyond maintaining a relaxed state, yet it provides in essence a snapshot in time of auditory processing that reflects both cognitive (auditory memory and attention) and sensory influences.

In a study of hearing-, age-, and sex-matched older adults (ages 60–73) with clinically normal hearing, the older adults with good speech-in-noise perception had more robust subcortical stimulus representation, with higher root-mean-square (RMS) and F_0 amplitudes compared to older adults with poor speech-in-noise perception (Figure 3) [38]. Perception of the F_0 is important for object identification and stream segregation, allowing us to attend to a single voice from a background of voices [50]; therefore, greater representation of the F_0 in subcortical responses may enhance one's ability to hear in noise. When we added noise (six-talker babble) to the presentation of the syllable, we found that the responses of individuals in the top speech-in-noise group were less degraded than in the bottom speech-in-noise group (Figure 3). These results are consistent with research from more than two decades documenting suprathreshold deficits

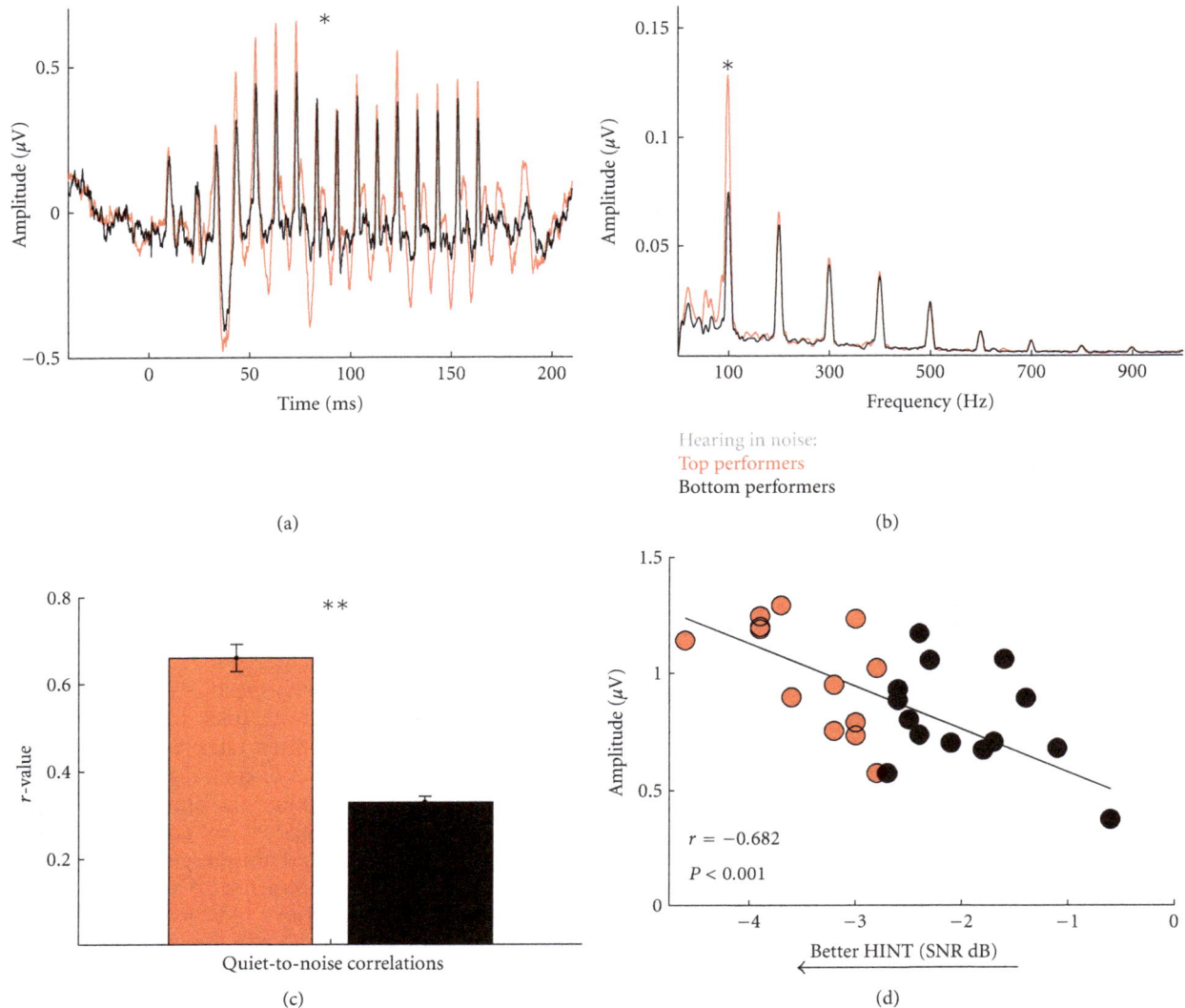

(a)

(b)

(c)

(d)

FIGURE 3: Responses to the syllable /da/ are more robust in older adults with good speech-in-noise perception compared to those with poor speech-in-noise perception, demonstrated by greater RMS amplitude (a) and amplitude of the F_0 in the good speech-in-noise group (b). The responses in the poor speech-in-noise group were more susceptible to the degrading effects of noise, as shown by greater differences in responses to the /da/ in quiet and noise (cross-correlations) (c). Relationship between speech-in-noise perception and the quiet-noise correlation (d). $^*P < 0.05$, $^{**}P < 0.01$. Modified from [38].

that cannot be identified by threshold testing [46, 47, 51–58]. Even in normal-hearing young adults, better speech-in-noise perception is related to more robust encoding of the F_0 in the cABR [53]. Furthermore, in a study with young adult participants, Ruggles et al. [51] found that spatial selective auditory attention performance correlates with the phase locking of the FFR to the speech syllable /da/. Furthermore, they found that selective attention correlates with the ability to detect frequency modulation but is not related to age, reading span, or hearing threshold.

The cABR provides evidence of age-related declines in temporal and spectral precision, providing a neural basis for speech-in-noise perception difficulties. In older adults, delayed neural timing is found in the region corresponding to the CV formant transition [59, 60], but timing in the

steady-state region remains unchanged. Importantly, age-related differences are seen in middle-aged adults as young as 45, indicating that declines in temporal resolution are not limited to the elderly population. Robustness of frequency representation also decreases with age, with the amplitude of the fundamental frequency declining in middle- and in older-aged adults. These results provide neural evidence for the finding of adults having trouble hearing in noise as soon as the middle-aged years [61].

What is the role of the cABR in clinical practice? The cABR can be collected in as little as 20 minutes, including electrode application. Nevertheless, even an additional twenty minutes would be hard to add to a busy practice. To be efficacious, the additional required time must yield information not currently provided by the existing protocol.

One of the purposes of an audiological evaluation is to determine the factors that contribute to the patient's self-perception of hearing ability. To evaluate the effectiveness of possible factors, we used multiple linear regression modeling to predict scores on the speech subtest of the Speech, Spatial, and Qualities Hearing Scale [62]. Pure-tone thresholds, speech-in-noise perception, age, and timing measures of the cABR served as meaningful predictors. Behavioral assessments predicted 15% of the variance in the SSQ score, but adding brainstem variables (specifically the onset slope, offset latency, and overall morphology) predicted an additional 16% of the variance in the SSQ (Figure 4). Therefore, the cABR can provide the clinician with unique information about biological processing of speech [43].

4. The cABR is Experience Dependent

As the site of intersecting afferent and efferent pathways, the inferior colliculus plays a key role in auditory learning. Indeed, animals models have demonstrated that the cortico-collicular pathway is essential for auditory learning [63, 64]. Therefore, it is reasonable to expect that the cABR reflects evidence of auditory training; in fact, the cABR shows influences of both life-long and short-term training. For example, native speakers of tonal languages have better brainstem pitch tracking to changing vowel contours than speakers of non-tonal languages [24]. Bilingualism provides another example of the auditory advantages conferred by language expertise. Bilingualism is associated with enhanced cognitive skills, such as language processing and executive function, and it also promotes experience-dependent plasticity in subcortical processing [65]. Bilingual adolescents, who reported high English and Spanish proficiency, had more robust subcortical encoding of the F_0 to a target sound presented in a noisy background than their age-, sex-, and IQ-matched monolingual peers. Within the bilingual group, a measure of sustained attention was related to the strength of the F_0; this relation between attention and the F_0 was not seen in the monolingual group. Krizman et al. [65] proposed that diverse language experience heightens directed attention toward linguistic inputs; in turn, this attention becomes increasingly focused on features important for speaker identification and stream segregation in noise, such as the F_0.

Musicianship, another form of auditory expertise, also extends to benefits of speech processing; musicians who are nontonal language speakers have enhanced pitch tracking to linguistically relevant vowel contours, similar to that of tonal language speakers [31]. Ample evidence now exits for the effects of musical training on the cABR [28, 60, 67–73]. The OPERA (Overlap, Precision, Emotion, Repetition, and Attention) hypothesis has been proposed as the mechanism by which music engenders auditory system plasticity [74]. For example, there is overlap in the auditory pathways for speech and music, explaining in part the musician's superior abilities for neural speech-in-noise processing. The focused attention required for musical practice and performance results in strengthened sound-to-meaning connections, enhancing top-down cognitive (e.g., auditory attention and memory) influences on subcortical processing [75].

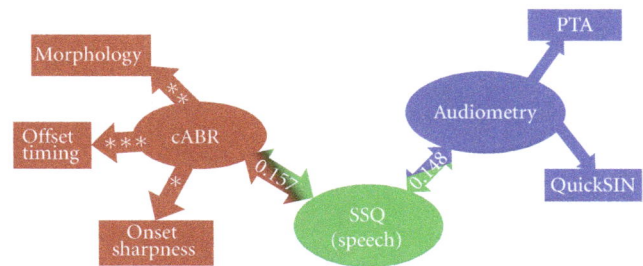

FIGURE 4: Self-perception of speech, assessed by the Speech Spatial Qualities Hearing scale (SSQ), is predicted by audiologic and cABR measures. The audiometric variables predict 15% of the variance in SSQ; the cABR variables predict an additional 16%. In the multiple linear regression model, only the contributions of the cABR onset time and morphology variables are significant. *$P < 0.05$, ***$P < 0.01$.

Musicians' responses to the cABR are more resistant to the degradative effects of noise compared to nonmusicians [68, 73]. Background noise delays and reduces the amplitude of the cABR [76]; however, musicianship mitigates the effects of six-talker babble noise on cABR responses in young adults, with earlier peak timing of the onset and the transition in musicians compared to nonmusicians. Bidelman and Krishnan [73] evaluated the effects of reverberation on the FFR and found that reverberation had no effect on the neural encoding of pitch but significantly degraded the representation of the harmonics. In addition, they found that young musicians had more robust responses in quiet and in most reverberation conditions. Benefits of musicianship have also been seen in older adults; when comparing effects of aging in musicians and nonmusicians, the musicians did not have the expected age-related neural timing delays in the CV transition indicating that musical experience offsets the effects of aging [60]. These neural benefits in older musicians are accompanied by better SIN perception, temporal resolution, and auditory memory [77].

But, what about the rest of us who are not able to devote ourselves full time to music practice—can musical training improve our auditory processing as well? Years of musical training in childhood are associated with more robust responses in adults [67], in that young adults with zero years of musical training had responses closer to the noise floor compared to groups of adults with one to five or six to eleven years of training who had progressively larger signal-to-noise ratios. In a structural equation model of the factors predicting speech-in-noise perception in older adults, two subsets were compared—a group who had no history of musical training and another group who had at least one year of musical training (range 1 year to 45 years). Cognitive factors (memory and attention) played a bigger role in speech-in-noise perception in the group with musical training, but life experience factors (physical activity and socioeconomic status) played a bigger role in the group with no experience. Subcortical processing (pitch encoding, harmonic encoding, and cross-correlations between responses in quiet and noise)

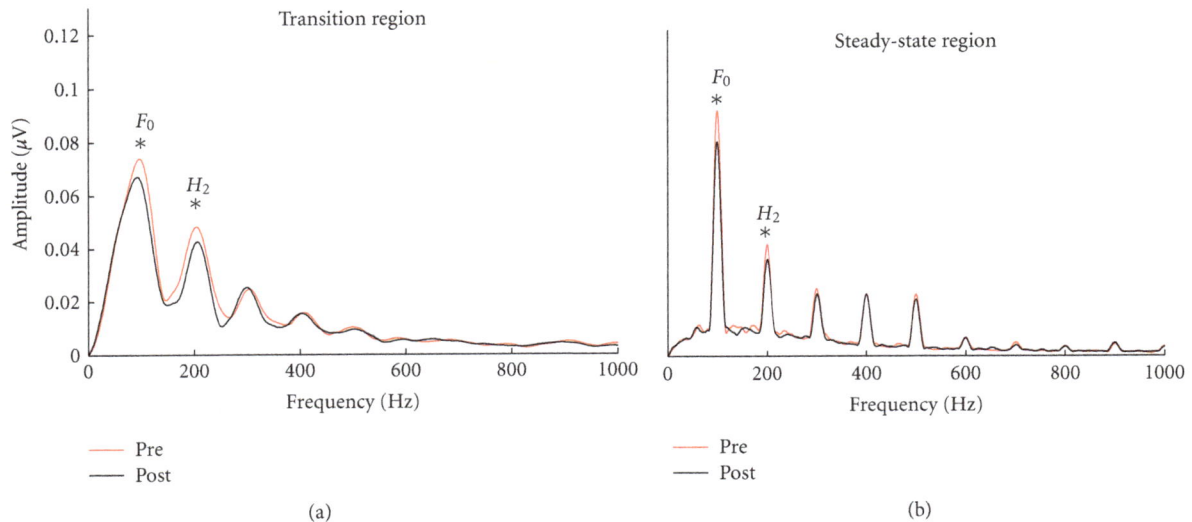

FIGURE 5: Young adults with normal hearing have greater representation of the F_0 in subcortical responses to /da/ presented in noise after undergoing LACE auditory training. The F_0 and the second harmonic have greater amplitudes in the postcondition when calculated over the transition (20–60 ms) (b) and the steady state (60–170 ms) (a). Modified from [66].

accounted for a substantial amount of the variance in both groups [78].

Short-term training can also engender subcortical plasticity. Carcagno and Plack [79] found changes in the FFR after ten sessions of pitch discrimination training that took place over the course of approximately four weeks. Four groups participated in the experiment: three experimental groups (static tone, rising tone, and falling tone) and one control group. Perceptual learning occurred for the three experimental groups, with effects somewhat specific to the stimulus used in training. These behavioral improvements were accompanied by changes in the FFR, with stronger phase locking to the F_0 of the stimulus, and changes in phase locking were related to changes in behavioral thresholds.

Just as long-term exposure to tonal language leads to better pitch tracking to changing vowel contours, just eight days of vocabulary training on words with linguistically relevant contours resulted in stronger encoding of the F_0 and decreases in the number of pitch-tracking errors [29]. The participants in this study were young adults with no prior exposure to a tonal language. Although the English language uses rising and falling pitch to signal intonation, the use of dipping tone would be unfamiliar to a native English speaker, and, interestingly, the cABR to the dipping tone showed the greatest reduction in pitch-tracking errors.

Training that targets speech-in-noise perception has also shown benefits at the level of the brainstem [80]. Young adults were trained to discriminate between CV syllables embedded in a continuous broad-band noise at a +10 dB signal-to-noise ratio. Activation of the medial olivocochlear bundle (MOCB) was monitored during the five days of training through the use of contralateral suppression of evoked otoacoustic emissions. Training improved performance on the CV discrimination task, with the greatest improvement occurring over the first three training days. A significant increase in

MOCB activation was found, but only in the participants who showed robust improvement (learners). The learners showed much weaker suppression than the nonlearners on the first day; in fact, the level of MOCB activation was predictive of learning. This last finding would be particularly important for clinical purposes—a measure predicting benefit would be useful for determining treatment candidacy.

There is renewed clinical interest in auditory training for the management of adults with hearing loss. Historically, attempts at auditory training had somewhat limited success, partly due to constraints on the clinician's ability to produce perceptually salient training stimuli. With the advent of computer technology and consumer-friendly software, auditory training has been revisited. Computer technology permits adaptive expansion and contraction of difficult-to-perceive contrasts and/or unfavorable signal-to-noise ratios. The Listening and Communication Enhancement program (LACE, Neurotone, Inc., Redwood City, CA) is an example of an adaptive auditory training program that employs top-down and bottom-up strategies to improve hearing in noise. Older adults with hearing loss who underwent LACE training scored better on the Quick Speech in Noise test (QuickSIN) [81] and the hearing-in-noise test (HINT) [82]; they also reported better hearing on self-assessment measures—the Hearing Handicap Inventory for the Elderly/Adults [83] and the Client Oriented Scale of Improvement [84, 85]. The control group did not show improvement on these measures.

The benefits on the HINT and QuickSIN were replicated in young adults by Song et al. [66]. After completing 20 hours of LACE training over a period of four weeks, the participants improved not only on speech-in-noise performance but also had more robust speech-in-noise representation in the cABR (Figure 5). They had training-related increases in the subcortical representation of the F_0 in response to speech sounds presented in noise but not in quiet. Importantly, the

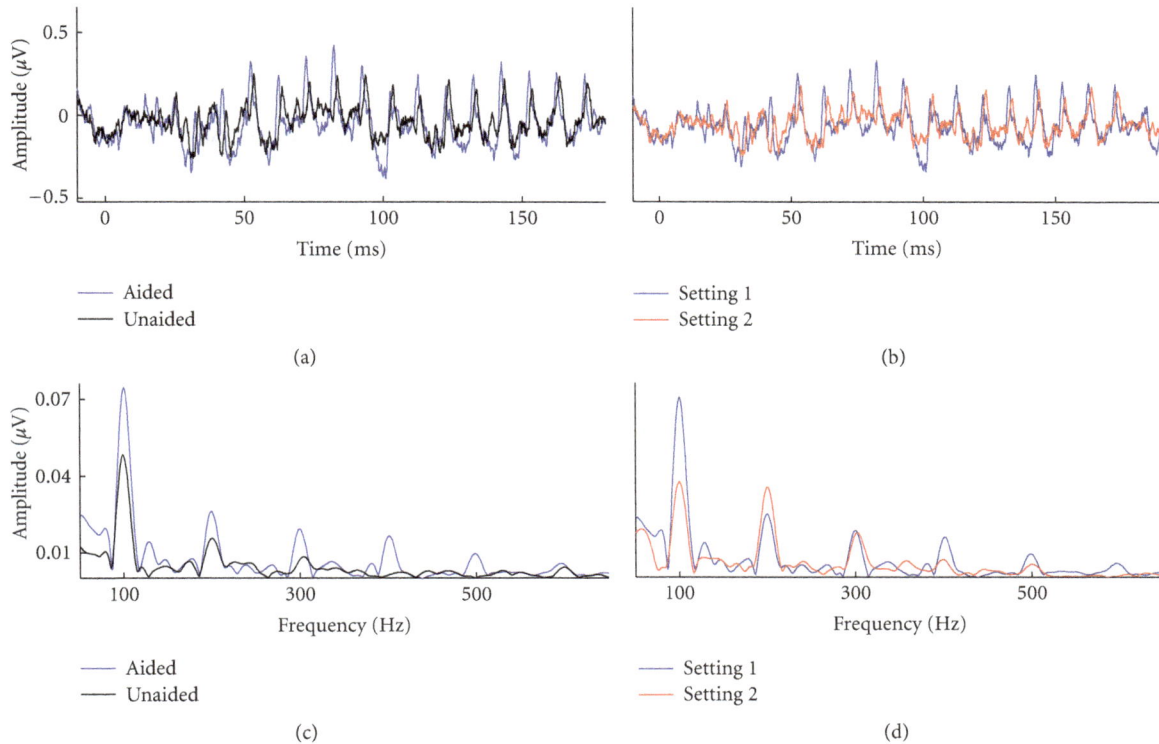

FIGURE 6: Responses were obtained to the stimulus /da/ presented at 80 dB SPL in sound field in aided (blue) versus unaided (black) conditions ((a) and (c)) and different settings in the same hearing aid ((b) and (d)). Responses show greater RMS and F_0 amplitudes in aided versus unaided conditions and for setting 1 versus setting 2.

amplitude of the F_0 at pretest predicted training-induced change in speech-in-noise perception. The advantages of computer-based auditory training for improved speech-in-noise perception and neural processing have also been observed in older adults [86]. Based on this evidence, the cABR may be efficacious for documenting treatment outcomes, an important component of evidence-based service.

5. The cABR and Hearing Aid Fitting

Any clinician who has experience with fitting hearing aids has encountered the patient who continues to report hearing difficulties, no matter which particular hearing aid or algorithm is tried. Although we have not yet obtained empirical evidence on the role of the cABR in the hearing aid fitting, we suggest that implementation of the cABR may enhance hearing aid fittings, especially in these difficult-to-fit cases. The clinician might be guided in the selection of hearing aid algorithms through knowledge of how well the brainstem encodes temporal and spectral information. For example, an individual who has impaired subcortical timing may benefit from slowly changing compression parameters in response to environmental changes.

We envision incorporating the cABR into verification of hearing aid performance. Cortical-evoked potentials have been used for verifying auditory system development after hearing aid or cochlear implant fitting in children [87–89].

In adults, however, no difference is noted in the cortical response between unaided and aided conditions, indicating that the cortical response may reflect signal-to-noise ratio rather than increased gain from amplification [90]. Therefore, cortical potentials may have limited utility for making direct comparisons between unaided and aided conditions in adults. We recently recorded the cABR in sound field and compared aided and unaided conditions and different algorithms in the aided condition. There is a marked difference in the amplitude of the waveform in response to an aided compared to an unaided condition. By performing stimulus-to-response correlations, it is possible to demonstrate that certain hearing aid algorithms resulted in a better representation of the stimulus than others (Figure 6). These preliminary data demonstrate the feasibility and possibility of using this approach. Importantly, these data also demonstrate meaningful differences easily observed in an individual.

6. Conclusions

With improvements in digital hearing aid technology, we are able to have greater expectations for hearing aid performance than ever before, even in noisy situations [91]. These improvements, however, do not address the problems we continue to encounter in challenging hearing aid fittings that leave us at a loss for solutions. The cABR provides an opportunity to evaluate and manage an often neglected part of hearing—the central auditory system—as well as the biological processing of key elements of sound. We envision future uses of the cABR to include assessment of central auditory function, prediction of treatment or hearing aid benefit, monitoring treatment or hearing aid outcomes, and assisting in hearing aid fitting. Because the cABR reflects both sensory and cognitive processes, we can begin to move beyond treating the ear to treating the person with a hearing loss.

Acknowledgments

The authors thank Sarah Drehobl and Travis White-Schwoch for their helpful comments on the paper. This work is supported by the NIH (R01 DC010016) and the Knowles Hearing Center.

References

[1] S. Gordon-Salant, P. J. Fitzgibbons, and S. A. Friedman, "Recognition of time-compressed and natural speech with selective temporal enhancements by young and elderly listeners," *Journal of Speech, Language, and Hearing Research*, vol. 50, no. 5, pp. 1181–1193, 2007.

[2] D. M. CasparyJ, J. C. Milbrand, and R. H. Helfert, "Central auditory aging: GABA changes in the inferior colliculus," *Experimental Gerontology*, vol. 30, no. 3-4, pp. 349–360, 1995.

[3] K. L. Tremblay, M. Piskosz, and P. Souza, "Effects of age and age-related hearing loss on the neural representation of speech cues," *Clinical Neurophysiology*, vol. 114, no. 7, pp. 1332–1343, 2003.

[4] K. C. Harris, M. A. Eckert, J. B. Ahlstrom, and J. R. Dubno, "Age-related differences in gap detection: effects of task difficulty and cognitive ability," *Hearing Research*, vol. 264, no. 1-2, pp. 21–29, 2010.

[5] J. P. Walton, "Timing is everything: temporal processing deficits in the aged auditory brainstem," *Hearing Research*, vol. 264, no. 1-2, pp. 63–69, 2010.

[6] M. K. Pichora-Fuller, B. A. Schneider, E. MacDonald, H. E. Pass, and S. Brown, "Temporal jitter disrupts speech intelligibility: a simulation of auditory aging," *Hearing Research*, vol. 223, no. 1-2, pp. 114–121, 2007.

[7] B. G. Shinn-Cunningham and V. Best, "Selective attention in normal and impaired hearing," *Trends in Amplification*, vol. 12, no. 4, pp. 283–299, 2008.

[8] M. K. Pichora-Fuller, "Cognitive aging and auditory information processing," *International Journal of Audiology*, vol. 42, no. S2, pp. 26–32, 2003.

[9] J. Hall, *New Handbook of Auditory Evoked Responses*, Allyn & Bacon, Boston, Mass, USA, 2007.

[10] S. Greenberg, *Neural Temporal Coding of Pitch and Vowel Quality: Human Frequency-Following Response Studies of Complex Signals*, Phonetics Laboratory, Department of Linguistics, UCLA, Los Angeles, Calif, USA, 1980.

[11] S. Greenberg, J. T. Marsh, W. S. Brown, and J. C. Smith, "Neural temporal coding of low pitch. I. Human frequency-following responses to complex tones," *Hearing Research*, vol. 25, no. 2-3, pp. 91–114, 1987.

[12] N. Kraus, "Listening in on the listening brain," *Physics Today*, vol. 64, no. 6, pp. 40–45, 2011.

[13] E. Skoe and N. Kraus, "Auditory brain stem response to complex sounds: a tutorial," *Ear and Hearing*, vol. 31, no. 3, pp. 302–324, 2010.

[14] B. Chandrasekaran and N. Kraus, "The scalp-recorded brainstem response to speech: neural origins and plasticity," *Psychophysiology*, vol. 47, no. 2, pp. 236–246, 2010.

[15] J. H. Song, K. Banai, N. M. Russo, and N. Kraus, "On the relationship between speech- and nonspeech-evoked auditory brainstem responses," *Audiology and Neurotology*, vol. 11, no. 4, pp. 233–241, 2006.

[16] G. A. Miller and P. E. Nicely, "An analysis of perceptual confusions among some English consonants," *Journal of the Acoustical Society of America*, vol. 27, no. 2, pp. 338–352, 1955.

[17] S. Anderson, E. Skoe, B. Chandrasekaran, and N. Kraus, "Neural timing is linked to speech perception in noise," *Journal of Neuroscience*, vol. 30, no. 14, pp. 4922–4926, 2010.

[18] M. Gorga, P. Abbas, and D. Worthington, "Stimulus calibration in ABR measurements," in *The Auditory Brainstem Response*, J. Jacobsen, Ed., pp. 49–62, College Hill Press, San Diego, Calif, USA, 1985.

[19] T. Campbell, J. R. Kerlin, C. W. Bishop, and L. M. Miller, "Methods to eliminate stimulus transduction artifact from insert earphones during electroencephalography," *Ear and Hearing*, vol. 33, no. 1, pp. 144–150, 2012.

[20] S. J. Aiken and T. W. Picton, "Envelope and spectral frequency-following responses to vowel sounds," *Hearing Research*, vol. 245, no. 1-2, pp. 35–47, 2008.

[21] J. Hornickel, S. Anderson, E. Skoe, H. G. Yi, and N. Kraus, "Subcortical representation of speech fine structure relates to reading ability," *NeuroReport*, vol. 23, no. 1, pp. 6–9, 2012.

[22] S. Anderson, E. Skoe, B. Chandrasekaran, S. Zecker, and N. Kraus, "Brainstem correlates of speech-in-noise perception in children," *Hearing Research*, vol. 270, no. 1-2, pp. 151–157, 2010.

[23] G. C. Galbraith, P. W. Arbagey, R. Branski, N. Comerci, and P. M. Rector, "Intelligible speech encoded in the human brain stem frequency-following response," *NeuroReport*, vol. 6, no. 17, pp. 2363–2367, 1995.

[24] A. Krishnan, Y. Xu, J. Gandour, and P. Cariani, "Encoding of pitch in the human brainstem is sensitive to language experience," *Cognitive Brain Research*, vol. 25, no. 1, pp. 161–168, 2005.

[25] N. Russo, T. Nicol, G. Musacchia, and N. Kraus, "Brainstem responses to speech syllables," *Clinical Neurophysiology*, vol. 115, no. 9, pp. 2021–2030, 2004.

[26] J. Hornickel, E. Skoe, T. Nicol, S. Zecker, and N. Kraus, "Subcortical differentiation of stop consonants relates to reading and speech-in-noise perception," *Proceedings of the National Academy of Sciences of the United States of America*, vol. 106, no. 31, pp. 13022–13027, 2009.

[27] E. Skoe, T. Nicol, and N. Kraus, "Cross-phaseogram: objective neural index of speech sound differentiation," *Journal of Neuroscience Methods*, vol. 196, no. 2, pp. 308–317, 2011.

[28] A. Parbery-Clark, A. Tierney, D. L. Strait, and N. Kraus, "Musicians have fine-tuned neural discrimination of speech syllables," *Neuroscience*, vol. 219, no. 2, pp. 111–119, 2012.

[29] J. H. Song, E. Skoe, P. C. M. Wong, and N. Kraus, "Plasticity in the adult human auditory brainstem following short-term linguistic training," *Journal of Cognitive Neuroscience*, vol. 20, no. 10, pp. 1892–1902, 2008.

[30] N. M. Russo, E. Skoe, B. Trommer et al., "Deficient brainstem encoding of pitch in children with Autism Spectrum Disorders," *Clinical Neurophysiology*, vol. 119, no. 8, pp. 1720–1731, 2008.

[31] P. C. M. Wong, E. Skoe, N. M. Russo, T. Dees, and N. Kraus, "Musical experience shapes human brainstem encoding of

linguistic pitch patterns," *Nature Neuroscience*, vol. 10, no. 4, pp. 420–422, 2007.

[32] G. Rance, "Auditory neuropathy/dys-synchrony and its perceptual consequences," *Trends in Amplification*, vol. 9, no. 1, pp. 1–43, 2005.

[33] A. Starr, T. W. Picton, Y. Sininger, L. J. Hood, and C. I. Berlin, "Auditory neuropathy," *Brain*, vol. 119, no. 3, pp. 741–753, 1996.

[34] N. Kraus, A. R. Bradlow, M. A. Cheatham et al., "Consequences of neural asynchrony: a case of of auditory neuropathy," *Journal of the Association for Research in Otolaryngology*, vol. 1, no. 1, pp. 33–45, 2000.

[35] J. Fell, "Cognitive neurophysiology: beyond averaging," *NeuroImage*, vol. 37, no. 4, pp. 1069–1072, 2007.

[36] S. Anderson, A. Parbery-Clark, T. White-Schwoch, and N. Kraus, "Aging affects neural precision of speech encoding," *The Journal of Neuroscience*, vol. 32, no. 41, pp. 14156–14164, 2012.

[37] C. Tallon-Baudry, O. Bertrand, C. Delpuech, and J. Pernier, "Stimulus specificity of phase-locked and non-phase-locked 40 Hz visual responses in human," *The Journal of Neuroscience*, vol. 16, no. 13, pp. 4240–4249, 1996.

[38] S. Anderson, A. Parbery-Clark, H. G. Yi, and N. Kraus, "A neural basis of speech-in-noise perception in older adults," *Ear and Hearing*, vol. 32, no. 6, pp. 750–757, 2011.

[39] J. H. Song, T. Nicol, and N. Kraus, "Test-retest reliability of the speech-evoked auditory brainstem response," *Clinical Neurophysiology*, vol. 122, no. 2, pp. 346–355, 2011.

[40] J. Hornickel, E. Knowles, and N. Kraus, "Test-retest consistency of speech-evoked auditory brainstem responses in typically-developing children," *Hearing Research*, vol. 284, no. 1-2, pp. 52–58, 2012.

[41] K. Banai, J. Hornickel, E. Skoe, T. Nicol, S. Zecker, and N. Kraus, "Reading and subcortical auditory function," *Cerebral Cortex*, vol. 19, no. 11, pp. 2699–2707, 2009.

[42] B. Wible, T. Nicol, and N. Kraus, "Atypical brainstem representation of onset and formant structure of speech sounds in children with language-based learning problems," *Biological Psychology*, vol. 67, no. 3, pp. 299–317, 2004.

[43] S. Anderson, A. Parbery-Clark, and N. Kraus, "Auditory brainstem response to complex sounds predicts self-reported speech-in-noise performance," *Journal of Speech, Language, and Hearing Research*. In press.

[44] M. Basu, A. Krishnan, and C. Weber-Fox, "Brainstem correlates of temporal auditory processing in children with specific language impairment," *Developmental Science*, vol. 13, no. 1, pp. 77–91, 2010.

[45] M. Killion and P. Niquette, "What can the pure-tone audiogram tell us about a patient's SNR loss?" *Hearing Journal*, vol. 53, no. 3, pp. 46–53, 2000.

[46] P. E. Souza, K. T. Boike, K. Witherell, and K. Tremblay, "Prediction of speech recognition from audibility in older listeners with hearing loss: effects of age, amplification, and background noise," *Journal of the American Academy of Audiology*, vol. 18, no. 1, pp. 54–65, 2007.

[47] S. E. Hargus and S. Gordon-Salant, "Accuracy of speech intelligibility index predictions for noise-masked young listeners with normal hearing and for elderly listeners with hearing impairment," *Journal of Speech and Hearing Research*, vol. 38, no. 1, pp. 234–243, 1995.

[48] B. R. Schofield, "Projections to the inferior colliculus from layer VI cells of auditory cortex," *Neuroscience*, vol. 159, no. 1, pp. 246–258, 2009.

[49] W. H. A. M. Mulders, K. Seluakumaran, and D. Robertson, "Efferent pathways modulate hyperactivity in inferior colliculus," *Journal of Neuroscience*, vol. 30, no. 28, pp. 9578–9587, 2010.

[50] A. J. Oxenham, "Pitch perception and auditory stream segregation: implications for hearing loss and cochlear implants," *Trends in Amplification*, vol. 12, no. 4, pp. 316–331, 2008.

[51] D. Ruggles, H. Bharadwaj, and B. G. Shinn-Cunningham, "Normal hearing is not enough to guarantee robust encoding of suprathreshold features important in everyday communication," *Proceedings of the National Academy of Sciences of the United States of America*, vol. 108, no. 37, pp. 15516–15521, 2011.

[52] S. A. Shamma, "Hearing impairments hidden in normal listeners," *Proceedings of the National Academy of Sciences*, vol. 108, no. 39, pp. 16139–16140, 2011.

[53] J. H. Song, E. Skoe, K. Banai, and N. Kraus, "Perception of speech in noise: neural correlates," *Journal of Cognitive Neuroscience*, vol. 23, no. 9, pp. 2268–2279, 2011.

[54] K. J. Cruickshanks, T. L. Wiley, T. S. Tweed et al., "Prevalence of hearing loss in older adults in Beaver dam, Wisconsin. The epidemiology of hearing loss study," *American Journal of Epidemiology*, vol. 148, no. 9, pp. 879–886, 1998.

[55] S. Gordon-Salant and P. J. Fitzgibbons, "Temporal factors and speech recognition performance in young and elderly listeners," *Journal of Speech and Hearing Research*, vol. 36, no. 6, pp. 1276–1285, 1993.

[56] J. R. Dubno, D. D. Dirks, and D. E. Morgan, "Effects of age and mild hearing loss on speech recognition in noise," *Journal of the Acoustical Society of America*, vol. 76, no. 1, pp. 87–96, 1984.

[57] S. Kim, R. D. Frisina, F. M. Mapes, E. D. Hickman, and D. R. Frisina, "Effect of age on binaural speech intelligibility in normal hearing adults," *Speech Communication*, vol. 48, no. 6, pp. 591–597, 2006.

[58] J. H. Lee and L. E. Humes, "Effect of fundamental-frequency and sentence-onset differences on speech-identification performance of young and older adults in a competing-talker background," *The Journal of the Acoustical Society of America*, vol. 132, no. 3, pp. 1700–1717, 2012.

[59] K. R. Vander Werff and K. S. Burns, "Brain stem responses to speech in younger and older adults," *Ear and Hearing*, vol. 32, no. 2, pp. 168–180, 2011.

[60] A. Parbery-Clark, S. Anderson, E. Hittner, and N. Kraus, "Musical experience offsets age-related delays in neural timing," *Neurobiol of Aging*, vol. 33, no. 7, pp. 1483.e1–1483.e4, 2012.

[61] K. S. Helfer and M. Vargo, "Speech recognition and temporal processing in middle-aged women," *Journal of the American Academy of Audiology*, vol. 20, no. 4, pp. 264–271, 2009.

[62] S. Gatehouse and W. Noble, "The speech, spatial and qualities of hearing scale (SSQ)," *International Journal of Audiology*, vol. 43, no. 2, pp. 85–99, 2004.

[63] V. M. Bajo, F. R. Nodal, D. R. Moore, and A. J. King, "The descending corticocollicular pathway mediates learning-induced auditory plasticity," *Nature Neuroscience*, vol. 13, no. 2, pp. 253–260, 2010.

[64] N. Suga and X. Ma, "Multiparametric corticofugal modulation and plasticity in the auditory system," *Nature Reviews Neuroscience*, vol. 4, no. 10, pp. 783–794, 2003.

[65] J. Krizman, V. Marian, A. Shook, E. Skoe, and N. Kraus, "Subcortical encoding of sound is enhanced in bilinguals and relates to executive function advantages," *Proceedings of the National Academy of Sciences*, vol. 109, no. 20, pp. 7877–7881, 2012.

[66] J. H. Song, E. Skoe, K. Banai, and N. Kraus, "Training to improve hearing speech in noise: biological mechanisms," *Cerebral Cortex*, vol. 22, no. 5, pp. 1180–1190, 2012.

[67] E. Skoe and N. Kraus, "A little goes a long way: how the adult brain is shaped by musical training in childhood," *Journal of Neuroscience*, vol. 32, no. 34, pp. 11507–11510, 2012.

[68] A. Parbery-Clark, E. Skoe, and N. Kraus, "Musical experience limits the degradative effects of background noise on the neural processing of sound," *Journal of Neuroscience*, vol. 29, no. 45, pp. 14100–14107, 2009.

[69] D. L. Strait, N. Kraus, E. Skoe, and R. Ashley, "Musical experience and neural efficiency—effects of training on subcortical processing of vocal expressions of emotion," *European Journal of Neuroscience*, vol. 29, no. 3, pp. 661–668, 2009.

[70] G. Musacchia, M. Sams, E. Skoe, and N. Kraus, "Musicians have enhanced subcortical auditory and audiovisual processing of speech and music," *Proceedings of the National Academy of Sciences of the United States of America*, vol. 104, no. 40, pp. 15894–15898, 2007.

[71] K. M. Lee, E. Skoe, N. Kraus, and R. Ashley, "Selective subcortical enhancement of musical intervals in musicians," *Journal of Neuroscience*, vol. 29, no. 18, pp. 5832–5840, 2009.

[72] G. M. Bidelman, J. T. Gandour, and A. Krishnan, "Cross-domain effects of music and language experience on the representation of pitch in the human auditory brainstem," *Journal of Cognitive Neuroscience*, vol. 23, no. 2, pp. 425–434, 2011.

[73] G. M. Bidelman and A. Krishnan, "Effects of reverberation on brainstem representation of speech in musicians and non-musicians," *Brain Research*, vol. 1355, pp. 112–125, 2010.

[74] A. D. Patel, "Why would musical training benefit the neural encoding of speech? The OPERA hypothesis," *Frontiers in Psychology*, vol. 2, article 142, 2011.

[75] N. Kraus and B. Chandrasekaran, "Music training for the development of auditory skills," *Nature Reviews Neuroscience*, vol. 11, no. 8, pp. 599–605, 2010.

[76] R. F. Burkard and D. Sims, "A comparison of the effects of broadband masking noise on the auditory brainstem response in young and older adults," *American Journal of Audiology*, vol. 11, no. 1, pp. 13–22, 2002.

[77] A. Parbery-Clark, E. Skoe, C. Lam, and N. Kraus, "Musician enhancement for speech-in-noise," *Ear and Hearing*, vol. 30, no. 6, pp. 653–661, 2009.

[78] S. Anderson, A. Parbery-Clark, T. White-Schwoch, and N. Kraus, "Sensory-cognitive interactions predict speech-in-noise perception: a structural equation modeling approach," in *Proceedings of the Cognitive Neuroscience Society Annual Meeting*, Chicago, Ill, USA, 2012.

[79] S. Carcagno and C. J. Plack, "Subcortical plasticity following perceptual learning in a pitch discrimination task," *Journal of the Association for Research in Otolaryngology*, vol. 12, no. 1, pp. 89–100, 2011.

[80] J. de Boer and A. R. D. Thornton, "Neural correlates of perceptual learning in the auditory brainstem: efferent activity predicts and reflects improvement at a speech-in-noise discrimination task," *Journal of Neuroscience*, vol. 28, no. 19, pp. 4929–4937, 2008.

[81] M. C. Killion, P. A. Niquette, G. I. Gudmundsen, L. J. Revit, and S. Banerjee, "Development of a quick speech-in-noise test for measuring signal-to-noise ratio loss in normal-hearing and hearing-impaired listeners," *The Journal of the Acoustical Society of America*, vol. 116, no. 4, pp. 2395–2405, 2004.

[82] M. Nilsson, S. D. Soli, and J. A. Sullivan, "Development of the hearing in noise test for the measurement of speech reception thresholds in quiet and in noise," *Journal of the Acoustical Society of America*, vol. 95, no. 2, pp. 1085–1099, 1994.

[83] C. W. Newman, B. E. Weinstein, G. P. Jacobson, and G. A. Hug, "Amplification and aural rehabilitation. Test-retest reliability of the hearing handicap inventory for adults," *Ear and Hearing*, vol. 12, no. 5, pp. 355–357, 1991.

[84] H. Dillon, A. James, and J. Ginis, "Client Oriented Scale of Improvement (COSI) and its relationship to several other measures of benefit and satisfaction provided by hearing aids," *Journal of the American Academy of Audiology*, vol. 8, no. 1, pp. 27–43, 1997.

[85] R. W. Sweetow and J. H. Sabes, "The need for and development of an adaptive listening and communication enhancement (LACE) program," *Journal of the American Academy of Audiology*, vol. 17, no. 8, pp. 538–558, 2006.

[86] S. Anderson, T. White-Schwoch, A. Parbery-Clark, and N. Kraus, "Reversal of age-related neural timing delays with training," *Proceedings of the National Academy of Sciences*. In press.

[87] A. Sharma, G. Cardon, K. Henion, and P. Roland, "Cortical maturation and behavioral outcomes in children with auditory neuropathy spectrum disorder," *International Journal of Audiology*, vol. 50, no. 2, pp. 98–106, 2011.

[88] A. Sharma, A. A. Nash, and M. Dorman, "Cortical development, plasticity and re-organization in children with cochlear implants," *Journal of Communication Disorders*, vol. 42, no. 4, pp. 272–279, 2009.

[89] W. Pearce, M. Golding, and H. Dillon, "Cortical auditory evoked potentials in the assessment of auditory neuropathy: two case studies," *Journal of the American Academy of Audiology*, vol. 18, no. 5, pp. 380–390, 2007.

[90] C. J. Billings, K. L. Tremblay, and C. W. Miller, "Aided cortical auditory evoked potentials in response to changes in hearing aid gain," *International Journal of Audiology*, vol. 50, no. 7, pp. 459–467, 2011.

[91] S. Kochkin, "MarkeTrak VIII Mini-BTEs tap new market, users more satisfied," *Hearing Journal*, vol. 64, no. 3, pp. 17–18, 2011.

16

A Prevalence Study of Hearing Loss among Primary School Children in the South East of Iran

Aqeel Absalan,[1] Ibrahim Pirasteh,[1] Gholam Ali Dashti Khavidaki,[2] Azam Asemi rad,[3] Ali Akbar Nasr Esfahani,[4] and Mohammad Hussein Nilforoush[5]

[1] *Audiology Department, Faculty of Rehabilitation, Zahedan University of Medical Sciences & Health Services, Zahedan, Iran*
[2] *Otolaryngology (ENT) Department, Zahedan University of Medical Sciences & Health Services, Zahedan, Iran*
[3] *Department of Anatomical Sciences, Shahid Beheshti University of Medical Sciences, Tehran, Iran*
[4] *Audiology Department, Faculty of Rehabilitation, Tehran University of Medical Sciences & Health Services, Tehran, Iran*
[5] *Audiology Department, Faculty of Rehabilitation, Isfahan University of Medical Sciences, Isfahan, Iran*

Correspondence should be addressed to Mohammad Hussein Nilforoush; mhnilforoush@rehab.mui.ac.ir

Academic Editor: Bill Yates

Hearing impairment substantially affects child's ability to normally acquire the spoken language. Such negative effects create problems for the child not only in terms of communication but also in terms of achievement in school as well as social and emotional growth. The aim of this research is to study the prevalence of hearing disorders and its relationship to age and gender among primary school students of Zahedan, Iran. In this cross-sectional and descriptive analytical study, 1500 students from elementary schools were screened for hearing loss. The selection of samples was performed using multistage sampling method. Primary information was obtained through direct observation, otoscopy, and audiometric and tympanometric screenings. Data was obtained and analyzed via ANOVA test. Statistical analysis showed a significant correlation between the age and the prevalence of middle ear abnormal function. Conductive hearing loss in males and females was 8.8% and 7.1%, respectively. In addition, 1% and 0.7% of male and female students, respectively, suffered from sensorineural hearing loss. Results indicated that 20.2% of students of elementary schools in Zahedan needed medical treatment for their problems. Therefore, it is recommended that the hearing screening of school-age children should be included in annual school health programs in this region.

1. Introduction

Hearing loss of even 15 dBHL can create hearing disability in children and consequently impairment in their mental growth [1–3]. Due to the occurrence of secreted middle ear otitis during a critical period (when the senses are emerging and adapting to the environment), these impairments can create various disabilities in children. These disabilities can cause behavioral complications in six functional areas: mental maturity, perception, speech and speaking, cognition and general intelligence, academic achievement, and interpersonal behaviors [4, 5]. One of the other impairments is unilateral hearing loss (UHL) that, if not examined, is normally detected later because one of the ears is healthy. For the impact of unilateral hearing loss on children's academic achievement, it was found that 30% of children with unilateral deafness lag at least 1.2 years behind their normal peers in terms of academic achievement [6]. Unilateral hearing loss has remarkable effects on academic achievement, language development, and children's auditory perception [7]. By considering the unpredictable difficulties, the best way to identify them would be individual assessment of children at risk. Due to the lack of knowledge and low cooperation of many parents, one of the appropriate times for prognosis, so-called screening, is the school age, because, at this age, the majority of children gather in academic centers and they can all be examined. According to the mentioned subjects and reasons, the Speech and Language Association of America (ASHA) has provided the following guidelines for screening [8].

(i) The program should be run annually for children aged 3–9 years.

(ii) After nine years of age, the program should be performed annually for children at risk.

TABLE 1: Results of direct observation and otoscopic examination based on gender.

Observation	Cerumen	External substance	Obstruction and narrowness of the canal	Eardrum rupture	Hearing aid
Male	65	4	1	2	4
Female	58	—	—	3	1

2. Subjects and Methods

In this cross-sectional and descriptive analytical study, 1,500 students from 30 elementary schools of Zahedan in the academic year 2010-2011 were screened for hearing loss. The selection of samples was performed through multistage sampling method. Out of 146 elementary schools in Zahedan, 30 schools were selected as follows: the schools of the city of Zahedan were divided into six regions based on two educational districts and 3 municipalities, and some schools were randomly selected from each region based on the relative frequency of the schools of that region. From each school, 50 students in 5-year range (6 to 10 years old) were selected randomly (10 persons from each age). In total, 300 males and females per age were included in the study. Physical environment in schools such as noise levels (inside and outside classes) was within the permissible level, and according to ANSI S12.602002, and weather temperature during testing was between 28 and 33°C. Primary information was obtained through direct observation, otoscopic examination, and audiometric and tympanometric screenings of every student. The rejected subjects were referred to for the full examination of hearing system that included complete medical history, pure tone and speech audiometric tests, and tympanometric as well as acoustic reflex assessments. The inclusion criteria for the specialized evaluation included the following.

(i) Presence of any structural and anatomic problems of auricle and the external ear canal.

(ii) Detection of abnormal cases of the ear canal and eardrum at the time of otoscopic examination.

(iii) No response of either ear to at least one of the experimental frequencies.

(iv) Detection of type B or C tympanogram.

In this study, the MT10 Audiometry and Tympanometry screening device was used for primary screening. The research results were collected by special forms, and the frequency distribution of different hearing impairments was obtained. Chi-square test was also used to compare the differences between both genders, and relationship between hearing impairment and students' age was evaluated by ANOVA test.

3. Results

The results of direct observation and otoscopic examination of students are presented in Table 1. The presence of excessive cerumen in canal in this stage of screening was the most common disorder in both genders and in all grades, as

the prevalence of this disorder was 8.7% in boys and 7.7% in girls. This difference was not statistically significant. In total, 8.2% of students suffered from this disorder. In tympanometric assessment, type C tympanogram was the most common disorder in all age groups and in both genders, whereas it was prevalent in 11.7% of boys and 6% of girls. The obtained results in this study suggested the influence of gender on the incidence of type C tympanogram, whereas the incidence of these disorders was more prevalent in boys ($z = 3.9057$). Other notable result of the tympanometry screening was the significant decrease of negative pressure incidences in the ear with an increase in age (Table 2). Using Spearman's correlation coefficient, a significant correlation was observed between school grade and the percentage of type C tympanogram ($P = 0.037$, $r = -0.9$), which suggests the decrease of type C tympanogram incidences with an increase in age. A particular correlation coefficient was obtained for the relationship between the amount of conductive problems cases and school grade of students at estimated value of $r = -0.972$, degree of freedom of $df = 3$, and confidence coefficient of $t = 19.331$, respectively. In other words, conductive problems are reduced with grade increase (Table 3). Table 4 shows the results of conductive hearing loss prevalence in terms of gender. The difference was not statistically significant. Table 5 shows the results of sensorineural hearing loss in terms of gender. The observed difference between the genders was not statistically significant.

4. Discussion

The frequency of different hearing losses in this study was obtained as 8.8%. Therefore, compared with the study conducted in Bangladesh (11.9%) [9] and in Turkey (10.4% and 9.8%) [10, 11], a lower percentage of students in Zahedan had suffered hearing loss. However, the percentage of conductive hearing loss (7.9%) had a higher rate compared with that in Thailand (6.8%) [12] and India (4.79) [13] and also is very close to the study in Egypt (8.5%) [14]. Compared with a study conducted on primary school children in Australia, the rate of mild and minimal hearing loss was far more (8.2% versus 3%) [15]. The annual organized screening programs as well as greater public awareness and information can also be the reason of lower incidence of conductive hearing loss in a country like Australia [16].

The results of this study had some similarity with behavioral test results of Poland study [17]. In Iran, some researches were done, compared with a study conducted on primary schools of Tehran, in which the prevalence of different hearing losses was shown to be 14.3% [18]; in the present study, this rate was 8.8% for Zahedan. Similarly, a lower value

TABLE 2: Frequency distribution of types of tympanogram based on school grade.

Tympanogram	Grade											
	6		7		8		9		10		Total	
	Fr.	Percent	Fr.	Percent	Fr.	Percent	Fr.	Percent	Fr.	Percent	Fr.	Percent
A	243	81%	266	88.7%	267	89%	275	91.7%	275	91.7%	1326	88.4%
B	12	4%	10	3.3%	6	2%	6	2%	6	2.3%	41	2.7%
C	45	15%	24	8%	27	9%	19	6.3%	18	6%	133	8.9%
Total	300	100%	300	100%	300	100%	300	100%	300	100%	1500	100%

*Fr.: frequency.

TABLE 3: Frequency distribution of conductive hearing loss based on grade.

Conductive hearing loss	Grade											
	1st grade		2nd grade		3rd grade		4th grade		5th grade		Total	
	Fr.	Percent	Fr.	Percent	Fr.	Percent	Fr.	Percent	Fr.	Percent	Fr.	Percent
Yes	30	11%	25	9%	20	7.3%	20	7.3%	14	5%	109	88.4%
No	243	89%	252	91%	253	92.7%	254	92.7%	268	95%	1270	2.7%
Total	273	100%	277	100%	273	100%	274	100%	282	100%	1379	100%

TABLE 4: Frequency distribution of conductive hearing loss based on gender.

Conductive hearing loss	Gender					
	Male		Female		Total	
	Fr.	Percent	Fr.	Percent	Fr.	Percent
Yes	59	8.8%	50	7.1%	109	7.9%
No	611	91.2%	659	92.9%	1270	92.1%
Total	670	100%	709	100%	1379	100%

TABLE 5: Frequency distribution of sensorineural hearing loss based on gender.

Sensorineural hearing loss	Gender					
	Male		Female		Total	
	Fr.	Percent	Fr.	Percent	Fr.	Percent
Yes	7	1%	5	0.7%	12	0.9%
No	663	99%	704	99.3%	1367	99.1%
Total	670	100%	709	100%	1379	100%

was obtained for this rate compared with the value obtained for the cities of Birjand (10.4%) [19], Islamabad (9.7%) [20], and Mahabad (18%) [21]. In contrast, compared with studies conducted in the cities of Nishapur (5.5%) [22], Isfahan (4.2%) [23] and Shiraz (6.5%) [24], prevalence of hearing loss types was obtained higher in primary schools of the city of Zahedan. It is necessary to mention that the time gap between this study and other studies conducted in the country is at least ten years. Therefore, given the growing trend of preschool assessments in the whole country, it is expected that these figures have experienced decreasing trends in various cities. Overall, 20.2% of students in this study needed treatment measures for problems including excessive wax, type B and C tympanograms and external substance. Compared with studies conducted in other cities, the rate was only lower than the rate obtained in the study conducted in Tehran. Shortage of specialized personnel, notifications, and public awareness can be factors contributing to this problem; meanwhile, economic issues cannot be ignored with respect to timely action to overcome the hearing loss. The rate of students who were in need of rehabilitation measures was 0.9%, which shows less prevalence only compared with the rate obtained in the study conducted in Birjand. In this study, we were faced with limitations such as inadequate cooperation of parents for diagnostic evaluations—despite necessary follow-ups and free-of-charge examinations—in such a way that, from a total number of 354 students referred to in the first phase, 121 subjects left the study. Consequently, the statistic associated with the types of hearing losses is calculated based on the number of referrers.

5. Conclusion

Hearing loss and its consequent difficulties on speech and language might be controlled and treated via appropriate hearing screening protocol and program in every educational setting; it is noteworthy that, according to the obtained results, the authors emphasize annual hearing screening programs for school-age children in order to promote health care and to prevent social and educational problems in this region, as these programs are being carried out in other areas.

References

[1] L. S. Eisenberg, K. C. Johnson, A. S. Martinez, L. Visser-Dumont, D. H. Ganguly, and J. F. Still, "Studies in pediatric hearing loss at the House Research Institute," *Journal of the American Academy of Audiology*, vol. 23, no. 6, pp. 412–421, 2012.

[2] M. A. Islam, M. S. Islam, M. A. Sattar, and M. I. Ali, "Prevalence and pattern of hearing loss," *Medicine Today*, vol. 23, no. 1, pp. 18–21, 2012.

[3] D. L. Sekhar, T. R. Zalewski, and I. M. Paul, "Variability of state school-based hearing screening protocols in the United States," *Journal of Community Health*, vol. 38, no. 3, pp. 569–574, 2013.

[4] D. C. Byrne, C. L. Themann, D. K. Meinke, T. C. Morata, and M. R. Stephenson, "Promoting hearing loss prevention in audiology practice," *Perspectives on Public Health Issues Related to Hearing and Balance*, vol. 13, no. 1, pp. 3–19, 2012.

[5] R. Müller, G. Fleischer, and J. Schneider, "Pure-tone auditory threshold in school children," *European Archives of Oto-Rhino-Laryngology*, vol. 269, no. 1, pp. 93–100, 2012.

[6] L. Turton and P. Smith, "Prevalence & characteristics of severe and profound hearing loss in adults in a UK National Health Service clinic," *International Journal of Audiology*, vol. 52, no. 2, pp. 92–97, 2013.

[7] J. E. C. Lieu, N. Tye-Murray, and Q. Fu, "Longitudinal study of children with unilateral hearing loss," *Laryngoscope*, vol. 122, no. 9, pp. 2088–2095, 2012.

[8] American Speech-Language-Hearing Association, *Guidelines for Audiologic Screening*, 1997, http://www.asha.org/policy/.

[9] M. M. Shaheen, A. Raquib, and S. M. Ahmad, "Chronic suppurative otitis media and its association with socio-econonic factors among rural primary school children of Bangladesh," *Indian Journal of Otolaryngology and Head and Neck Surgery*, vol. 64, no. 1, pp. 36–41, 2012.

[10] O. C. Erdivanli, Z. O. Coskun, K. C. Kazikdas, and M. Demirci, "Prevalence of Otitis Media with Effusion among Primary School Children in Eastern Black Sea, in Turkey and the Effect of Smoking in the Development of Otitis Media with Effusion," *Indian Journal of Otolaryngology and Head and Neck Surgery*, vol. 64, no. 1, pp. 17–21, 2012.

[11] M. Kırıs, T. Muderris, T. Kara, S. Bercin, H. Cankaya, and E. Sevil, "Prevalence and risk factors of otitis media with effusion in school children in Eastern Anatolia," *International Journal of Pediatric Otorhinolaryngology*, vol. 76, no. 7, pp. 1030–1035, 2012.

[12] M. Mahadevan, G. Navarro-Locsin, H. K. K. Tan et al., "A review of the burden of disease due to otitis media in the Asia-Pacific," *International Journal of Pediatric Otorhinolaryngology*, vol. 76, no. 5, pp. 623–635, 2012.

[13] S. Chadha, A. Sayal, V. Malhotra, and A. Agarwal, "Prevalence of preventable ear disorders in over 15 000 schoolchildren in northern India," *Journal of Laryngology & Otology*, vol. 127, no. 1, pp. 28–32, 2013.

[14] G. Yamamah, A. Mabrouk, E. Ghorab, M. Ahmady, and H. Abdulsalam, "Middle ear and hearing disorders of schoolchildren aged 7–10 years in South Sinai, Egypt," *Eastern Mediterranean Health Journal*, vol. 18, no. 3, pp. 255–260, 2012.

[15] V. Yiengprugsawan, A. Hogan, and L. Strazdins, "Longitudinal analysis of ear infection and hearing impairment: findings from 6-year prospective cohorts of Australian children," *BMC Pediatrics*, vol. 13, no. 1, article 28, 2013.

[16] M. Wake and Z. Poulakis, "Slight and mild hearing loss in primary school children," *Journal of Paediatrics and Child Health*, vol. 40, no. 1-2, pp. 11–13, 2004.

[17] L. Śliwa, S. Hatzopoulos, K. Kochanek, A. Piłka, A. Senderski, and P. H. Skarżyński, "A comparison of audiometric and objective methods in hearing screening of school children. A preliminary study," *International Journal of Pediatric Otorhinolaryngology*, vol. 75, no. 4, pp. 483–488, 2011.

[18] A. Mousavi and M. Sedaie, "Hearing screening of school age children (aged between 7–12 years old)," *Audiology*, vol. 4, no. 1-2, pp. 5–9, 1996 (Persian).

[19] F. Sokhdari, *Determination of frequency distribution of hearing loss incidences in 7-12 years old students of Birjand public primary schools [M.S. thesis]*, Tehran University of Medical Sciences, Tehran, Iran, 2008.

[20] A. Qasem Pour, *Determination of frequency distribution of hearing loss incidences among students of West Islamabad public primary schools [M.S. thesis]*, Iran University of Medical Sciences, Tehran, Iran, 2005.

[21] M. Abdollahi, *Frequency distribution of hearing loss incidences in school children of Mahabad [M.S. thesis]*, University of Welfare Sciences, Tehran, Iran, 2007.

[22] J. Shahzadeh, *Determination of frequency distribution of hearing loss incidences among students in public primary schools of Neishabur [M.S. thesis]*, Iran University of Medical Sciences, Tehran, Iran, 2003.

[23] M. Mirlohyan, *Determination of frequency distribution of hearing loss incidences among 7-12 years of age students of Isfahan public primary schools [M.S. thesis]*, Iran University of Medical Sciences, Tehran, Iran, 2000.

[24] M. Parhizgar, *Determination of frequency distribution of types of hearing losses among 7–12 years old primary school students of Shiraz [M.S. thesis]*, Tehran University of Medical Sciences, Tehran, Iran, 2002.

17

Comparison of Pediatric and Adult Tonsillectomies Performed by Thermal Welding System

Tolga Ersözlü,[1] Yavuz Selim Yıldırım,[2] and Selman Sarica[3]

[1] *Department of Otorhinolaryngology Head and Neck Surgery, Elbistan State Hospital, 46300 Kahramanmaras, Turkey*
[2] *Department of Otorhinolaryngology and Head and Neck Surgery, Faculty of Medicine, Bezmialem Vakif University, Adnan Menderes Bulvarı, Vatan Caddesi Fatih, 34093 Istanbul, Turkey*
[3] *Department of Otorhinolaryngology Head and Neck Surgery, Afşin State Hospital, 46300 Kahramanmaras, Turkey*

Correspondence should be addressed to Yavuz Selim Yıldırım; dryavuzselim@yahoo.com

Academic Editor: Charles Monroe Myer

Objective. To compare pediatric and adult age groups in terms of postoperative bleeding and pain following tonsillectomy performed by thermal welding system (TWS). *Method.* The study consisted of 213 patients, of whom 178 were children and 35 were adults. The mean age of the pediatric patients (81 girls and 97 females) was 6.7 ± 2.4 years (range 3–13 years) and the mean age of the adults (20 males and 15 females) was 21.8 ± 7.07 years (range 15–41 years). All of the patients were evaluated in terms of postoperative bleeding and pain following tonsillectomy performed by TWS. *Results.* Bleeding was detected in the late postoperative period in 11 pediatric and 7 adult patients and of them 2 pediatric and 3 adult patients controlled under general. Postoperative bleeding was significantly less prevalent in the pediatric age group compared to the adult age group ($P = 0.04$). Likewise, postoperative pain was significantly less prevalent in the pediatric age group as compared to the adult age group ($P < 0.001$). *Conclusion.* Both postoperative bleeding and pain following tonsillectomy performed by TWS were more prevalent in the adult age group compared to the pediatric age group.

1. Introduction

Tonsillectomy is the most common surgical procedure performed in the ear, nose, and throat practice. It is most frequently performed via cold dissection both in the pediatric and adult age group worldwide. Many hot dissection methods have been defined as an alternative to the cold dissection. Hot dissection methods include bipolar and/or monopolar electrocautery, radiofrequency, harmonic scalpel, coblator, and thermal welding system (TWS) [1]. Previous studies have reported and compared the outcomes of radiofrequency, TWS, cold knife, or monopolar electrocautery in terms of posttonsillectomy bleeding and pain [2]. Thermal welding is the technique that simultaneously uses heat and pressure to provide coagulation. In a study conducted on adults, tonsillectomies performed by TWS and bipolar electrocautery were compared in terms of intraoperative bleeding, operation duration, postoperative pain, time to regain normal diet, and postoperative bleeding [3, 4]. Multiparametric studies

comparing a few methods have been conducted also in the pediatric age group [5]. However, studies comparing adult and pediatric patients in terms of postoperative bleeding and pain following tonsillectomy performed by TWS are limited. The aim of the present study was to investigate and compare the postoperative bleeding and pain following tonsillectomy performed by TWS in the pediatric and adult patients.

2. Materials and Method

The present prospective study included 213 pediatric and adult patients that underwent only tonsillectomy and/or adenotonsillectomy under general anesthesia by thermal welding device in Elbistan State Hospital Ear-Nose-Throat clinic between February 2008 and June 2012. Of the patients, 178 were children aged between 3 and 13 years and 35 were adults aged between 15 and 41 years. The indications for tonsillectomy were recurrent tonsillitis and/or tonsillar

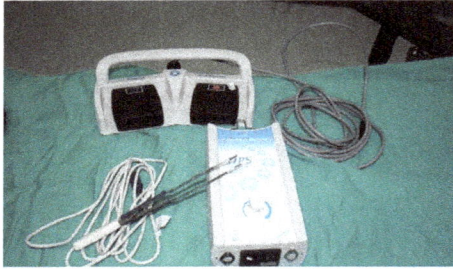

FIGURE 1: Thermal welding system (TWS) device.

TABLE 1: The ages and visual analogue scale scores of the patients.

	Mean ± SD	95% CI	RSD	Median	Min–Max
Pediatric patients ($n = 178$)					
Age	6.7 ± 2.40	6.3–7.0	0.35	6	2–13
VAS score	7.3 ± 1.15	7.2–7.5	0.15	8	6–10
Adult patients ($n = 35$)					
Age	21.8 ± 7.07	19.4–24.3	0.32	21	15–41
VAS score	85.6 ± 5.80	83.6–87.6	0.067	85	70–95

VAS: visual analogue scale; SD: standard deviation; CI: confidence interval; RSD: relative standard deviation; Min–Max: minimum–maximum.

hypertrophy in the pediatric patients and chronic tonsillitis in the adult patients.

Patients with history for penicillin allergy, coagulation disorder and/or abnormal elevated prothrombin time, and activated partial thromboplastin time were excluded from the study. All of the patients were operated by the same surgeon (Togla Ersözlü) under general anesthesia with endotracheal intubation. One hour prior to the surgical procedure, the pediatric patients were given 500 mg ampicillin/sulbactam intravenously, whereas the adult patients were given 1000 mg ampicillin/sulbactam intravenously. Both pediatric and adult patients received 0.5 mg/kg methylprednisolone intraoperatively. After the surgery, patients in the pediatric age group received amoxicillin/clavulanate and paracetamol suspension two times a day for ten days and the patients in the adult age group received amoxicillin/clavulanate and paracetamol tablets two times a day with ten days.

2.1. Surgical Technique. TWS consists of a single-use probe (ENTceps), double-controlled foot switch, and a universal power supply (UPS). The energy from the universal power supply turns into thermal energy in the heating wire (nichrome) at the distal end of the thermal welding probe and causes coagulation by simultaneous pressure that occurs as the probe is closed by the silicone boot at the other distal end [6, 7]. Nichrome wire at the ends of the probe cannot be activated via left foot switch unless completely squeezed by hands. Tissue-cutting is performed by clamping the coagulated tissue between the ends of the probe and activating via the right side of the foot switch (Figure 1).

In the present study, we performed extracapsular tonsillectomy with TWS using a probe with a power setting of "3" after placing the mouth gag. While the tonsil was retracted medially using allis clamp, dissection was made via tonsil probe at the upper pole of the tonsil by clamping the anterior pillar mucosal tissue. The tissue was activated with the foot switch and clamped between the ends of the tonsil probe for approximately 6 seconds and coagulation was performed. Thereafter, cutting procedure was performed by activating with the right foot switch for approximately two seconds. Dissection was extended from the upper pole to the lower pole by exposing the tonsil capsule. Tonsil tissue was coagulated for the last time at the lower pole and removed from the surgical area. This technique was performed for both tonsils. Tonsil bed was postoperatively monitored for

bleeding. Surgical area was washed with normal saline. Cold diet was initiated both to the pediatric group and adult group 3 hours after the surgery. All of the patients were discharged on the postoperative 2nd day.

Pain was questioned by nurse on the 1st, 3rd, 7th, and 10th postoperative days via faces pain scale under the assistance of the families of the children younger than 8 years [8], whereas it was evaluated via visual analogue scale (VAS) in the patients older than 8 years [1]. Postoperative bleeding was monitored and recorded if any.

2.2. Statistical Analysis. Data were evaluated using the MedCalc statistics program version 11.5.1 (MedCalc Software, Mariakerke, Belgium). The Chi-square test was used to compare the categorical variables, whereas Mann-Whitney U-test and independent samples t-test were used to determine intergroup differences. The data were expressed as mean ± standard deviation. A P value <0.05 was considered significant. Comparison of two groups proportions, minimally required sample size per group 13.

3. Results

The present study included 213 patients, of whom 178 were pediatric and 35 were adult. The pediatric age group comprised 80 girls and 98 boys with a mean age of 6.7 ± 2.4 years (range 3–13 years). The adult age group comprised 20 male and 15 female patients with a mean age of 21.8 ± 7.07 years (range 15–41 years). Of the pediatric patients, 11 developed postoperative bleeding in the late term (1–10 days); bleeding was controlled under general anesthesia in two patients. Postoperative bleeding was developed in 7 of 35 adult patients in the late term, and the bleeding was controlled under general anesthesia in 3 patients. Postoperative bleeding was significantly less prevalent in the pediatric age group compared to the adult age group ($P = 0.04$). Moreover, postoperative pain was significantly less prevalent in the pediatric age group as compared to the adult age group ($P < 0.001$). Ages and postoperative pain in the pediatric and adult age groups are presented in Table 1.

4. Discussion

Tonsillectomy techniques have been compared through various parameters in the previous studies. These comparisons have been performed only among pediatric and/or adult age groups [3–5]. There have also been studies comparing various techniques in both age groups [2, 9]. However, limited number of studies in the literature has compared adult and pediatric patients in terms of the same technique. In the present study, we compared the adult and pediatric patients in terms of postoperative bleeding and pain following tonsillectomy performed TWS.

Karatzias et al. [9] reported no postoperative bleeding after tonsillectomy performed by TWS in the adult and pediatric patients. Moreover, operation duration was shorter in the pediatric patients than in the adults. In that particular study, 3 adult patients developed intraoperative bleeding from the tonsillar artery in the inferior pole region and the bleeding was controlled by bipolar electrocautery. In the present study, postoperative bleeding was developed in both groups, being significantly more prevalent in the adult age group. Karatzias et al. [9] mentioned that intraoperative bleeding requires additional coagulation of the large vessels and additional suture techniques particularly in the adult patients. This result was consistent with the result of the present study, which revealed more prevalent postoperative bleeding among adult patients.

Stavroulaki et al. [1] compared cold dissection and TWS in the adult patients and showed significantly lower pain scores in the TWS group particularly within the first four postoperative days. In the present study, pain scores were found higher in the adult age group as compared to the pediatric age group. Stavroulaki et al. [1] attributed this result to the fact that TWS was simple and faster and produced much lower collateral thermal damage as compared to the monopolar or bipolar electrocautery. They found no significant difference between these two techniques in terms of postoperative bleeding. Postoperative bleeding was observed only in 3 patients in the cold dissection group, of whom 2 had a history of peritonsillar abscess.

Karatzanis et al. [10] performed a comparative study in the adults using TWS and LigaSure method and found no difference between the techniques in terms of the intraoperative bleeding and mean operation duration. On the other hand, the mean pain score was significantly lower in the TWS group on each postoperative day as compared to that in the LigaSure group. Moreover, they noted late postoperative bleeding in 1 patient in the TWS group and in 2 patients in the LigaSure group. Thus, they concluded that both techniques provide adequate homeostasis in the adult patients. The present study showed higher incidence of postoperative bleeding among adult patients as compared to that in the TWS group of Karatzanis et al. [10].

In their comparative study conducted on adult patients using TWS and bipolar electrocautery, Karatzias et al. [3] reported that 9 patients presented with late postoperative bleeding, of whom 4 were in the TWS group and 5 were in the bipolar electrocautery group. They noted no bleeding in the mouths or pharynxes of 2 patients in the TWS group and

3 patients in the bipolar electrocautery group, and the patients were discharged. The remaining 1 (1.2%) patient in the TWS group and 3 (4.3%) patients in the bipolar electrocautery group were hospitalized because of bleeding in the oral cavity. Bleeding was controlled under general anesthesia in 1 patient in the bipolar electrocautery group. In the present study, postoperative bleeding was observed in 7 adult patients, of whom 4 (11.4%) were hospitalized due to bleeding in the oral cavity and were discharged without any intervention. Bleeding was controlled under general anesthesia in the remaining 3 (8.5%) patients.

In their multiparametric study, Chimona et al. [5] compared cold knife, radiofrequency, and TWS in the children undergoing tonsillectomy, and they reported that postoperative pain was significantly lower in the cold knife procedure. They found no significant difference between these three methods in terms of late postoperative bleeding. In that particular study, the incidence of postoperative bleeding was 2.23%, whereas, it was 6.18% among pediatric age group in the present study. Of the pediatric patients with postoperative bleeding, 2 (1.12%) required bleeding control under general anesthesia. Chimona et al. [5] indicated that the incidence of posttonsillectomy bleeding was low in their study and they attributed this result to the experience of the surgeons whom performed the procedure, as well as to the time that they recommended to the children to start their normal diet and activity.

Michel et al. [2] conducted a study on 100 patients and divided them into two subgroups according to their ages; patients between 2 and 12 years of age constituted younger group and patients between 13 and 47 years of age constituted older group. This study, which is the only study in the literature similar to the present study, introduced the preliminary results about safety, efficacy, and morbidity of TWS used for tonsillectomy and compared the results with those of other total tonsillectomy techniques in the literature. In that particular study, the mean pain score during healing was 2.0 in the younger group and 3.1 in the older group. These results were consistent with the results of the present study; the postoperative pain score was significantly lower in the pediatric patients compared to that in the adults. Moreover, in that particular study, the incidence of late postoperative bleeding was the same both in the younger and older groups (2%). The incidence of late postoperative bleeding in the present study was 6.18% in the pediatric age group and 20% in the adult age group.

In the literature, Lee et al. [11] reported that there was no difference between cold and hot dissections in terms of the incidence of secondary bleeding in the pediatric age group. Nevertheless, in their study Michel et al. [2] performed a literature review and reported the incidences of late postoperative bleeding for different techniques as follows: 8.6% ($n = 1455$) for electrodissection, 3.9% ($n = 1829$) for coblation, 2.8% ($n = 468$) for harmonic scalpel, and 1.5% ($n = 1610$) for cold knife. In the present study, the incidence of late postoperative bleeding was 6.18% in the pediatric age group and 20% in the adult age group.

The present study evaluated postoperative bleeding and pain following tonsillectomy performed by TWS in the pediatric and adult age groups and revealed higher incidences of postoperative bleeding and pain in the late term in the adult age group compared to those in the pediatric age group. Large-scale studies comparing different tonsillectomy techniques in adult and pediatric age groups are needed.

Conflict of Interests

The authors declare that they have no conflict of interests.

References

[1] P. Stavroulaki, C. Skoulakis, E. Theos, N. Kokalis, and D. Valagianis, "Thermal welding versus cold dissection tonsillectomy: a prospective, randomized, single-blind study in adults patients," *Annals of Otology, Rhinology and Laryngology*, vol. 116, no. 8, pp. 565–570, 2007.

[2] R. G. Michel, B. I. Weinstock, and K. Tsau, "Safety and efficacy of pressure-assisted tissue-welding tonsillectomy: a preliminary evaluation," *Ear, Nose and Throat Journal*, vol. 87, no. 2, pp. 100–105, 2008.

[3] G. T. Karatzias, V. A. Lachanas, and V. G. Sandris, "Thermal welding versus bipolar tonsillectomy: a comparative study," *Otolaryngology—Head and Neck Surgery*, vol. 134, no. 6, pp. 975–978, 2006.

[4] J. Silvola, A. Salonen, J. Nieminen, and H. Kokki, "Tissue welding tonsillectomy provides an enhanced recovery compared to that after monopolar electrocautery technique in adults: a prospective randomized clinical trial," *European Archives of Oto-Rhino-Laryngology*, vol. 268, no. 2, pp. 255–260, 2011.

[5] T. Chimona, E. Proimos, C. Mamoulakis, M. Tzanakakis, C. E. Skoulakis, and C. E. Papadakis, "Multiparametric comparison of cold knife tonsillectomy, radiofrequency excision and thermal welding tonsillectomy in children," *International Journal of Pediatric Otorhinolaryngology*, vol. 72, no. 9, pp. 1431–1436, 2008.

[6] B. I. Weinstock, "An improved method for tonsillectomy using thermal welding technology," http://www.hakermedikal.com/doc/Advances%20in%20Otolaryngologyhs_Tonsillectomy.pdf.

[7] H. Yaşar, H. Özkul, and A. Verim, "Comparison of the thermal welding technique and cold dissection for pediatric tonsillectomy," *Trakya Üniversitesi Tıp Fakültesi Dergisi*, vol. 26, no. 4, pp. 326–330, 2009.

[8] D. Bieri, R. A. Reeve, G. D. Champion, L. Addicoat, and J. B. Ziegler, "The faces pain scale for the self-assessment of the severity of pain experienced by children: development, initial validation, and preliminary investigation for ratio scale properties," *Pain*, vol. 41, no. 2, pp. 139–150, 1990.

[9] G. T. Karatzias, V. A. Lachanas, S. M. Papouliakos, and V. G. Sandris, "Tonsillectomy using the thermal welding system," *ORL, Journal of Oto-Rhino-Laryngology and Its Related Specialties*, vol. 67, no. 4, pp. 225–229, 2005.

[10] A. Karatzanis, C. Bourolias, E. Prokopakis, I. Panagiotaki, and G. Velegrakis, "Thermal welding technology vs ligasure tonsillectomy: a comparative study," *The American Journal of Otolaryngology*, vol. 29, no. 4, pp. 238–241, 2008.

[11] M. S. W. Lee, M.-L. Montague, and S. S. M. Hussain, "Post-tonsillectomy hemorrhage: cold versus hot dissection," *Otolaryngology—Head and Neck Surgery*, vol. 131, no. 6, pp. 833–836, 2004.

18

The Need for Improved Detection and Management of Adult-Onset Hearing Loss in Australia

Catherine M. McMahon,[1,2] Bamini Gopinath,[3] Julie Schneider,[4] Jennifer Reath,[5] Louise Hickson,[2,6] Stephen R. Leeder,[4] Paul Mitchell,[3] and Robert Cowan[2,7]

[1] Centre for Language Sciences, Australian Hearing Hub, 16 University Dve, Macquarie University, North Ryde, NSW 2109, Australia
[2] HEARing Cooperative Research Centre, 550 Swanston St, Audiology, Hearing and Speech Sciences University of Melbourne, VIC 3010, Australia
[3] Centre for Vision Research, Department of Ophthalmology and Westmead Millennium Institute, The University of Sydney, Westmead Hospital, Westmead, NSW 2145, Australia
[4] Menzies Centre for Health Policy, Victor Coppleson Building, The University of Sydney, NSW 2006, Australia
[5] School of Medicine, University of Western Sydney, Penrith, NSW 2751, Australia
[6] School of Health and Rehabilitation Sciences, St Lucia Campus, University of Queensland, Brisbane, QLD 4072, Australia
[7] School of Audiology, 550 Swanston St, Audiology, Hearing and Speech Sciences, University of Melbourne, VIC 3010, Australia

Correspondence should be addressed to Catherine M. McMahon; cath.mcmahon@mq.edu.au

Academic Editor: Charles Monroe Myer

Adult-onset hearing loss is insidious and typically diagnosed and managed several years after onset. Often, this is after the loss having led to multiple negative consequences including effects on employment, depressive symptoms, and increased risk of mortality. In contrast, the use of hearing aids is associated with reduced depression, longer life expectancy, and retention in the workplace. Despite this, several studies indicate high levels of unmet need for hearing health services in older adults and poor use of prescribed hearing aids, often leading to their abandonment. In Australia, the largest component of financial cost of hearing loss (excluding the loss of well-being) is due to lost workplace productivity. Nonetheless, the Australian public health system does not have an effective and sustainable hearing screening strategy to tackle the problem of poor detection of adult-onset hearing loss. Given the increasing prevalence and disease burden of hearing impairment in adults, two key areas are not adequately met in the Australian healthcare system: (1) early identification of persons with chronic hearing impairment; (2) appropriate and targeted referral of these patients to hearing health service providers. This paper reviews the current literature, including population-based data from the Blue Mountains Hearing Study, and suggests different models for early detection of adult-onset hearing loss.

1. Introduction

Adult-onset hearing loss is a highly prevalent yet relatively underrecognised health problem in the older adult Australian population [1, 2]. Because hearing loss is often progressive and gradual in its onset in most individuals, it is typically diagnosed and managed several years after its onset, often only after having led to multiple negative consequences including effects on employment, poor quality of life, social isolation, depressive symptoms, increased mortality risk, and reduced independence [3–9]. It is one of the leading causes of burden of disease prior to older age, for ages 45–64 years,

in men and women [9]. Further, as hearing loss interferes with so many of life's activities, it may prove to be a major impediment to society's need to have people remain longer in the workforce as the proportion of "working age" people in developed countries shrinks [10]. In Australia, the annual cost of lost earnings due to workplace separation and early retirement from hearing loss was estimated at $6.7 billion, which is over half of the calculated economic impact of hearing loss ($11.75 billion, representing 1.4% of GDP) [11]. Therefore there is a need to better understand the barriers that may exist to help seek an effective remediation for hearing loss in this population.

Hearing loss is a chronic problem and, contrary to current community perception and funding models of hearing services, hearing aids are typically a part of a rehabilitation program rather than provide a single and simple restorative solution to hearing loss [12]. As such, hearing loss needs to be effectively managed under a biopsychosocial model of care [13], following the framework for intervention and treatment of the International Classification of Functioning Disability, and Health model [14]. This framework not only considers the impairment *per se*, but also the impact that it has on the individual in terms of activity limitations (such as inability to perceive speech in noisy environments) and participation restrictions (such as the ability to fully participate in communication and conversational activities) [15]. Nonetheless, hearing aid use is a measurable quantity and, therefore, the majority of studies that have evaluated functional and quality-of-life outcomes of rehabilitation programs for individuals with hearing loss have used this as a marker. Multiple studies have identified that rehabilitation interventions can effectively address many of the difficulties associated with impaired hearing [16–20]. Importantly, evidence shows that the later hearing rehabilitation occurs in the course of hearing loss, the less likely older adults are to continue to use and derive benefit from hearing aids [21]. Despite this, several studies [22, 23] indicate high levels of unmet need for hearing health services and poor use of prescribed hearing aids. "Denial" or nonacceptance of hearing loss and the stigma associated with hearing loss are factors associated with this reluctance to seek help. Other reasons include an underestimation of the negative impacts of hearing impairment on overall health by general practitioners (GPs) and older adults, leading to poor referral to appropriate medical and allied health practitioners, such as ear, nose, and throat specialists and audiologists [24].

To date, the Australian public health system does not have an effective and sustainable hearing loss screening strategy for late-onset hearing loss in adults to manage this problem. This paper aims to review the current pathway of detection, referral, and management of late-onset adult hearing loss in Australia and to identify an alternative, more effective pathway for the future.

2. Prevalence, Incidence, and Risk Factors of Adult-Onset Hearing Loss in Australia

Australian population-based data describing prevalence, incidence, and risk factors for hearing loss have been identified in the Blue Mountains Hearing Study (BMHS) in 1997–2000 among 2956 participants of the Blue Mountains Eye Study (BMES) cohort (an overall response rate of 75.5% for the cross-section) [25, 26]. Of these, 870 participants without hearing loss and 439 with hearing loss were reexamined during 2002–2004. Hearing thresholds were measured in audiometric soundproof rooms by qualified audiologists and bilateral hearing loss was described by the pure-tone average of air-conduction thresholds at octave frequencies between 500 and 4000 Hz ($PTA_{0.5-4\,kHz}$) in the better ear. Any hearing

loss was defined as $PTA_{0.5-4\,kHz} > 25$ dBHL. Risk factors measured (either via self-report or practitioner measurement) included self-reported health, noise exposure, and family history of hearing loss. In this study, we identified that a 33.0% prevalence of bilateral hearing loss existed in persons aged 50+ years (51% showed hearing loss in the worse ear) consistent with that measured in the US-based Epidemiology of Hearing Loss Study (EHLS) [27]. More specifically, mild hearing loss was present in 22.4% of participants, moderate in 8.9% and severe in 1.7% participants. For each decade beyond age 50, prevalence of hearing loss doubled. Men were 40% more likely to have hearing loss than women. Further, a history of having worked in a noisy environment predicted a 70% increased likelihood of any hearing loss, whereas family history predicted a 68% increased risk of hearing loss, which increased with greater magnitudes of loss [28]. The overall 5-year progression of hearing loss, defined as a difference in PTA > 10 dB, was moderately high at 15.7%, with the highest rate being evident in adults aged 80 years or older [26]. Additionally, for each decade of age over 60 years, the risk of incident hearing loss increased threefold.

As well as health-related influences, our epidemiological study also assessed quality-of-life and mental health factors, such as cognitive function and depression. BMHS-I data showed that bilateral hearing loss was associated with poorer SF-36 scores in both physical and mental domains (decrease in physical component score (PCS) of 1.4 points, $P = 0.025$; decrease in mental component score (MCS) of 1.0 point, $P = 0.13$); with poorer scores associated with more severe levels of impairment (PCS $P_{trend} = 0.04$, MCS $P_{trend} = 0.003$) [3]. BMHS participants with any hearing loss were 64% more likely to have depressive symptoms [4]. Persons with moderate-to-severe hearing loss had slightly lower mean cognitive function scores than those without hearing loss ($P < 0.001$) [29]. Therefore, while milder levels of hearing losses were significantly more common in working-aged older adults, a lack of responsiveness to manage this early can lead to significant negative effects on quality of life, personal relationships, and ability to continue to work effectively. As the risk of hearing loss increases with advancing age, it seems that early detection and management would be critical to minimising any longer-term effects.

3. Poor Recognition and Uptake of Hearing Services

Stephens et al. [30] suggest that the average consumer presenting at a hearing aid or rehabilitation clinic for the first time is aged ~70 years and has had hearing problems for about 10 years. As hearing loss significantly impacts on communication ability [31] and communication is necessary for developing and maintaining effective relationships [32], it is likely that within this prolonged timeframe the individual and his/her family have experienced considerable frustration from the disability [33]. Hearing aids and associated rehabilitation programs have been shown to minimise such impacts. The US National Council on Aging survey of 2069 hearing-impaired individuals and 1710 of family and

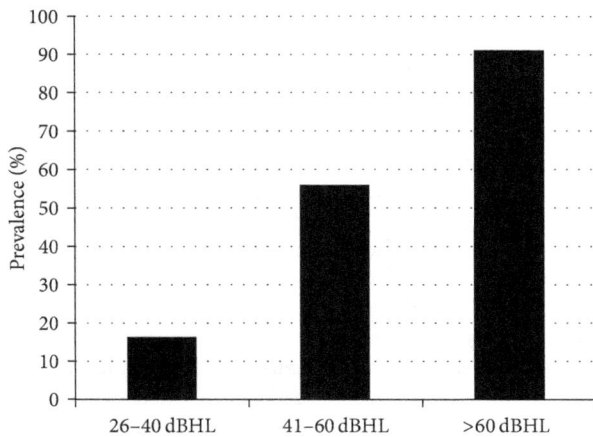

FIGURE 1: Prevalence of hearing aid ownership for individuals with a mild (26–45 dBHL), moderate (46–60 dBHL), and sever-profound (>60 dBHL) hearing loss. Data from Hartley et al. [35].

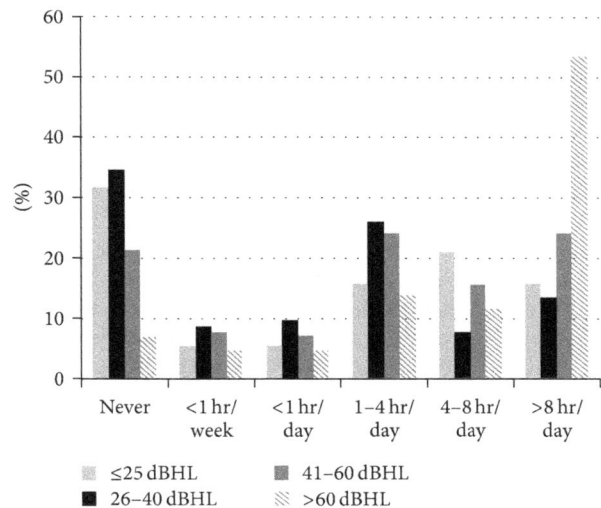

FIGURE 2: Percentage of time spent wearing hearing aids by magnitude of hearing loss in the better ear. Amended from Hartley et al. [35].

friends demonstrated that hearing aid use is associated with lesser degrees of anger and frustration reported by family members [12]. Further, Stark and Hickson [34] demonstrated benefits in hearing-related quality-of-life scales for both the individual with hearing loss and their significant other after hearing aid fitting, despite only 1/3 of the individuals with hearing loss showing initial motivation to attend the hearing appointment. Certainly, we found that BMHS participants who used their hearing aid at least 1 hour/day or more were only one-third as likely to report depressive symptoms as infrequent users, multivariate adjusted OR 0.32 (95% CI 0.14–0.76) [4]. Despite this, BMHS findings [34] showed that of 33.0% persons with measured bilateral hearing loss, only 33% owned hearing aids and, of these, only 25% used them habitually [3], similar to the rates of use reported in the EHLS study [27]. When stratified into magnitudes of hearing loss, BMHS data showed that hearing aids were owned by only 16.4% of individuals with a mild loss, compared with 55.8% with a moderate loss and 91.3% with a severe-profound loss (Figure 1) [35], suggesting that either there is a critical unmet need for hearing services in individuals with mild-moderate levels of hearing loss or that hearing aids are not needed for all individuals with lower magnitudes of loss or that the technology is too difficult to manage in this population. Nonetheless, BMHS data showed that 33.4% of older adults with average hearing levels greater than 40 dBHL in the better ear did not own a hearing aid [35]. While milder forms of hearing loss may be less correlated with hearing disability, Dillon [10] showed that more significant losses do show higher levels of benefit. Further, BMHS data demonstrate that 53.5% of older adults with severe losses wear their hearing aids for over 8 hours per day compared to 24% of those with moderate losses and 13.5% with mild losses [35], suggesting an increased need for amplification for greater magnitudes of loss (Figure 2).

Low rates for use of hearing services and hearing aids highlight barriers including cost [36] and/or reluctance by many to accept their hearing loss (or those without self-perceived hearing disability) [37]. However, similar low rates of hearing service uptake and device use have been observed in the Australian Federal Government Office of Hearing Services program [10], where hearing services are largely provided free of charge to eligible older adults. Therefore, we assume that under use of fitted aids by older adults in Australia may suggest either poor targeting of individuals with hearing loss or fitting at too late a stage for derived benefit. Substantial delays in accessing hearing services may impact effective hearing aid use because advancing age is associated with poorer auditory and cognitive processing, physical dexterity, and learning abilities making it more challenging to perceive sounds in competing noise environments, position a hearing aid in the ear, and to learn how to use new technology [38–41]. Additionally, there is an increased likelihood of other health problems coexisting so that the management of hearing loss may be considered less of a priority and prove to be burdensome. As the consequences of the hearing loss are more significant, this may lead to poorer motivation to manage the impairment and/or its impacts.

4. GP Hearing Screening Strategies

There remains a large proportion of hearing-impaired adults who would benefit from hearing aids but who decide not to seek help [21]. Further, while BMHS showed that approximately one-third of people aged ≥50 years with measured bilateral hearing loss reported seeking help from their general practitioner (GP), a random cross-sectional survey of GP activity in Australia between 2003 and 2008 identified that only approximately 3/1000 consultations for older adults included hearing loss management [24]. Similar studies of GPs undertaken in UK identified that the chance of referral to hearing services for older adults who reported hearing loss was only about 50% [42]. Screening and intervention programmes have been recommended to improve this situation [21, 43]. Screening programs are not systematically implemented throughout the Australian population, their success at meeting the needs of the target population is not assured, and they have no automatic link to action if the need for action is detected [44]. Audiograms conducted by trained audiologists in soundproof booths, are currently used to diagnose hearing impairment and largely determine whether or not an individual is offered hearing rehabilitation. Audiometry is expensive and may not necessarily be accessible to those needing it. Particularly for late-onset hearing loss, it provides little information about effects of hearing loss on everyday functioning [45, 46]. It is important to note that while hearing impairment is extremely common in older adults, not all are significantly disturbed by this. The BMHS findings collectively show that severe hearing disability is strongly associated with measured hearing loss, poorer QOL, and probable depression. This suggests that identifying hearing-related activity limitations and participation restrictions could potentially be effective in identifying persons more likely to have suffered an important impact from their hearing impairment and, thus, would be most likely to benefit most from using hearing aids. Self-perception of a hearing disability (e.g., increasing social isolation) can often be an important reason to seek aural rehabilitation. In fact, Dillon [10] showed that the benefits reported by individuals with hearing aids appear to be only weakly correlated with hearing loss, particularly for mild-moderate losses. This may in part explain why at least 20% of individuals fitted with hearing aids do not wear them. On the other hand, benefits are actually more highly correlated with initial motivation and perceived listening difficulty [10, 47, 48]. Thus, greater engagement by GPs in hearing health could potentially be a cost-saving strategy, as GPs are ideally placed to better motivate and identify older people with hearing loss disability, that is, those likely to benefit the most from a hearing aid, thereby improving the targeting of hearing-impaired patients for rehabilitation.

There exists a need for a readily accessible screening test assessing hearing disability which could more accurately identify rehabilitation need, rather than just measurement of hearing loss. Validated, self-administered questionnaires about hearing disability have been shown to detect functional hearing impairment accurately and, so, have been recommended as potential screening tools [49–52]. These can also be administered quickly without specialised training [53]. In particular, it has been suggested that primary care services could cost-effectively be used to identify hearing disability using targeted questions, possibly alongside other screening interventions [21, 43]. Previous work through UK GP-based case finding, which targeted people in the 50–65-year age group, showed that effective hearing aid use can be at least tripled [30, 54]. One study assessed the patient's take-up of hearing disability screening and the subsequent take-up of hearing aids as an intervention for hearing disability. Substantial benefits were reported in hearing aid benefit outcome inventories and moderate benefits in health utilities

index and quality-of-life scores from amplification for this target group [21]. Another UK study of 604 GP patients, aged 50–65 years [30], showed that the first posting of hearing disability questionnaires detected 78% of those prepared to accept hearing aids for the first time. The possession of hearing aids rose from 7% (at baseline) to 24% (after intervention), and 6 months later the hearing aids were being used regularly. The authors concluded that simple questionnaires are effective in detecting hearing disability in older adults and that this intervention was acceptable by many of those reporting significant hearing difficulties.

Given the pivotal role of the GP in the early identification and management of chronic health problems, at least in Australia, the implementation of a GP-based hearing screening program for adults >50 years of age would be beneficial in addressing this problem. Further, with the inadequacies of the medical model in the treatment of chronic health conditions and the move towards a model of patient-centred care, GPs are effectively placed to assist with the minimisation of the stigma associated with hearing loss and enhancing patient self-motivation to manage this [55]. Current research identifies a critical role for GPs in both detection and appropriate referral of many other disorders/diseases such as obesity [56–58]. However, several such studies identified that the knowledge and attitudes of GPs can be a major barrier to effective intervention within this process [38]. Hence, underlying reasons for low rates of GP involvement in hearing health could include lack of awareness/understanding of (a) simple tools to identify hearing loss and associated disability; (b) risk factors for age-related hearing loss and ways to use this information to identify at-risk patients; (c) adverse impacts caused by hearing loss on the mental and physical well-being of older adults (i.e., disability); and (d) the benefits of aural rehabilitation.

Given the increasing prevalence and disease burden of undetected hearing loss in older adults and the availability of effective interventions (e.g., hearing aids and/or assisted listening devices), there are 3 potential critical roles for the GP in hearing health: (1) early identification of patients with age-related hearing loss, as well as recognition of whether any negative consequences/disability has resulted; (2) assistance in reducing the stigma of hearing loss and motivating patients to seek further help; and (3) appropriate referral of these patients to hearing health providers. This could be achieved by sensitising GPs to recognise at-risk individuals and providing targeted questions to identify hearing loss disability.

We have identified an important role of GPs in the process of targeting individuals with late-onset hearing loss and referral; however, the challenge that remains is how to effectively increase GPs knowledge and practice behaviour in this area. Possibly the most obvious method is through development of a continuing medical education (CME) program that targets the impacts of hearing loss and remediation and provides a reliable method of hearing screening in adults. The evidence for good outcomes of CMEs measured by factors including increased knowledge and skills as well as altered attitudes and practice behaviours is varied and possibly depends partly on the learners and learning context [59]. A review of the literature has identified that while the quality of evidence is not high, generally CME provides a strategy that increases knowledge and may elicit a change in practice behaviour [60]. However, in a meta-analysis of the CME literature, Forsetlund and colleagues [61] report that education meetings are likely to only have a moderate effect on professional practice and a smaller improvement on patient outcomes. Despite this, Cook et al. [59] demonstrated that while Internet-based programs have a significant effect on knowledge and behaviour compared with no-intervention, there is limited evidence to suggest that it is superior to other methods of delivery of learning materials. Therefore it is possible that both educational meetings and Internet-based programs will have only a moderate impact in enhancing referrals to hearing healthcare providers.

5. Telephone/Internet Screening Programs

An alternative method of screening of hearing loss and disability which does not require GP involvement is telephone and/or Internet screening using digits in noise [62–64], which provides a quick, effective, and relatively inexpensive technique to detect hearing loss in adults [62, 63]. In addition, this presumably has a broader reach than GP screening because of the program's accessibility to individuals in rural and remote areas where worldwide shortages of healthcare professionals and services exist [65]. Further, it provides information about the individual's hearing to the significant proportion of individuals who were not intending to see a GP or hearing healthcare provider (as shown in [64]). Smits and colleagues [62, 64] developed the first telephone screening test which was introduced into The Netherlands in 2003 as the National Hearing Test. The screening test used 23 monosyllabic digit triplets presented by a female speaker, adaptively varying in level by 4 dB (to determine audibility) and then 2 dB (to seek threshold) and embedded in a 73 dBA speech noise, shaped to match the long-term average speech spectrum. They estimated the average signal-to-noise ratio (SNR) for speech reception threshold (SRT; 50% correctly identified) and characterised normal hearing using a criterion of −4.1 dB SNR, insufficient hearing between −4.1 and −1.4 dB SNR, and poor hearing >−1.4 dB SNR. In 38 participants with varying levels of hearing [62], this screening test showed excellent test-retest reliability (<1 dB error), sensitivity (0.91), and specificity (0.93) when compared to an equivalent speech-in-noise test conducted under headphones and took approximately 3 minutes to complete. A similar telephone screening test "Telscreen" using digit triplets embedded in spectrally shaped noise was developed and implemented in Australia in 2007 [63]. The noise was amplitude modulated by a 20 Hz sinusoid and had gaps in the frequency spectrum to increase the sensitivity of this test to identify sensorineural hearing losses (described in [63]). Significant correlations were found between Telscreen and the individual's four-frequency pure-tone average ($r = 0.77$, $P < 0.001$) and Telscreen and the presence of subjectively rated disability ($r = 0.65$, $P < 0.001$).

Smits and colleagues [64] demonstrated that over 50% of those referred to medical or other professional hearing healthcare in The Netherlands were compliant in following this advice. On the other hand, Meyer and colleagues [63] showed that only 36% of the 193 individuals who failed the Telscreen in Australia went on to receive medical or other professional support. It is not clear whether such differences in health-seeking behaviour are explained by cultural, social, or economic factors.

6. Speech-in-Noise Tests

Another hearing screening program is the use of an automated face-to-face monosyllabic speech-in-noise test which aims to evaluate hearing disability in adults. The speech understanding in noise (SUN) test was developed by Paglialonga and colleagues [66, 67] and has been evaluated in multiple nonclinical sites with varying levels of ambient noise showing good sensitivity up to 65 dBA. The SUN test presents monosyllabic vowel-consonant-vowel sounds in a 3-alternative forced-choice paradigm. The response is provided through a touch screen, thereby avoiding tester scoring errors, and takes approximately 2 minutes to evaluate both ears. Good associations were found between pure-tone audiometry and referral on the SUN test [66] which indicates the benefit of this test as a screening test for adult hearing loss.

7. Conclusions

Given the ageing demographic and increasing average life span in Western countries, chronic hearing loss is projected to increase. A renewed focus on targeting the provision of hearing rehabilitation to people with self-perceived hearing disability, rather than those with only measured hearing loss, may lead to better long-term retention and use of aids. Therefore, over time the costs saved by provision of an effective and better-targeted health intervention enabling improved daily functioning among older adults will no doubt demonstrate this strategy and will provide "value for money."

Acknowledgment

The authors acknowledge the financial support of the HEARing CRC, established and supported under the Cooperative Research Centres Program—an initiative of the Australian Government.

References

[1] M. A. Gratton and A. E. Vazquez, "Age-related hearing loss: current research," *Current Opinion in Otolaryngology & Head and Neck Surgery*, vol. 11, pp. 367–371, 2003.

[2] D. B. Reuben, K. Walsh, A. A. Moore, M. Damesyn, and G. A. Greendale, "Hearing loss in community-dwelling older persons: national prevalence data and identification using simple questions," *Journal of the American Geriatrics Society*, vol. 46, no. 8, pp. 1008–1011, 1998.

[3] E. M. Chia, J. J. Wang, E. Rochtchina, R. R. Cumming, P. Newall, and P. Mitchell, "Hearing impairment and health-related quality of life: the blue mountains hearing study," *Ear and Hearing*, vol. 28, no. 2, pp. 187–195, 2007.

[4] B. Gopinath, J. J. Wang, J. Schneider et al., "Depressive symptoms in older adults with hearing impairments: the blue mountains study: letters to the editor," *Journal of the American Geriatrics Society*, vol. 57, no. 7, pp. 1306–1308, 2009.

[5] I. Appollonio, C. Carabellese, E. Magni, L. Frattola, and M. Trabucchi, "Sensory impairments and mortality in an elderly community population: a six-year follow-up study," *Age and Ageing*, vol. 24, no. 1, pp. 30–36, 1995.

[6] B. E. Weinstein and I. M. Ventry, "Hearing impairment and social isolation in the elderly," *Journal of Speech and Hearing Research*, vol. 25, no. 4, pp. 593–599, 1982.

[7] M. J. Karpa, B. Gopinath, K. Beath et al., "Associations between hearing impairment and mortality risk in older persons: the blue mountains hearing study," *Annals of Epidemiology*, vol. 20, no. 6, pp. 452–459, 2010.

[8] J. Schneider, B. Gopinath, M. J. Karpa et al., "Hearing loss impacts on the use of community and informal supports," *Age and Ageing*, vol. 39, no. 4, pp. 458–464, 2010.

[9] S. Begg, T. Vos, B. Barker, C. Stevenson, L. Stanley, and A. D. Lopez, *The Burden of Disease and Injury in Australia 2003*, PHE 82, Australian Institute of Health and Welfare, Canberra, Australia, 2007.

[10] H. Dillon, *The 2006 Libby Harricks Memorial Oration: Hearing Loss: The Silent Epidemic. Who, Why, Impact and What Can we Do about it*, ACT, Deafness Forum Limited, 2006.

[11] "Listen Hear! The economic impact and cost of hearing loss in Australia," CRC for Cochlear Implant and Hearing Aid Innovation and Vicdeaf, Access Economics Pty Limited, Vicdeaf, Australia, 2006.

[12] M. L. Hyde and K. Riko, "A decision-analytic approach to audiological rehabilitation," *Academy of Rehabilitative Audiology*, vol. 27, supplement, pp. 337–374, 1994.

[13] J. P. Gagnè, "What is treatment evaluation research? What is its relationship to the goals of audiological rehabilitation? Who are the stakeholders of this type of research?" *Ear and Hearing*, vol. 21, no. 4, supplement, pp. 60S–73S, 2000.

[14] World Health Organisation, *International Classification of Impairments, Disability and Health*, Geneva, Switzerland, 2001.

[15] H. B. Abrams, T. H. Chisolm, and R. McArdle, "Health-related quality of life and hearing aids: a tutorial," *Trends in Amplification*, vol. 9, no. 3, pp. 99–109, 2005.

[16] I. Appollonio, C. Carabellese, L. Frattola, and M. Trabucchi, "Effects of sensory aids on the quality of life and mortality of elderly people: a multivariate analysis," *Age and Ageing*, vol. 25, no. 2, pp. 89–96, 1996.

[17] S. Kochkin and C. M. Rogin, "Quantifying the obvious: the impact of hearing instruments on quality of life," *Hearing Review*, vol. 7, no. 1, pp. 6–34, 2000.

[18] T. H. Chisolm, H. B. Abrams, and R. McArdle, "Short- and long-term outcomes of adult audiological rehabilitation," *Ear and Hearing*, vol. 25, no. 5, pp. 464–477, 2004.

[19] S. M. Cohen, R. F. Labadie, M. S. Dietrich, and D. S. Haynes, "Quality of life in hearing-impaired adults: the role of cochlear implants and hearing aids," *Otolaryngology*, vol. 131, no. 4, pp. 413–422, 2004.

[20] H. Tsuruoka, S. Masuda, K. Ukai, Y. Sakakura, T. Harada, and Y. Majima, "Hearing impairment and quality of life for the elderly in nursing homes," *Auris Nasus Larynx*, vol. 28, no. 1, pp. 45–54, 2001.

[21] A. Davis, P. Smith, M. Ferguson, D. Stephens, and I. Gianopoulos, "Acceptability, benefit and costs of early screening for hearing disability: a study of potential screening tests and models," *Health Technology Assessment*, vol. 11, no. 42, pp. 1–294, 2007.

[22] J. Jee, J. J. Wang, K. A. Rose, R. Lindley, P. Landau, and P. Mitchell, "Vision and hearing impairment in aged care clients," *Ophthalmic Epidemiology*, vol. 12, no. 3, pp. 199–205, 2005.

[23] D. S. Dalton, K. J. Cruickshanks, B. E. K. Klein, R. Klein, T. L. Wiley, and D. M. Nondahl, "The impact of hearing loss on quality of life in older adults," *Gerontologist*, vol. 43, no. 5, pp. 661–668, 2003.

[24] J. M. Schneider, B. Gopinath, C. M. McMahon et al., "Role of general practitioners in managing age-related hearing loss," *Medical Journal of Australia*, vol. 192, no. 1, pp. 20–23, 2010.

[25] B. Gopinath, E. Rochtchina, J. J. Wang, J. Schneider, S. R. Leeder, and P. Mitchell, "Prevalence of age-related hearing loss in older adults: blue mountains study," *Archives of Internal Medicine*, vol. 169, no. 4, pp. 415–416, 2009.

[26] P. Mitchell, B. Gopinath, J. J. Wang et al., "Five-year incidence and progression of hearing impairment in an older population," *Ear and Hearing*, vol. 32, no. 2, pp. 251–257, 2011.

[27] M. M. Popelka, K. J. Cruickshanks, T. L. Wiley, T. S. Tweed, B. E. K. Klein, and R. Klein, "Low prevalence of hearing aid use among older adults with hearing loss: the epidemiology of hearing loss study," *Journal of the American Geriatrics Society*, vol. 46, no. 9, pp. 1075–1078, 1998.

[28] C. M. McMahon, A. Kifley, E. Rochtchina, P. Newall, and P. Mitchell, "The contribution of family history to hearing loss in an older population," *Ear and Hearing*, vol. 29, no. 4, pp. 578–584, 2008.

[29] T. Tay, J. W. Jie, A. Kifley, R. Lindley, P. Newall, and P. Mitchell, "Sensory and cognitive association in older persons: findings from an older Australian population," *Gerontology*, vol. 52, no. 6, pp. 386–394, 2006.

[30] S. D. G. Stephens, D. E. Callaghan, S. Hogan, R. Meredith, A. Rayment, and A. C. Davis, "Hearing disability in people aged 50–65: effectiveness and acceptability of rehabilitative intervention," *British Medical Journal*, vol. 300, no. 6723, pp. 508–511, 1990.

[31] S. Arlinger, "Negative consequences of uncorrected hearing loss—a review," *International Journal of Audiology*, vol. 42, no. 2, pp. S17–S20, 2003.

[32] M. I. Wallhagen, W. J. Strawbridge, S. J. Shema, and G. A. Kaplan, "Impact of self-assessed hearing loss on a spouse: a longitudinal analysis of couples," *Journals of Gerontology B*, vol. 59, no. 3, pp. S190–S196, 2004.

[33] R. Hetu, L. Jones, and L. Getty, "The impact of a acquired hearing impairment on intimate relationships: implications for rehabilitation," *Audiology*, vol. 32, no. 6, pp. 363–381, 1993.

[34] P. Stark and L. Hickson, "Outcomes of hearing aid fitting for older people with hearing impairment and their significant others," *International Journal of Audiology*, vol. 43, no. 7, pp. 390–398, 2004.

[35] D. Hartley, E. Rochtchina, P. Newall, M. Golding, and P. Mitchell, "Use of hearing aids and assistive listening devices in an older australian population," *Journal of the American Academy of Audiology*, vol. 21, no. 10, pp. 642–653, 2010.

[36] J. R. Franks and N. J. Beckmann, "Rejection of hearing aids: attitudes of a geriatric sample," *Ear and Hearing*, vol. 6, no. 3, pp. 161–166, 1985.

[37] D. C. Garstecki and S. F. Erler, "Hearing loss, control, and demographic factors influencing hearing aid use among older

adults," *Journal of Speech, Language, and Hearing Research*, vol. 41, no. 3, pp. 527–537, 1998.

[38] D. N. Brooks, "Factors relating to the under-use of postaural hearing aids," *British Journal of Audiology*, vol. 19, no. 3, pp. 211–217, 1985.

[39] P. B. Kricos, "Audiologic management of older adults with hearing loss and compromised cognitive/psychoacoustic auditory processing capabilities," *Trends in Amplification*, vol. 10, no. 1, pp. 1–28, 2006.

[40] P. A. Gosselin and J. P. Gagné, "Older adults expend more listening effort than young adults recognizing speech in noise," *Journal of Speech, Language, and Hearing Research*, vol. 54, no. 3, pp. 944–958, 2011.

[41] A. J. Chaffin and S. D. Harlow, "Cognitive learning applied to older adult learners and technology," *Educational Gerontology*, vol. 31, no. 4, pp. 301–329, 2005.

[42] C. Humphrey, K. G. Herbst, and S. Faurqi, "Some characteristics of the hearing-impaired elderly who do not present themselves for rehabilitation," *British Journal of Audiology*, vol. 15, no. 1, pp. 25–30, 1981.

[43] B. Yueh, N. Shapiro, C. H. MacLean, and P. G. Shekelle, "Screening and management of adult hearing loss in primary care: scientific review," *Journal of the American Medical Association*, vol. 289, no. 15, pp. 1976–1985, 2003.

[44] J. L. Smith, P. Mitchell, J. J. Wang, and S. R. Leeder, "A health policy for hearing impairment in older Australians: what should it include?" *Australia and New Zealand Health Policy*, vol. 2, no. 1, article 31, 2005.

[45] B. E. Weinstein and I. M. Ventry, "Audiometric correlates of the hearing handicap inventory for the elderly," *Journal of Speech and Hearing Disorders*, vol. 48, no. 4, pp. 379–384, 1983.

[46] G. A. Gates, M. Murphy, T. S. Rees, and A. Fraher, "Screening for handicapping hearing loss in the elderly," *Journal of Family Practice*, vol. 52, no. 1, pp. 56–62, 2003.

[47] L. Hickson, L. Hamilton, and S. P. Orange, "Factors associated with hearing aid use," *Australian Journal of Audiology*, vol. 8, no. 2, pp. 37–41, 1986.

[48] L. Hickson, M. Timm, L. Worrall, and K. Bishop, "Hearing aid fitting: outcomes for older adults," *Australian Journal of Audiology*, vol. 21, no. 1, pp. 9–21, 1999.

[49] E. Ciurlia-Guy, M. Cashman, and B. Lewsen, "Identifying hearing loss and hearing handicap among chronic care elderly people," *Gerontologist*, vol. 33, no. 5, pp. 644–649, 1993.

[50] M. J. Lichtenstein, F. H. Bess, and S. A. Logan, "Validation of screening tools for identifying hearing-impaired elderly in primary care," *Journal of the American Medical Association*, vol. 259, no. 19, pp. 2875–2878, 1988.

[51] I. M. Ventry and B. E. Weinstein, "Identification of elderly people with hearing problems," *American Speech-Language-Hearing Association*, vol. 25, no. 7, pp. 37–42, 1983.

[52] M. J. Lichtenstein, F. H. Bess, and S. A. Logan, "Diagnostic performance of the hearing handicap inventory for the elderly (screening version) against differing definitions of hearing loss," *Ear and Hearing*, vol. 9, no. 4, pp. 208–211, 1988.

[53] B. Yueh, M. P. Collins, P. E. Souza et al., "Long-term effectiveness of screening for hearing loss: the screening for auditory impairment—which hearing assessment test (SAI-WHAT) randomized trial," *Journal of the American Geriatrics Society*, vol. 58, no. 3, pp. 427–434, 2010.

[54] A. Davis, D. Stephens, A. Rayment, and K. Thomas, "Hearing impairments in middle age: the acceptability, benefit and cost

of detection (ABCD)," *British Journal of Audiology*, vol. 26, no. 1, pp. 1–14, 1992.

[55] C. May, G. Allison, A. Chapple et al., "Framing the doctor-patient relationship in chronic illness: a comparative study of general practitioners' accounts," *Sociology of Health and Illness*, vol. 26, no. 2, pp. 135–158, 2004.

[56] E. L. Harvey, A. Glenny, S. F. Kirk, and C. D. Summerbell, "Improving health professionals' management and the organisation of care for overweight and obese people," *Cochrane Database of Systematic Reviews*, no. 2, Article ID CD000984, 2001.

[57] R. M. Puhl and C. A. Heuer, "The stigma of obesity: a review and update," *Obesity*, vol. 17, no. 5, pp. 941–964, 2009.

[58] L. Epstein and J. Ogden, "A qualitative study of GPs' views of treating obesity," *British Journal of General Practice*, vol. 55, no. 519, pp. 750–754, 2005.

[59] D. A. Cook, A. J. Levinson, S. Garside, D. M. Dupras, P. J. Erwin, and V. M. Montori, "Internet-based learning in the health professions: a meta-analysis," *Journal of the American Medical Association*, vol. 300, no. 10, pp. 1181–1196, 2008.

[60] S. S. Marinopoulos, T. Dorman, N. Ratanawongsa et al., "Effectiveness of continuing medical education," *Evidence Report/Technology Assessment*, no. 149, pp. 1–69, 2007.

[61] L. Forsetlund, A. Bjørndal, A. Rashidian et al., "Continuing education meetings and workshops: effects on professional practice and health care outcomes," *Cochrane Database of Systematic Reviews*, no. 2, Article ID CD003030, 2009.

[62] C. Smits, T. S. Kapteyn, and T. Houtgast, "Development and validation of an automatic speech-in-noise screening test by telephone," *International Journal of Audiology*, vol. 43, no. 1, pp. 15–28, 2004.

[63] C. Meyer, L. Hickson, A. Khan, D. Hartley, H. Dillon, and J. Seymour, "Investigation of the actions taken by adults who failed a telephone-based hearing screen," *Ear and Hearing*, vol. 32, no. 6, pp. 720–731, 2011.

[64] C. Smits, P. Merkus, and T. Houtgast, "How we do it: the Dutch functional hearing-screening tests by telephone and internet," *Clinical Otolaryngology*, vol. 31, no. 5, pp. 436–440, 2006.

[65] N. W. Wilson, I. D. Couper, E. De Vries, S. Reid, T. Fish, and B. J. Marais, "A critical review of interventions to redress the inequitable distribution of healthcare professionals to rural and remote areas," *Rural and Remote Health*, vol. 9, no. 2, p. 1060, 2009.

[66] A. Paglialonga, G. Tognola, and F. Grandori, "Pilot initiatives of adult hearing screening in Italy," *Audiology Research*, vol. 1, no. 1, article e17, 2011.

[67] A. Paglialonga, G. Tognola, and F. Grandori, "SUN-test (Speech Understanding in Noise): a method for hearing disability screening," *Audiology Research*, vol. 1, no. 1, article e13, 2011.

19

Allergic Sensitization to Perennial Allergens in Adults and Children Sensitized to Japanese Cedar or Japanese Cypress Pollen in Japan

Masafumi Ohki[1] and Masanobu Shinogami[2]

[1] Department of Otolaryngology, Saitama Medical Center, 1981 Kamoda, Kawagoe-shi, Saitama 350-8550, Japan
[2] Department of Otolaryngology, Tokyo Metropolitan Police Hospital, 4-22-1 Nakano, Nakano-ku, Tokyo 164-8541, Japan

Correspondence should be addressed to Masafumi Ohki; m-ohki@umin.ac.jp

Academic Editor: Charles Monroe Myer

In Japan, seasonal allergic rhinitis in the spring due to exposure to Japanese cedar or Japanese cypress pollen is common. However, the allergic profile for perennial allergens in spring pollinosis remains unclear. Therefore, in this study, we investigated the allergic profiles of 652 patients with rhinitis. Total serum IgE, serum-specific IgE, and blood eosinophil counts were measured. Allergic sensitization, determined by the serum allergen-specific IgE level, did not always correspond with the patient's symptoms. Only 27% of patients with allergic symptoms in response to spring pollens were sensitized to these allergens alone; 31% of patients were also sensitized to perennial allergens, even without symptoms due to perennial allergens. Total serum IgE and eosinophil cell counts were significantly elevated in patients sensitized to perennial allergens and spring pollens, as compared to patients sensitized only to spring pollens. Most children sensitized to spring pollen (84%) were sensitized to perennial allergens, at a higher rate than adults (49%). Patients sensitized to spring pollens are likely to be latently sensitized to perennial allergens. This is especially true for children and should be monitored closely. Improvement in seasonal allergic conditions, including latent perennial allergy, is important to prevent symptoms that could advance to asthma.

1. Introduction

Seasonal allergic rhinitis caused by either Japanese cedar or Japanese cypress pollen is common in Japan. And Japanese cedar pollinosis is the most prevalent allergy in Japan [1]. In 2003, the prevalence of Japanese cedar pollinosis was reported to be 19.4% [2]. Such patients often complain that their symptoms occur only during the spring. However, patients may be sensitized to other allergens as well, despite being asymptomatic. Allergy is a systemic disorder that can affect the respiratory tract, eyes, skin, and gastrointestinal tract [3] and can cause asthma as well as allergic rhinitis. Perennial allergens such as mites, fungal spores, and domestic animals are considered important risk factors for the development of other allergic disorders such as asthma [4]. To control allergic diseases and prevent allergic rhinitis from progressing to other allergic disorders, it is important

for patients to know their allergic profile, that is, the type and seriousness of their allergy. Therefore, we investigated the allergic profiles and sensitization to other allergens in patients sensitized to either Japanese cedar or Japanese cypress pollens.

2. Materials and Methods

This study was conducted on 652 consecutive outpatients (284 males, 368 females) with rhinitis, from January 2004 to March 2005. Patients enrolled were aged 2–87 years (median age, 44 years) and consisted of 544 adults above 18 years of age (225 men and 319 women; age range, 18–87 years) and 108 children below 18 years of age (59 boys and 49 girls; age range, 2–17 years). Patients with acute rhinosinusitis, common cold, and flu were excluded from the study. None of the patients had been treated previously with any specific immunotherapy. In addition to the standard otorhinolaryn-gological examination, we measured total serum IgE, serum-specific IgE levels (Cap-RAST (Radioallergosorbent test), Bio Medical Laboratories, Inc., Tokyo, Japan), and blood eosinophil counts. These serum tests were done at the time when rhinitis symptoms appeared. Serum-specific IgE was measured for the following allergens: Japanese cedar (*Cryptomeria japonica*), Japanese cypress (*Chamaecyparis obtusa*), grass (*Dactylis glomerata*, *Phleum pratense*, and *Ambrosia artemisiifolia*), cat dandruff, dog dandruff, molds (*Alternaria alternata*, *Aspergillus*, and *Candida*), and mites (*Dermatophagoides pteronyssinus* and *Dermatophagoides fari-nae*). In Japan, pollens of Japanese cedar and Japanese cypress are released mainly in spring [1]. In contrast, pollens of *Dactylis glomerata* and *Phleum pretense* peak in summer, and pollen of *Ambrosia artemisiifolia* is most prevalent in fall. These allergens were classified into three types: spring pollens, summer/fall pollens, and perennial allergens. Spring pollens included Japanese cedar and Japanese cypress. The summer/fall pollen examined was grass. Perennial allergens were cat and dog dandruff, *A. alternata*, *Aspergillus*, *Candida*, and mites. The cutoff value for serum-specific IgE levels was defined as 0.35 kUA/L. The diagnosis of Japanese cedar or Japanese cypress pollinosis is done by otorhinolaryn-gologist according to clinical history, nasal findings, and serum-specific IgE levels. Patients, whose serum-specific IgE levels were more than 0.35 kUA/L, were defined as having sensitization to specific allergens. Asthma is diagnosed by pulmonologists or pediatricians, according to clinical history and physical findings suggesting recurrent episodes of airflow obstruction, and spirometry to demonstrate obstruction and assess reversibility.

The statistical methods used included chi-square tests for trend assessment, the Mann-Whitney U test for assessments of differences between two groups. All reported P values were two-tailed. Statistical analyses were performed using the Ekuseru-Toukei 2012 software (Social Survey Research Information Co. Ltd., Tokyo, Japan).

This study was approved by the local ethics committee and was performed in accordance with the Helsinki Decla-ration (JAMA 2000; 284: 3043-3049). Informed consent was obtained from all patients or their parents.

3. Results

3.1. Sensitization in Patients Symptomatic Only to Japanese Cedar and/or Japanese Cypress.
One hundred and thirty-five patients had allergic symptoms in response to only spring allergens, that is, Japanese cedar and/or Japanese cypress. Only 27% (36/135) of these patients showed allergic sensi-tization exclusively to these allergens, while 34% (46/135) of patients were also sensitized to perennial allergens (31%, 42/135) or summer/fall allergens (3%, 4/135) without allergic symptoms. In addition, 32% (43/135) of patients showed no sensitization to any allergen, despite the presence of allergic symptoms. Of the total, 7% (10/135) of patients were not sensitized to cedar and/or cypress pollen, but only to

TABLE 1: Allergic sensitization.

	Adults	Children	Total
Only spring pollens	93	5	98
Only fall pollens	7	1	8
Only perennial allergens	51	15	66
Spring and fall pollens	17	1	18
Spring pollens and perennial allergens	59	16	75
Fall pollens and perennial allergens	2	0	2
Spring and fall pollens and perennial allergens	47	15	62
No sensitization	268	55	323

summer/fall pollens (1%, 2/135) or perennial allergens (6%, 8/135).

3.2. Allergic Sensitization in Adults and Children.
Three hundred and twenty-nine (50%) of the 652 patients showed allergic sensitization in our study. One hundred and twenty-three of these patients were sensitized only to seasonal allergens (spring (18%, 115/652) or summer/fall pollen (4%, 26/652)), while 21% (137/652) of patients were sensitized to both spring pollens and perennial allergens (Table 1). Ten percent of patients (68/652) were sensitized to perennial allergens but not to spring pollens.

Two hundred and sixteen (40%) of 544 adult patients were sensitized to spring pollens. One hundred and six (49%) of 216 adults were sensitized to perennial allergens as well as spring pollens, while 43% (93/216) of adult patients showed sensitization only to spring pollens, and 8% (17/216) did only to spring and summer/fall pollen. Thirty-seven (34%) of 108 children were sensitized to spring pollens. However, only 5 of 37 children (14%) were sensitized only to spring pollens. Hence, most children (84%; 31/37) sensitized to spring pollens were also sensitized to perennial allergens.

Children were significantly more likely than adults to be sensitized to perennial allergens in addition to spring pollens ($P = 0.0001$, chi-square test). The rate of sensitization to spring pollens gradually increased with the patient's age and peaked in the early 20s (Figure 1) and then fell gradually with age after that. A similar tendency was shown in perennial allergens (mites) although the rate of sensitization peaked at ages 15–17, unlike with spring pollens. In children aged 15–17, the rate of sensitization to perennial allergens (mites) was higher than it was to spring allergens. After patients reached their 20s, the rate of sensitization to spring pollens was higher than perennial allergens (mites).

3.3. Total Serum IgE.
The mean total serum IgE level ± S.E. was 118 ± 16 IU/mL in the 98 patients sensitized only to spring pollen and 609 ± 104 IU/mL in the 137 patients sensi-tized to both perennial allergens and spring pollens (Table 2). Mean total serum IgE level was significantly elevated in patients sensitized to both perennial allergens and spring pollens, as compared to patients sensitized only to spring pollens ($P < 0.0001$, Mann-Whitney U test) (Figure 2(a)).

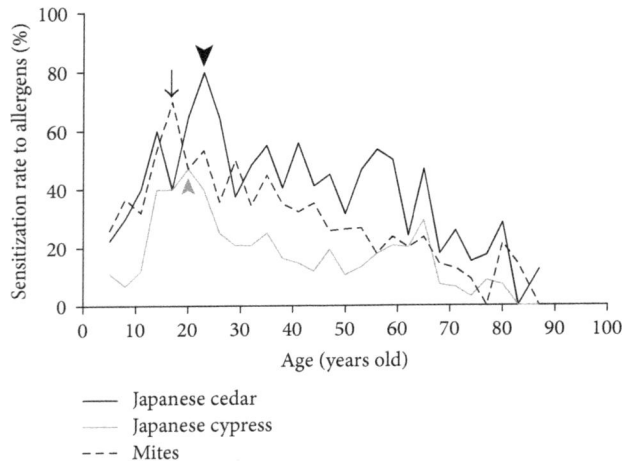

FIGURE 1: The rate of sensitization (determined by RAST) to Japanese cedar, Japanese cypress, and mites was affected by the patient's age. Black arrow head, gray arrow head, and black arrow show the peaks of each rate, respectively.

TABLE 2: Serum total IgE and blood cell eosinophil.

	Total IgE (IU/mL)	Eosinophil cell proportion (%)
Only spring pollens	118 ± 16	4.5 ± 0.4
Only fall pollens	172 ± 93	3.7 ± 1.4
Only perennial allergens	288 ± 51	3.2 ± 0.4
Spring and fall pollens	174 ± 30	5.2 ± 0.9
Spring pollens and perennial allergens	391 ± 67	5.4 ± 0.5
Fall pollens and perennial allergens	—	—
Spring and fall pollens and perennial allergens	878 ± 213	6.1 ± 0.6
No sensitization	120 ± 15	3.1 ± 0.2

The average of total serum IgE levels was highest in 8-17-year olds and decreased with age (Figure 3(a)).

3.4. Blood Cell Eosinophil Count.

The blood cell eosinophil count was also compared between groups. The eosinophil cell proportion was $4.5 \pm 0.4\%$ in patients sensitized only to spring pollens, while it was significantly higher ($5.7 \pm 0.4\%$) in patients sensitized to both perennial allergens and spring pollens ($P = 0.0146$, Mann-Whitney U test) (Figure 2(b), Table 2). The blood cell eosinophil count showed the same reductive tendency (Figure 3(b)).

3.5. Allergic Sensitization in Asthma.

Fifty-nine patients (46 adults, 13 children) had been previously diagnosed with asthma. The remaining 593 patients had not been diagnosed with asthma. Sensitization to any allergen was detected in 58% of patients with asthma (34/59). Twenty-six (44%) of 59 patients were sensitized to spring pollens (Table 3). Approximately half of the asthma patients (51%; 30/59) were sensitized to perennial allergens. Seven percent of patients with asthma (4/59) were sensitized only to spring

TABLE 3: Allergic sensitization in asthma.

Only spring pollens	4
Only fall pollens	0
Only perennial allergens	7
Spring and fall pollens	0
Spring pollens and perennial allergens	14
Fall pollens and perennial allergens	1
Spring and fall pollens and perennial allergens	8
No sensitization	25

pollen, while 16% (94/593) in patients without asthma were sensitized exclusively to these allergens. Thirty-seven percent of patients with a previous asthma diagnosis (22/59) were sensitized to both spring and perennial allergens, which was significantly higher than that observed in patients without asthma (20%; 117/593) ($P = 0.0017$, chi-square test).

Mean total serum IgE levels in patients with asthma were 477 ± 89 IU/mL, while those in patients without asthma were 224 ± 27 IU/mL ($P = 0.0001$ compared to patients with asthma, Mann-Whitney U test). Blood eosinophil cell proportion in patients with asthma was $5.4 \pm 0.6\%$. In patients without asthma, the proportion was $3.9 \pm 0.2\%$. Blood eosinophil cell proportion in patients with asthma was significantly higher than those in patients without asthma ($P = 0.008$, Mann-Whitney U test).

4. Discussion

Allergic sensitization, as diagnosed by the serum allergen-specific IgE level, does not always correspond with the patient's symptoms. We found that approximately twice as many patients were sensitized to both spring pollens and perennial allergens compared to patients sensitized only to spring pollens. However, many patients were asymptomatic to perennial allergens. Exposure to perennial allergens, such as house dust mite and cat and dog dandruff, is an important predisposing risk factor for asthma [4]. Previous diagnosis of asthma was largely related to serum IgE levels and blood eosinophil counts [5–7]. Even in nonasthmatic patients, airway responsiveness (assessed using methacholine [8]) is increased in some cases of allergic rhinitis, indicating an increased risk for asthma [9–11]. Sensitization to cat dandruff, dust mite, cockroach, and ragweed is an important predictor of airway hyperresponsiveness [12]. Airway hyperresponsiveness is strongly related to elevated total serum IgE levels, even in asymptomatic patients [5, 13]. In other words, total serum IgE level is considered an indicator of probable airway hyperresponsiveness or asthma. In our study, total serum IgE levels and blood cell eosinophil counts were significantly elevated in patients sensitized to both spring pollens and perennial allergens, as compared to patients sensitized only to spring pollens. Therefore, patients sensitized to both spring pollens and perennial allergens might be at greater risk of developing airway hyperresponsiveness or asthma.

Compared to adults, fewer children were sensitized only to spring pollens. Most children (approximately 80%) had

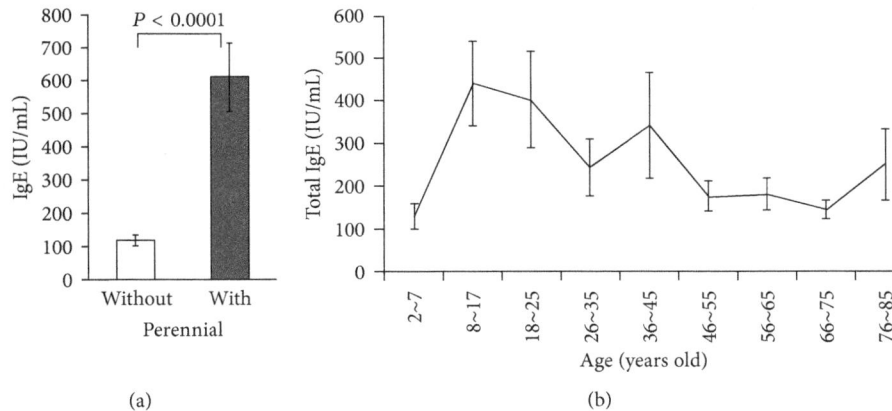

FIGURE 2: (a) Total serum IgE levels were significantly elevated in 137 patients sensitized to both perennial allergens and spring pollens (609 ± 104 IU/mL) compared to 98 patients sensitized only to spring pollens (118 ± 16 IU/mL; $P < 0.0001$, Mann-Whitney U test). (b) Variation of eosinophil cell count with age. This parameter was highest in children 9–17 years of age.

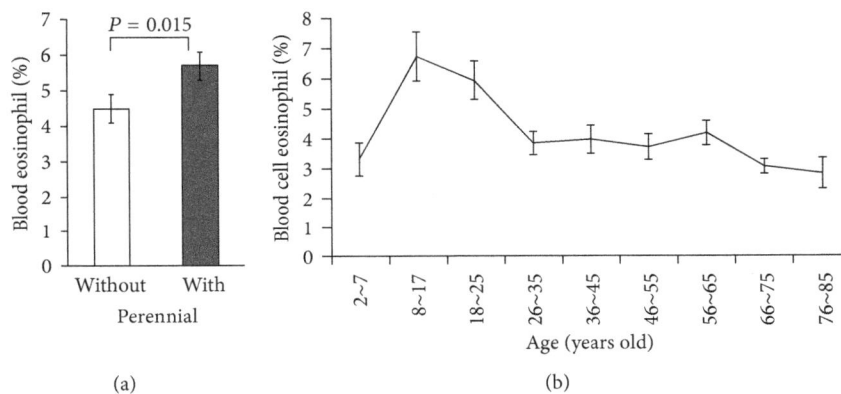

FIGURE 3: (a) Eosinophil cell count was significantly higher in patients sensitized to both perennial allergens and spring pollens (5.7% ± 0.4%) than in patients sensitized only to spring pollens (4.5% ± 0.4%; $P = 0.146$, Mann-Whitney U test). (b) Variation of serum total IgE levels with age. This parameter was highest in children 9–17 years of age.

perennial allergen sensitization as well as spring pollen sensitization if exposed previously, whereas for adults, the proportion was approximately 50%. Early childhood is a critical factor for determining whether a child will be predisposed to asthma later in life [4, 13, 14]. Sensitization to perennial allergens early in life can lead to chronic asthma, characterized by airway hyperresponsiveness and impairment of lung function [14, 15]. In addition, exposure to high levels of perennial allergens aggravates this process, while sensitization to seasonal allergens has not been shown to be important [14]. Therefore, patients with allergic rhinitis caused by spring pollen include those at high risk for developing asthma, since approximately two-thirds of individuals are concomitantly sensitized to perennial allergens without symptoms. Uncontrolled allergic rhinitis may cause the condition of patients with coexisting asthma to deteriorate [16]. On the other hand, seasonal allergens may affect asthma to some degree, considering that patients with hay fever demonstrate airway hyperresponsiveness during pollen season [10]. In addition, disease control by pollen immunotherapy could

help prevent the development of asthma in children with seasonal allergic rhinitis [17]. Improvement in seasonal allergic conditions, including covert perennial allergy, is important for preventing the progression of allergic rhinitis to asthma. In particular, children with seasonal allergic rhinitis should avoid exposure to perennial allergens as well as spring pollens to prevent them from developing asthma. As we found in this study, the majority of children with seasonal allergic rhinitis are also sensitized to perennial allergens. Even children who are not allergic may benefit from minimal exposure to perennial allergens to prevent sensitization. Improvement of allergic conditions is considered important to prevent airway hyperresponsiveness and the development of asthma.

5. Conclusion

Patients who have been sensitized to spring pollen are also likely to have been covertly sensitized to perennial allergens. This is especially true for children. Improvement in the seasonal allergic conditions, including covert perennial allergy, is considered important for preventing the development of asthma.

Conflict of Interests

The authors declare that there is no conflict of interests regarding the publication of this paper.

References

[1] N. Maeda, N. Inomata, A. Morita, M. Kirino, and Z. Ikezawa, "Correlation of oral allergy syndrome due to plant-derived foods with pollen sensitization in Japan," *Annals of Allergy, Asthma and Immunology*, vol. 104, no. 3, pp. 205–210, 2010.

[2] M. Okuda, "Epidemiology of Japanese cedar pollinosis throughout Japan," *Annals of Allergy, Asthma and Immunology*, vol. 91, no. 3, pp. 288–296, 2003.

[3] G.-J. Braunstahl, "The unified immune system: respiratory tract-nasobronchial interaction mechanisms in allergic airway disease," *Journal of Allergy and Clinical Immunology*, vol. 115, no. 1, pp. 142–148, 2005.

[4] R. Sporik, S. T. Holgate, T. A. E. Platts-Mills, and J. J. Cogswell, "Exposure to house-dust mite allergen (Der p I) and the development of asthma in childhood. A prospective study," *New England Journal of Medicine*, vol. 323, no. 8, pp. 502–507, 1990.

[5] M. R. Sears, B. Burrows, E. M. Flannery, G. P. Herbison, C. J. Hewitt, and M. D. Holdaway, "Relation between airway responsiveness and serum IgE in children with asthma and in apparently normal children," *New England Journal of Medicine*, vol. 325, no. 15, pp. 1067–1071, 1991.

[6] B. Burrows, F. D. Marinez, M. Halonen, R. A. Barbee, and M. G. Cline, "Association of asthma with serum IgE levels and skin-test reactivity to allergens," *New England Journal of Medicine*, vol. 320, no. 5, pp. 271–277, 1989.

[7] M. Kerkhof, J. P. Schouten, and J. G. R. De Monchy, "The association of sensitization to inhalant allergens with allergy symptoms: the influence of bronchial hyperresponsiveness and blood eosinophil count," *Clinical and Experimental Allergy*, vol. 30, no. 10, pp. 1387–1394, 2000.

[8] R. G. Townley, U. Y. Ryo, B. M. Kolotkin, and B. Kang, "Bronchial sensitivity to methacholine in current and former asthmatic and allergic rhinitis patients and control subjects," *Journal of Allergy and Clinical Immunology*, vol. 56, no. 6, pp. 429–442, 1975.

[9] S. S. Braman, A. A. Barrows, B. A. DeCotiis, G. A. Settipane, and W. M. Corrao, "Airway hyperresponsiveness in allergic rhinitis. A risk factor for asthma," *Chest*, vol. 91, no. 5, pp. 671–674, 1987.

[10] E. Madonini, G. Briatico-Vangosa, A. Pappacoda, G. Maccagni, A. Cardani, and F. Saporiti, "Seasonal increase of bronchial reactivity in allergic rhinitis," *Journal of Allergy and Clinical Immunology*, vol. 79, no. 2, pp. 358–363, 1987.

[11] E. H. Ramsdale, M. M. Morris, R. S. Roberts, and F. E. Hargreave, "Asymptomatic bronchial hyperresponsiveness in rhinitis," *Journal of Allergy and Clinical Immunology*, vol. 75, no. 5, pp. 573–577, 1985.

[12] E. C. Tepas, A. A. Litonjua, J. C. Celedón, D. Sredl, and D. R. Gold, "Sensitization to aeroallergens and airway hyperresponsiveness at 7 years of age," *Chest*, vol. 129, no. 6, pp. 1500–1508, 2006.

[13] B. Burrows, M. R. Sears, E. M. Flannery, G. P. Herbison, and M. D. Holdaway, "Relationships of bronchial responsiveness assessed by methacholine to serum IgE, lung function, symptoms, and diagnoses in 11-year-old New Zealand children," *Journal of Allergy and Clinical Immunology*, vol. 90, no. 3, pp. 376–385, 1992.

[14] S. Illi, E. von Mutius, S. Lau, B. Niggemann, C. Grüber, and U. Wahn, "Perennial allergen sensitisation early in life and chronic asthma in children: a birth cohort study," *The Lancet*, vol. 368, no. 9537, pp. 763–770, 2006.

[15] O. Linna, J. Kokkonen, and M. Lukin, "A 10-year prognosis for childhood allergic rhinitis," *Acta Paediatrica*, vol. 81, no. 2, pp. 100–102, 1992.

[16] F. E. R. Simons, "Allergic rhinobronchitis: the asthma-allergic rhinitis link," *Journal of Allergy and Clinical Immunology*, vol. 104, no. 3, pp. 534–540, 1999.

[17] C. Möller, S. Dreborg, H. A. Ferdousi et al., "Pollen immunotherapy reduces the development of asthma in children with seasonal rhinoconjunctivitis (the PAT-Study)," *Journal of Allergy and Clinical Immunology*, vol. 109, no. 2, pp. 251–256, 2002.

20

Clinical Predictors for Successful Uvulopalatopharyngoplasty in the Management of Obstructive Sleep Apnea

Aamir Yousuf, Zafarullah Beigh, Raja Salman Khursheed, Aleena Shafi Jallu, and Rafiq Ahmad Pampoori

Department of ENT and HNS, Government Medical College, Srinagar, Jammu and Kashmir 190001, India

Correspondence should be addressed to Aamir Yousuf; miraamir_83@yahoo.com

Academic Editor: David W. Eisele

Objective. To assess the clinical parameters for successful uvulopalatopharyngoplasty in the management of obstructive sleep apnoea syndrome documented with pre- and postoperative polysomnography. *Materials and Methods.* A study group of 50 patients diagnosed as having OSA by full night polysomnography were assessed clinically and staged on basis of Friedman staging system. BMI and neck circumference were considered, and videoendoscopy with Muller's maneuver was done in all to document the site of obstruction. The study group divided into surgical and nonsurgical ones. Twenty-two patients out of fifty were then selected for uvulopalatopharyngoplasty. The selection of surgical group was done primarily on basis of clinical parameters like neck circumference, Friedman stage of the patient and site, and/or level of obstruction of patient. Postoperative polysomnography was done six months after surgery to document the change in AHI score. *Result.* The study group consists of fifty patients with mean age of 44.4 ± 9.3 years. UPPP was done in twenty-two, and the result of the surgery as defined by 50% reduction in preoperative AHI with postoperative AHI < 20/h was seen to be 95.2%. Postoperative change in AHI done after 6-month interval was seen to be statistically significant with P value < 0.001. *Conclusion.* UPPP is ideal option for management of obstructive sleep apnoea syndrome in properly selected patients on the basis of Friedman stage and site of obstruction detected by videoendoscopy with Muller's maneuver.

1. Introduction

Obstructive sleep apnea (OSA) is a common condition, affecting 4% of men and 2% of women [1]. Currently the condition is diagnosed by history, physical examination, imaging studies, and polysomnography. Common symptoms of the condition have limited predictive value in identifying patients with OSA. The upper airway is the main anatomical site responsible for OSA. Clinical examination may point to severe retrognathia, hypertrophic tonsils, macroglossia and redundant pillars, elongated uvula, and a crowded oropharynx [2]. Endoscopic investigations have been performed in awake as well as in sleeping patients, with the pharynx in relaxed or active states, but their predictive value remains limited, both for diagnostic purposes and for identifying patients who may benefit from surgery [3]. The otolaryngologist has the unique opportunity to examine the palate, pharynx, and neck of the patient and suspect OSA when appropriate. Diagnosis of a disease is based on clinical symptoms and physical findings and is corroborated by laboratory examinations. Polysomnography remains the standard in the diagnosis of sleep-related breathing disorders [2, 4]. Continuous positive airway pressure (CPAP), a technique that pneumatically supports the upper airway, is a therapeutic mainstay for OSA, other options for patients with OSA, including risk factor modification such as weight loss, oral appliances that advance the mandible or tongue during sleep, or a variety of surgical procedures to bypass or expand the upper airway [5]. The most common surgical procedure performed for OSA is uvulopalatopharyngoplasty (UPPP) Introduced by Fujita et al. in 1981; UPPP involves tonsillectomy (if not previously performed), trimming and reorientation of the posterior and anterior tonsillar pillars, and excision of the uvula and posterior palate. Often, UPPP is combined with other nasopharyngeal or oropharyngeal procedures. The reported success of UPPP as a treatment of OSA is between 16% and 83%, depending on the definition of a positive outcome and selection of patients. Some authors have defined surgical success or cure after UPPP as a 50% reduction in the AHI, whereas others combine this criterion with an absolute AHI of 20 or less [3, 6–8].

2. Materials and Methods

This study was conducted in Department of Otorhinolaryngology and Head Neck Surgery, Government Medical College Srinagar, Jammu and Kashmir, India, from January 2010 to June 2011 and was approved by institutional ethics committee. Any patient who came to our department directly or had been referred from other centres with one or more complaints of excessive daytime somnolence (EDS), snoring, or observed apnoea was identified as high risk and underwent full assessment. The study group of total 50 patients was selected among those most high risk patients for OSAS and was analysed thoroughly and properly diagnosed as obstructive sleep apnoea using full night polysomnography. The sleep study (in hospital full night polysomnography) of all the patient was done in order to objectively quantify any sleep apnoea using Embletta Gold device, and the data was analysed by using Remlogic software. The parameters considered were electroencephalography, electrocardiography, abdominal movements, thoracic movements, snore nasal pressure by nasal thermistor, Spo2 level (pulse oximeter), Pulse rate, Body position, and flow pressure (nasal cannula). On the basis of these parameters apnea, hypopneas, snore level, and oxygen deasturation level were noticed, and patients were classified on the basis of their AHI (apnea/hypopnea index). The various events/indexes of sleep-related breathing disorders, apnea, is defined as reduction in airflow greater than $\geq 90\%$ as recorded by oronasal thermistors or nasal pressure cannulas lasting ≥ 10 sec. Hypopnea is defined as reduction in airflow $\geq 30\%$ as recorded by nasal pressure cannulas or alternatively by induction of plethysmography or oronasal thermistors lasting ≥ 10 sec with reduction in saturation at least $\geq 4\%$ from baseline SpO2% prior to the event. Apnea-hypopnea index (AHI) is defined as the number of apneas and hypopneas per hour of sleep, confirmed by electroencephalogram (EEG) [2]. All the essential anthropometric measurements like neck circumference and body mass index were tabulated. The clinical assessment of the upper airway was done for any abnormality that could contribute to airway narrowing, such as a deviated nasal septum or a small oropharyngeal airway and tonsil size, and tongue/palatal position was considered [7, 9]. The Friedman tongue position is based on visualization of structures in the mouth with the mouth open widely without protrusion of the tongue. Palate Grade I allows the observer to visualize the entire uvula and tonsils. Palate Grade II allows visualization of the uvula but not the tonsils. Palate Grade III allows visualization of the soft palate but not the uvula. Palate Grade IV allows visualization of the hard palate. All the patients were then staged on the basis of Friedman staging system that includes tonsil size, Friedman tongue position, and BMI of patients. In all patients videoendoscopy with Muller's maneuver was done, and site of obstruction was documented. Videoendoscopy was done using fiberoptic laryngoscope, and the patients were explained to inspire forcibly against closed mouth and nose,

TABLE 1: Age wise distribution of patients ($n = 50$).

Age (year)	n	% age
≤30	4	8.0
31 to 40	12	24.0
41 to 50	22	44.0
51 to 60	12	24.0
mean ± SD		44.4 ± 9.3 (18, 60)

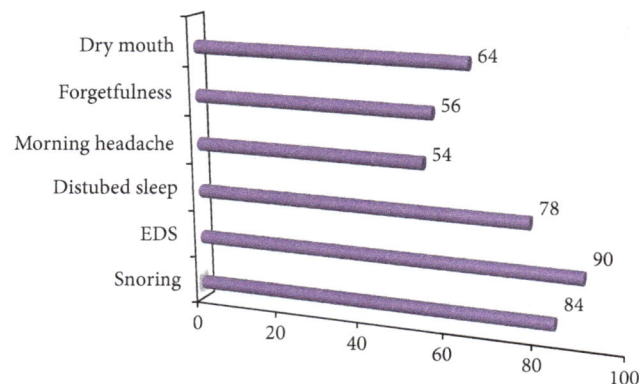

FIGURE 1: Distribution of presenting complaints.

and collapse of upper airway was documented at retropalatal, retrolingual, and hypopharyngeal levels [3, 10]. The study group of fifty was then divided into surgical and nonsurgical groups. Twenty-two patients out of fifty were selected for uvulopalatopharyngoplasty. The selection of surgical group was done primarily on the basis of clinical parameters like neck circumference, BMI and Friedman stage of the patient, and site and/or level of obstruction of the patient [10, 11]. Patients with Friedman stage I and II along with unilevel obstruction mostly at retropalatal level and with less neck circumference were selected for surgery.

3. Results

The study group comprises of total fifty patients of mean age 44.4 ± 9.3 years with 56% males and 44% females Table 1. The most common presenting complaints of our patients were snoring seen in 84% and excessive day time sleepiness seen in 90% (Figure 1). All the patients were thoroughly evaluated, and neck circumference and body mass index (BMI) were considered. The neck circumference ranges from 24 cm to 42 cm with mean 36.6 cm, and the BMI ranges from 27 kg/m² to 40 kg/m² with mean 34.7 kg/m². The mean AHI of all the patients was 53/h that ranges from 22 to 81/h. In our study group all the fifty patients were grouped on the basis of Friedman tongue position as I, II, III, and IV with 0%, 28%, 46%, and 26%, respectively. On basis of tonsil size of patients, it was seen that 30% of the patients had Grade 2 and 26% and 24% patients had Grade 1 and grade 3 tonsillar enlargement, respectively, and grade 0 was seen in 12% and grade 4 in 8% of patients. Grouping together these characteristics, all the patients were graded on Friedman staging system as stage I,

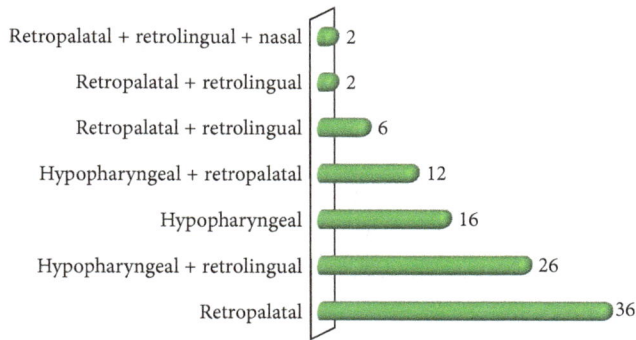

FIGURE 2: Site of obstruction seen by videoendoscopy with Muller's maneuver.

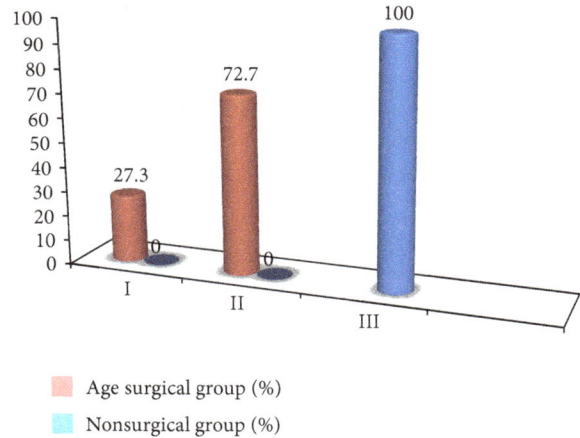

Age surgical group (%)

Nonsurgical group (%)

FIGURE 3: Comparison of surgical and nonsurgical group of patients on the basis of friedman stage.

II, and III. Friedman stage I constitutes 12%, stage II, 32%, and stage III, 56% of patients. For determining the exact site of obstruction in study group patients, videoendoscopy with Mueller's maneuver was done (Figure 3). In 36% of the patients only retropalatal obstruction was seen and in 16% only hypopharyngeal. The rest of the patients have multilevel obstruction with 26% having hypopharyngeal and retrolingual and 12% with hypopharyngeal and retropalatal. 6% of the patients had retropalatal and retrolingual; retropalatal, retrolingual, and nasal in 2%; and retropalatal, nasal in 2% of patients as shown in Table 2 and Figure 2. The degree of collapse of upper airway was graded as 1+ minimal collapse, 2+ is 50% collapse, 3+ is 75% collapse, and 4+ is obliteration of the airway. The study group of fifty patients was then divided into surgical and nonsurgical groups. The surgical group selected was entirely on clinical parameters like neck circumference, BMI, tonsil grade, tongue position, and level of upper airway collapse. There was significant (P value < 0.001) difference of these parameters among surgical and nonsurgical groups of patients as shown in Table 3. On the basis of tonsil grade criteria, the surgical group was selected with higher grade of tonsil (54.5% had Grade 3 and 27.3% had Grade 2); lesser tonsil grade patients were kept in nonsurgical group (Grade 1 in 46.4% and Grade 2 in 32.1%) as shown in Table 4. This was seen to be statistically significant with P value of <0.001. On the basis of Friedman tongue position, the patients with lower FTP were selected for surgical group (Grade 2,54.5% and Grade 3,45.5%) as compared to nonsurgical group where patients with higher FTP were kept like Grade 3 (56.6%) and Grade 4 (46.4%). This difference was statistically significant with P value of <0.001 as shown in Table 5. Among the surgical group of 22 patients, 77.3% of the patients had only retropalatal obstruction, and in 13.6% of patients retropalatal and retrolingual obstruction was seen; retropalatal, retrolingual, and nasal obstruction was seen in 4.5%; and retropalatal and nasal in 4.5% of patients as shown in Tables 6 and 7. This group of patients was selected for UPPP, and the result of the surgery as defined by 50% reduction in preoperative AHI with postoperative AHI < 20/h was seen to be 95.2%. Significant change in major presenting symptoms was documented six months after surgery as shown in Table 9. Postoperative change in

TABLE 2: Site of obstruction seen by videoendoscopy with Muller's maneuver.

Site of obstruction	No. of patients	Percentage
Hypopharyngeal	8	16
Retropalatal	18	36
Hypopharyngeal + retropalatal	6	12
Hypopharyngeal + retrolingual	13	26
Retropalatal + retrolingual	3	6
Retropalatal + nasal	1	2
Retropalatal + retrolingual + nasal	1	2
Total	50	100

TABLE 3: Comparative analysis of surgical and nonsurgical groups on physical parameters.

Physical parameter	Surgical group Mean ± SD	Non surgical group Mean ± SD	P value
Neck size cm	32.2 ± 3.2	40.0 ± 1.9	<0.001 (Sig)
BMI (wt/h m²)	31.7 ± 2.9	37.0 ± 1.8	<0.000 (Sig)

AHI done after 6-month interval was seen to be statistically significant with P value < 0.00 as shown in Table 8 and Figure 4.

4. Discussion

Uvulopalatopharyngoplasty is the most common surgical procedure performed for the management of OSAS, but the success rate and the role of UPPP in the management of OSA remain unclear because most studies are limited by small sample size, lack of consensus on a clear definition of surgical success, and an inability to compare UPPP in a blinded

TABLE 4: Comparison of surgical and nonsurgical group on the basis of tonsil grade.

Tonsil grade	Surgical group (n = 22)		Non surgical group (n = 28)		P value
	n	% age	n	% age	
0	0	0.0	6	21.4	
1	0	0.0	13	46.4	
2	6	27.3	9	32.1	<0.001 (sig)
3	12	54.5	0	0.0	
4	4	18.2	0	0.0	

χ^2 test analysis.

TABLE 5: Comparison of surgical and non surgical patient groups on the basis of Friedman tongue position.

FTP	Surgical group (n = 22)		Non surgical group (n = 28)		P value
	n	%	n	%	
2	12	54.5	0	0.00	
3	10	45.5	15	56.6	<0.001 (sig)
4	0	0.00	13	46.4	
Total	22	100	28	100	

χ^2 test analysis.

TABLE 6: Distribution of patients in surgical group on site of obstruction (n = 22).

Site of obstruction	No. of patients	Percentage
Retropalatal	17	77.3
Retropalatal + retrolingual	3	13.6
Retropalatal + retrolingual	1	4.5
Retropalatal + retrolingual + nasal	1	4.5
Total	22	100

TABLE 7: Distribution of patients on site of obstruction surgical versus nonsurgical groups.

Site of obstruction	Surgical group		Non surgical group		P value
	n	Percentage	n	Percentage	
Single	17	77.3	9	32.1	0.002 (sig)
Multiple	5	22.7	19	67.9	
Total	22	100	28	100	

χ^2 test analysis.

TABLE 8: Preoperative and postoperative AHI of surgical group.

	Mean	SD	P value
Pre-Op PSG AHI score/Hr	43.1	16.4	<0.001 (Sig)
Post-Op PSG AHI score/Hr	13.2	4.1	

TABLE 9: Preoperative and postoperative comparison of symptoms.

Symptoms	Preoperative		Postoperative		P value
	n	%	n	%	
Snoring	18	81.8	3	13.6	<0.001 (Sig)
EDS	20	90.9	2	9.1	<0.001 (sig)
Disturbed Sleep	18	81.8	4	18.2	<0.001 (Sig)
Morning Headache	9	40.9	2	9.1	0.020 (Sig)
Forgetfulness	8	36.4	4	18.2	0.157 (NS)
Dry Mouth	11	50.0	4	18.2	0.008 (Sig)

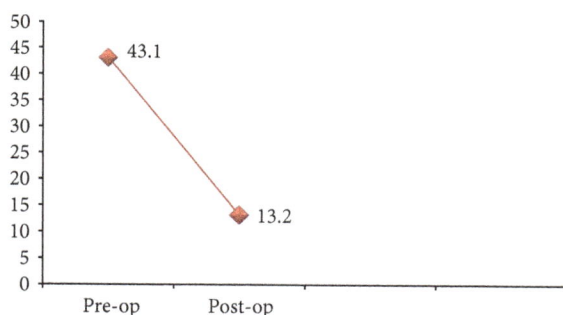

FIGURE 4: Preoperative and Postoperative AHI of surgical group.

manner with CPAP [1, 2, 7]. The main goal of this study was to redefine the ideal clinical parameters to identify those patients with high likelihood of successful UPPP and separate them from those with high likelihood of failure, thus guiding patient selection and improving outcome. Traditionally, a successful outcome of UPPP has been defined as achieving a reduction in AHI of at least 50% and/or a residual AHI of 20 or less. The study format analysing clinical parameters like neck circumference, level/site of obstruction in addition to BMI, tonsil grade, and Friedman palatal position have augmented the guiding criteria for improving the successful result of UPPP in the management of OSAS. Friedman stage I and II were considered for surgery, and stage III was compared as nonsurgical group. Friedman stage was also seen to be significantly correlated with the AHI severity of patient, so the patients in the surgical group were having lesser severity of disease on the basis of AHI as compared to the nonsurgical group. The neck size and BMI of patients in surgical group were seen to be significantly less as compared to nonsurgical group [7, 11, 12]. On the basis of site of obstruction as seen with videoendoscopy with Mueller's manoeuvre, patients with retropalatal and retrolingual were only considered for surgery and all the hypopharyngeal and multilevel obstruction patients were excluded to increase surgical outcome rates. So the videoendoscopy is a complementary diagnostic tool that can be easily performed, especially for surgeons who need to know where and how the obstruction occurs [3, 7, 13]. The successful outcome of the surgery as defined by 50% reduction in preoperative AHI with postoperative AHI < 20/h was seen to be 95.2% as shown in Figure 4. In almost all previous studies done for UPPP, utmost 80% successful treatment outcome was achieved as in all these level/site of obstruction was neglected. As most of the patients have multilevel obstruction with hypopharyngeal as one of the component, UPPP that corrects retropalatal and retrolingual obstruction only is not sufficient treatment. This improved successful treatment goal with UPPP is possible only through proper selection of patients on merits of neck size and site of obstruction in addition to Friedman staging system [7, 8, 11, 13]. In addition, there was no craniofacial abnormality in our selected group, hypopharyngeal obstruction was not considered, and the sample size, once stratified, was relatively small. One of the strengths of the our study is the assessment of pre-UPPP and post-UPPP symptomatology changes in

major symptoms as measured by working questionnaires which may strengthen interpretation of the surgical results. Significant changes were noted in major symptoms after surgery. While success rates are slightly higher than those published by Friedman and colleagues, the response seen with this anatomic staging system suggests that this is an effective method for stratifying surgical OSA patients for possible successful UPPP surgery.

5. Conclusion

This study redefines the clinical assessment parameters of OSAS patients for successful outcome of the UPPP. UPPP is a better option for management of obstructive sleep apnoea syndrome in properly selected patients on the basis of Friedman stage and site of obstruction detected by videoendoscopy with muller's maneuver. All cases of obstruction at the palatal level can be addressed by UPPP with satisfactory success rate.

References

[1] C. Guilleminault and V. C. Abad, "Obstructive sleep apnea syndromes," *The Medical Clinics of North America*, vol. 88, no. 3, pp. 611–630, 2004.

[2] W. T. McNicholas, "Diagnosis of obstructive sleep apnea in adults," *Proceedings of the American Thoracic Society*, vol. 5, no. 2, pp. 154–160, 2008.

[3] U. Tunçel, H. M. Inançli, S. S. Kürkçüoğlu, and M. Enöz, "Can the Müller maneuver detect multilevel obstruction of the upper airway in patients with obstructive sleep apnea syndrome?" *Kulak Burun Boğaz Ihtisas Dergisi*, vol. 20, no. 2, pp. 84–88, 2010.

[4] E. M. Weaver, V. Kapur, and B. Yueh, "Polysomnography versus aelf-reported measures in patients with sleep apnea," *Archives of Otolaryngology*, vol. 130, no. 4, pp. 453–458, 2004.

[5] M. A. D. O. Almeida, A. O. D. B. Teixeira, L. S. Vieira, and C. C. A. Quintão, "Treatment of obstructive sleep apnea and hipoapnea syndrome with oral appliances," *Brazilian Journal of Otorhinolaryngology*, vol. 72, no. 5, pp. 699–703, 2006.

[6] A. Khan, K. Ramar, S. Maddirala, O. Friedman, J. F. Pallanch, and E. J. Olson, "Uvulopalatopharyngoplasty in the management of obstructive sleep apnea: the mayo clinic experience," *Mayo Clinic Proceedings*, vol. 84, no. 9, pp. 795–800, 2009.

[7] R. P. Millman, C. C. Carlisle, C. Rosenberg, D. Kahn, R. McRae, and N. R. Kramer, "Simple predictors of uvulopalatopharyngoplasty outcome in the treatment of obstructive sleep apnea," *Chest*, vol. 118, no. 4, pp. 1025–1030, 2000.

[8] J. D. Harwick, "Preface," *Otolaryngologic clinic of North America*, vol. 40, pp. 11–12, 2007.

[9] D. Schlosshan and M. W. Elliott, "Sleep·3: clinical presentation and diagnosis of the obstructive sleep apnoea hypopnoea syndrome," *Thorax*, vol. 59, no. 4, pp. 347–352, 2004.

[10] L. Valera Veloro, "Michael alexius adea sarte, samantha soriano castaneda. Collar size as predictor of sleep apnoea," *Phillipine Journal of Otolaryngology*, vol. 23, no. 2, pp. 14–16, 2008.

[11] A. I. Zonato, L. R. Bittencourt, F. L. Martinho, J. Ferreira Santos Jr., L. C. Gregório, and S. Tufik, "Association of systematic head and neck physical examination with severity of obstructive sleep apnea-hypopnea syndrome," *The Laryngoscope*, vol. 113, no. 6, pp. 973–980, 2003.

[12] A. Dreher, R. de la Chaux, C. Klemens et al., "Correlation between otorhinolaryngologic evaluation and severity of
obstructive sleep apnea syndrome in snorers," *Archives of Otolaryngology*, vol. 131, no. 2, pp. 95–98, 2005.

[13] M. Friedman, H. Tanyeri, M. la Rosa et al., "Clinical predictors
of obstructive sleep apnea," *The Laryngoscope*, vol. 109, no. 12,
pp. 1901–1907, 1999.

21

Utility of Intraoperative Frozen Sections during Thyroid Surgery

Russel Kahmke,[1] Walter T. Lee,[1,2] Liana Puscas,[1,2] Richard L. Scher,[1] Michael J. Shealy,[3] Warner M. Burch,[4] and Ramon M. Esclamado[1]

[1] *Division of Otolaryngology-Head and Neck Surgery, Department of Surgery, Duke University Medical Center, Duke University, Durham, NC 27710, USA*
[2] *Section of Otolaryngology-Head and Neck Surgery, Department of Surgery, Durham VA Medical Center, Durham, NC 27705, USA*
[3] *Division of Pathology Clinical Services, Department of Pathology, Duke University Medical Center, Duke University, Durham, NC 27710, USA*
[4] *Division of Endocrinology, Metabolism, and Nutrition, Department of Medicine, Duke University Medical Center, Duke University, Durham, NC 27710, USA*

Correspondence should be addressed to Walter T. Lee; walter.lee@duke.edu

Academic Editor: Richard L. Doty

Objective. To describe the usefulness of intraoperative frozen section in the diagnosis and treatment of thyroid nodules where fine needle aspirate biopsies have evidence of follicular neoplasm. *Study Design.* Retrospective case series. *Methods.* All patients have a fine needle aspirate biopsy, an intraoperative frozen section, and final pathology performed on a thyroid nodule after initiation of the Bethesda System for Reporting Thyroid Cytopathology in 2009 at a single tertiary referral center. Sensitivity, specificity, positive predictive value, and negative predictive value are calculated in order to determine added benefit of frozen section to original fine needle aspirate data. *Results.* The sensitivity and specificity of the frozen section were 76.9% and 67.9%, respectively, while for the fine needle aspirate were 53.8% and 74.1%, respectively. The positive and negative predictive values for the fine needle aspirates were 25% and 90.9%, respectively, while for the frozen sections were 27.8% and 94.8%, respectively. There were no changes in the operative course as a consequence of the frozen sections. *Conclusion.* Our data does not support the clinical usefulness of intraoperative frozen section when the fine needle aspirate yields a Bethesda Criteria diagnosis of follicular neoplasm, suspicious for follicular neoplasm, or suspicious for malignancy at our institution.

1. Introduction

The incidence of thyroid cancer increased 2.4-fold from 3.6 to 8.7 per 100,000 Americans [1] over a thirty-year period ending in 2002. The annual incidence of palpable thyroid nodules in North America is 0.1% [2] and most of those under 1 cm cannot be detected by physical exam alone [3]. The introduction of high resolution ultrasound technology has increased our ability to diagnose thyroid nodules [4]. A patient of male gender, aged <20 years or >70 years, with a family history of medullary thyroid carcinoma (MTC) or multiple endocrine neoplasia (MEN), rapid nodular growth, a firm or fixed nodule, a history of head and neck irradiation, a nodule that is >4 cm or is partially cystic, or a compressive sensation should raise increased suspicion for thyroid carcinoma [5].

In 2009, the Bethesda Criteria for Reporting Thyroid Cytopathology were published to create a common language by which multidisciplinary teams could accurately discuss the diagnosis and implications of a fine needle aspiration (FNA) biopsy [6]. The six categories found within the Bethesda Criteria each implies a different malignancy risk (Table 1) and treatment approaches ranging from watchful waiting to total thyroidectomy with postoperative radioactive iodine.

FNA biopsies with a diagnosis of follicular neoplasm, suspicious for follicular neoplasm, or suspicious for malignancy carry a 15–75% chance of malignancy [6]. Unfortunately, it is difficult to distinguish between follicular adenoma and follicular carcinoma based solely on an FNA biopsy because histologic evidence of capsular and/or vascular invasion is required to determine malignancy for a follicular lesion [7]. Approximately 30% of these FNA biopsies showing follicular

TABLE 1: Fine needle aspiration biopsy diagnostic categories, adapted from Cibas and Ali (The Bethesda System for Thyroid Cytopathology) [6].

Diagnostic category	Risk of malignancy (%)
Nondiagnostic or unsatisfactory	1–4
Benign	0–3
Atypia or follicular lesion of undetermined significance	5–15
Follicular neoplasm or suspicious for follicular neoplasm	15–30
Suspicious for malignancy	60–75
Malignant	97–99

TABLE 2: Stratification of fine needle aspiration biopsies according to Bethesda system.

Diagnostic category	Number of samples
Non-diagnostic or unsatisfactory	0
Benign	34
Atypia or follicular lesion of undetermined significance	32
Follicular neoplasm or suspicious for follicular neoplasm	26
Suspicious for malignancy	2
Malignant	0

lesions prove to be malignant on histologic examination [8]. A diagnostic thyroid lobectomy provides the tissue necessary for a pathologic diagnosis.

In thyroid surgery, intraoperative FS is used to assist in further surgical treatment at this point in care, with good concordance rates between FNA results and FS in the setting of papillary thyroid carcinoma [9]. However, FS is usually insufficient to determine true capsular or vascular invasion and deferral to a final pathologic diagnosis is often necessary in the setting of a follicular lesion [10]. The use of intraoperative FS has long been debated secondary to concerns about increased cost and operative time without a true consensus [11].

The overall objective of this study was to describe the usefulness of intraoperative FS in the diagnosis and treatment of thyroid nodules where FNA biopsies have evidence of follicular neoplasm. This was achieved by (1) determining the sensitivity and specificity of FS with both FNA and final pathology, (2) assessing the added benefit of FS to information obtained from the FNA, and (3) calculating the positive predictive value (PPV) and negative predictive value (NPV) of FS as a tool for intraoperative decision making.

2. Materials and Methods

This retrospective chart review was approved by the Duke University School of Medicine Institutional Review Board. The review was performed on patients who have been evaluated and treated for a thyroid nodule within the Duke University Health System after the initiation of the Bethesda System for Reporting Thyroid Cytopathology in 2009. Our inclusion criteria required that a fine needle aspiration biopsy and an operative procedure with intraoperative frozen section and final pathology be performed at our tertiary care center. Our exclusion criteria included an FNA biopsy diagnostic of malignancy (e.g., papillary carcinoma), nondiagnostic/unsatisfactory FNA samples, FNA reports not in congruence with the Bethesda Criteria, and a history of irradiation to the head and neck.

FNA and intraoperative FS results were compared with final pathology. An FNA specimen was considered "suggests negative" if it was reported as "benign", "negative," or of "undetermined significance." An FNA specimen was "suggests positive" if it showed "follicular neoplasm", "suspicious for follicular neoplasm," or "suspicious for malignancy". Reports showing "Hurthle cell" within the description were considered to be part of the "follicular neoplasm" category. An FS specimen was considered "suggests negative" if the pathologist reported "benign", "adenoma", "negative for malignancy", "nodular hyperplasia", or "goiter". An FS specimen was considered "suggests positive" for reports of "follicular lesion", "follicular neoplasm", "suspicious for carcinoma/malignancy", "atypical features", or "defer". Final pathology was deemed positive if malignancy was found, regardless of size (i.e., incidentally found microcarcinoma). Sensitivity, specificity, positive predictive value (PPV), and negative predictive value (NPV) were calculated.

3. Results and Discussion

A total of 93 patients met inclusion criteria with 72 females (77.4%) and 21 males (22.6%). Median age was 51.9 years with a range between 9 and 76. One patient had two suspicious lesions which were analyzed, resulting in 94 thyroid nodules available for statistical analysis.

Table 2 shows the stratification of FNA results that were available for analysis. No patients had FNA reporting malignancy or nondiagnostic/unsatisfactory per study design. There were 32 samples that were read as atypia or follicular lesion of undetermined significance and 26 samples read as follicular neoplasm or suspicious for follicular neoplasm. The rest were read as either benign or suspicious for malignancy (34 and 2 samples, resp.). Despite the 0–3% risk of malignancy for benign diagnostic category, there were additional indications for surgery including suspicious ultrasound findings, compressive symptoms, persistent growth, or even patient preference. There were four patients noted to have nondiagnostic/insufficient FNA biopsies, one with a negative FS and positive final pathology (papillary carcinoma), two with FS suggesting positive although final pathology was negative, and one with both negative FS and final pathology. There were 2 patients who were diagnostic malignancy where their FS and final pathology were both positive (papillary carcinoma and metastatic melanoma).

Table 3 shows each patient and the correlation between the FNA Bethesda Criteria, FS, and final pathology. The

TABLE 3: Fine needle aspiration (FNA) Bethesda Criteria and frozen section (FS) compared with final pathology.

FNA	Frozen section	Final pathology		
Benign	Negative	Negative	19	
		Positive	1	FVPC
	Positive	Negative	12	
		Positive	2	FVPC ×2
AUS/FLUS	Negative	Negative	19	
		Positive	1	Follicular ca
	Positive	Negative	10	
		Positive	3	Follicular ca, FVPC, micropapillary ca
FN/SFN	Negative	Negative	14	
		Positive	1	Micropapillary ca
	Positive	Negative	6	
		Positive	5	Papillary ca, micropapillary ca ×2, FVPC, Hurthle cell ca
SM	Negative	Negative	1	
		Positive	0	
	Positive	Negative	1	
		Positive	0	

AUS/FLUS: atypia/follicular lesion of undetermined significance; FN/SFN: follicular neoplasm or suspicious for follicular neoplasm; SM: suspicious for malignancy; FNA: fine needle aspiration biopsy; FVPC: follicular variant of papillary carcinoma; ca: carcinoma.

sensitivity and specificity of FS were 76.9% and 67.9%, respectively. This is compared to the sensitivity and specificity for FNA, which were 53.8% and 74.1%, respectively. The PPV and NPV for FS were 27.8% and 94.8%, respectively. In comparison, FNA demonstrated a PPV of 25% and NPV of 90.9%. There were no changes in operative course as a consequence of a FS result.

Our study did not demonstrate added information when intraoperative FS was used in patients with an FNA of benign, follicular neoplasm, suspicious for follicular neoplasm, or suspicious for malignancy reading. With this information, patients can be scheduled for a thyroid lobectomy with the knowledge that a diagnosis of malignancy will not be obtained until final pathologic analysis is completed. If malignancy is determined, a completion thyroidectomy can then be scheduled. The time and expense of intraoperative FS and scheduling operating room time for a total thyroidectomy, when it is not initially indicated, can therefore be spared.

The initiation of the Bethesda Criteria for Reporting Thyroid Cytopathology has greatly improved our ability to have accurate and meaningful conversations with our patients about their thyroid disease. In our case series, the sensitivity of FS was 76.9% compared to 53.8% for FNA, which is lower than previously published data [9, 12, 13]. However, these publications were performed prior to the Bethesda Criteria and this may account for these differences. Even when evaluating only patients with a diagnosis of malignancy, Makay et al. observed FS to only have a 72% sensitivity [14]. The PPV of both the FS and FNA biopsy were 27.8% and 25%, respectively. The challenges of FNA interpretation are well known and documented. Chang and colleagues [13] showed that when there was discrepancy between the FNA and FS, the FS was shown to be more accurate (78.9% versus 21.1%).

Our results indicate that the addition of an FS does not allow for a more accurate and predictive result. There were no instances within our series where the FS altered the clinical course (i.e., conversion to a total thyroidectomy). There were no false positive results of malignancy for our FSs while there were two false negatives, one with a papillary microcarcinoma and the other a follicular carcinoma.

Future directions for the diagnosis and treatment of thyroid nodules should include addressing highly variable language used among pathologists in regard to thyroid intraoperative FS reporting; diagnosis may benefit from a more uniform language akin to that instituted for FNA biopsies. A standardized language may assist pathologists in their assessment as well as helping surgeons make decisions while in the operative theatre.

4. Conclusion

Our data does not support the clinical usefulness of FS for FNA biopsies with the diagnosis of follicular neoplasm, suspicious for follicular neoplasm, or suspicious for malignancy at our institution. As such, decision for completion thyroidectomy should be determined by the final pathology. This data is useful for both counseling patients with thyroid lesions and subsequent surgical planning.

Conflict of Interests

The authors declare that they have no conflict of interests.

References

[1] L. Davies and H. G. Welch, "Increasing incidence of thyroid cancer in the United States, 1973–2002," *Journal of the American Medical Association*, vol. 295, no. 18, pp. 2164–2167, 2006.

[2] G. Popoveniuc and J. Jonklass, "Thyroid nodules," *Medical Clinics of North America*, vol. 96, no. 2, pp. 329–349, 2012.

[3] G. H. Tan and H. Gharib, "Thyroid incidentalomas: management approaches to nonpalpable nodules discovered incidentally on thyroid imaging," *Annals of Internal Medicine*, vol. 126, no. 3, pp. 226–231, 1997.

[4] P. W. Wiest, M. F. Hartshorne, P. D. Inskip et al., "Thyroid palpation versus high-resolution thyroid ultrasonography in the detection of nodules," *Journal of Ultrasound in Medicine*, vol. 17, no. 8, pp. 487–496, 1998.

[5] L. Hegedus, "Clinical Practice. The thyroid nodule," *The New England Journal of Medicine*, vol. 351, no. 17, pp. 1764–1771, 2004.

[6] E. S. Cibas and S. Z. Ali, "The bethesda system for reporting thyroid cytopathology," *Thyroid*, vol. 19, no. 11, pp. 1159–1165, 2009.

[7] T. Davidov, S. Z. Trooskin, B. A. Shanker et al., "Routine second-opinion cytopathology review of thyroid fine needle aspiration biopsies reduces diagnostic thyroidectomy," *Surgery*, vol. 148, no. 6, pp. 1294–1299, 2010.

[8] Z. W. Baloch, S. Fleisher, V. A. LiVolsi, and P. K. Gupta, "Diagnosis of 'follicular neoplasm': a gray zone in thyroid fine-needle aspiration cytology," *Diagnostic Cytopathology*, vol. 26, no. 1, pp. 41–44, 2002.

[9] B. Cetin, S. Aslan, C. Hatiboglu et al., "Frozen section in thyroid surgery: is it a necessity?" *Canadian Journal of Surgery*, vol. 47, no. 1, pp. 29–33, 2004.

[10] V. A. LiVolsi and Z. W. Baloch, "Use and abuse of frozen section in the diagnosis of follicular thyroid lesions," *Endocrine Pathology*, vol. 16, no. 4, pp. 285–294, 2005.

[11] M. C. Miller, C. J. Rubin, M. Cunnane et al., "Intraoperative pathologic examination: cost effectiveness and clinical value in patients with cytologic diagnosis of cellular follicular thyroid lesion," *Thyroid*, vol. 17, no. 6, pp. 557–565, 2007.

[12] D. L. Mandell, E. M. Genden, J. I. Mechanick, D. A. Bergman, H. F. Biller, and M. L. Urken, "Diagnostic accuracy of fine-needle aspiration and frozen section in nodular thyroid disease," *Otolaryngology—Head and Neck Surgery*, vol. 124, no. 5, pp. 531–536, 2001.

[13] H. Y. Chang, J. D. Lin, J. F. Chen et al., "Correlation of fine needle aspiration cytology and frozen section biopsies in the diagnosis of thyroid nodules," *Journal of Clinical Pathology*, vol. 50, no. 12, pp. 1005–1009, 1997.

[14] O. Makay, G. Icoz, B. Gurcu et al., "The ongoing debate in thyroid surgery: should frozen section analysis be omitted?" *Endocrine Journal*, vol. 54, no. 3, pp. 385–390, 2007.

22

A Clinical Prediction Formula for Apnea-Hypopnea Index

Mustafa Sahin,[1] Cem Bilgen,[2] M. Sezai Tasbakan,[3] Rasit Midilli,[2] and Ozen K. Basoglu[3]

[1] *Department of Otorhinolaryngology, Diskapi Yildirim Beyazit Research and Training Hospital, Irfan Bastug Street,*
Dıskapi, 06110 Ankara, Turkey
[2] *Department of Otorhinolaryngology, Ege University School of Medicine, İzmir, Turkey*
[3] *Department of Chest Diseases, Ege University School of Medicine, İzmir, Turkey*

Correspondence should be addressed to Mustafa Sahin; iskebaha@gmail.com

Academic Editor: David W. Eisele

Objectives. There are many studies regarding unnecessary polysomnography (PSG) when obstructive sleep apnea syndrome (OSAS) is suspected. In order to reduce unnecessary PSG, this study aims to predict the apnea-hypopnea index (AHI) via simple clinical data for patients who complain of OSAS symptoms. *Method.* Demographic, anthropometric, physical examination and laboratory data of a total of 390 patients (290 men, average age 50 ± 11) who were subject to diagnostic PSG were obtained and evaluated retrospectively. The relationship between these data and the PSG results was analyzed. A multivariate linear regression analysis was performed step by step to identify independent AHI predictors. *Results.* Useful parameters were found in this analysis in terms of body mass index (BMI), waist circumference (WC), neck circumference (NC), oxygen saturation measured by pulse oximetry (SpO_2), and tonsil size (TS) to predict the AHI. The formula derived from these parameters was the predicted $AHI = (0.797 \times BMI) + (2.286 \times NC) - (1.272 \times SpO_2) + (5.114 \times TS) + (0.314 \times WC)$. *Conclusion.* This study showed a strong correlation between AHI score and indicators of obesity. This formula, in terms of predicting the AHI for patients who complain about snoring, witnessed apneas, and excessive daytime sleepiness, may be used to predict OSAS prior to PSG and prevent unnecessary PSG.

1. Introduction

OSAS is one of the most significant health problems in middle-aged people and leads to daytime sleepiness and cognitive deficiencies as well as many systemic diseases. It is a highly prevalent disorder, and at least 4% of middle-aged males and 2% of middle-aged females are estimated to be affected [1]. Diagnosis of OSAS is essentially performed via patient history, clinical examination, and some anthropometric measurements. Polysomnography (PSG) helps to establish a definite diagnosis. Overnight in-laboratory PSG is used most widely to confirm or to refute a suspected OSAS. However, in-lab PSG's limited availability, its high cost, and time- and labor-consuming nature are its disadvantages. The waiting lists of sleep clinics for PSG are quite long, and it is difficult to perform PSG on all patients suspected of OSAS [2]. Thus, many studies that aim to diagnose OSAS via clinical findings and easily applicable tests have been carried out. To this aim, multivariate clinical prediction formulas have been developed using mathematical modeling to assess ambulatory PSG, nap or half night PSG, morphometric analysis, self-reported symptoms, and questionnaires. While declared prediction models using logistic regression have high sensitivity (more than 85%), their specificity is low (less than 55%) [3]. Because a low cost and less time-consuming diagnostic method is needed, this study aims to evaluate the predictive values of symptoms and anthropometric, laboratory, and physical examination findings in order to determine a formula to detect OSAS in patients earlier and to reduce the constantly increasing PSG density in our sleep centers.

2. Material and Methods

2.1. Methods

2.1.1. Study Population.
In this observational study, we retrospectively evaluated 390 consecutive, unselected subjects who were referred to the sleep laboratory of a university hospital to

evaluate presumed sleep-disordered breathing and who had undergone PSG. Each individual included in this study was referred to sleep laboratory by otolaryngology department after detailed ear, nose, and throat examination which was performed by the same specialist. Demographic data (age, gender, smoking history, and alcohol and psychotropic drug use), anthropometric measurements (height, weight, body mass index, and circumferences of neck, waist, and hip), and medical history were evaluated.

BMI, the most commonly used method to measure obesity, was calculated by dividing weight in kilograms by the square of height in meters (kg/m^2). Neck circumference was measured in centimeters at the level of the cricothyroid membrane. Waist circumference was measured in centimeters at the level above the iliac crest. Hip circumference was measured in centimeters while patients were standing still and their feet were fairly close and at the level of the point where the maximum circumference over the buttocks was measured.

After asking patients about their complaints, the following parameters emerged: snoring, witnessed apnea, the existence of nasal obstruction, smoking, and alcohol use. Subjective daytime sleepiness was assessed by using the Turkish version of the Epworth Sleepiness Scale (ESS). Scores higher than 10 were considered to be sleepiness. Pulmonary function tests (including spirometry and flow volume curves), chest X-rays, pulse oximeters in polyclinics to evaluate peripheral oxygen saturation (plus MED-pulse oximeter, plus 50-DL, Contec Medical Systems), arterial blood gas analysis, and a full-night in-laboratory PSG were performed on all subjects.

2.1.2. Ear Nose Throat Examination. Detailed otolaryngologic physical examinations were performed by the same specialist. Parameters obtained in these examinations were included in statistical evaluations and included the following: protrusion and retrusion of the mandibles, tonsil sizes, the relationship between the soft palate and the neutral position of the tongue, the tongue-base size, nasal septum deviation, the inferior turbinate size, the endoscopic nasal cavity, and nasopharynx examinations using a 0° rigid endoscope, endoscopic larynx, and hypopharynx examinations using a 70° rigid endoscope (4 mm, 18 cm, Korl Storz Hopkins, Tuttlingen, Germany).

Mandibular retrognathism was evaluated in accordance with the position of the pogonion when the virtual imaginary line between the vermilion line and the chin on a patient sitting in a Frankfort horizontal position is taken into consideration. The examinations of the oral cavity started with an inspection of the relative position of the hard and of the soft palate to the tongue inside the mouth, without protrusion using the modified Mallampati index (MMI), ranging from Class I to Class IV, with Class I representing the highest visibility (the tonsils, the pillars, and the soft palate being visible) and Class IV representing the lowest level of visibility (only the hard palate being visible) of the posterior oropharynx [4]. The tonsils were classified by degree in accordance with hypertrophy, from Degree I to Degree IV as follows: tonsils in the tonsillary fossa and they are barely seen behind the anterior pillars were Grade I,

tonsils that occupied 25% of the oropharynx were Grade II, tonsils that occupied 50% of the oropharynx were Grade III, and tonsils that occupied at least 75% of the oropharynx were Grade IV, if they meet in the midline. Tongue-base sizes were ranked between Grades 1 and 3. The tongue was classified as Grade 1 when the vallecula was partially visible in an examination using a 70° rigid endoscope, while the tongue was in an easy position within the mouth; it was classified as Grade 2 when the vallecula was invisible and the tongue base touched the epiglottis; and when the tongue base pushed the epiglottis, it was classified as Grade 3. Nasal examinations were performed via anterior rhinoscopy and a 0° rigid endoscope, and internal nasal pathways were evaluated following research on pathology, such as septum deviation, turbinate hypertrophy, and intranasal obstructive lesions, such as polypus. The movement of obstructive lesions and the vocal cords in the larynx and in the hypopharynx was evaluated following a larynx examination via a 70° rigid endoscope.

2.1.3. Polysomnography. All subjects underwent a full overnight in-laboratory diagnostic PSG (Compumedics E Series, Australia or Alice 5 Diagnostic Sleep System, Philips, Respironics, USA). Electroencephalography electrodes were positioned according to the international 10–20 system. PSG consisted of monitoring of sleep by electroencephalography, electrooculography, electromyography, airflow, and respiratory muscle effort and included measures of electrocardiographic rhythm and blood oxygen saturation. Thoracoabdominal plethysmograph, oronasal temperature thermistor, and nasal-cannula pressure transducer system were used to identify apneas and hypopneas. Transcutaneous finger pulse oximeter was used to measure oxygen saturation. Sleep was recorded and scored according to the standard method [5]. AHI was the sum of the number of apneas and hypopneas per hour of sleep. OSAS was defined as an AHI of 5 events/h and the presence of clinical symptoms, for example, excessive daytime sleepiness, loud snoring, witnessed apneas, and nocturnal choking, or AHI of 15 events/h without any OSAS symptoms [6]. Besides, an AHI of <5 events/h was considered within normal limits. No split-night studies were performed.

2.1.4. Statistical Analysis. SPSS version 17.0 was used for statistical analysis. First, the correlation between the AHI and all of the variables included in the study was analyzed in order to identify variables to be used to predict the AHI. Mann-Whitney U test was performed to evaluate the statistical difference between AHI values of men and women. Following this test it was not a statistically significant difference between men and women according to AHI values ($P = 0.190$). Therefore different models were not developed regarding the gender. Prior to the correlation analysis, we identified whether these variables provided parametric assumptions. We found in the results of the Kolmogorov-Smirnov test that variables did not demonstrate normal distribution. Spearman's rank order correlation analysis was performed because variables did not provide normal distribution as required. Following this analysis, variables that were identified to have had a correlation with the AHI were integrated into the

TABLE 1: Characteristics of the study population.

Variables	Study population (n = 390)
Age (year)*	50.1 ± 11.1
Sex (n, %)	Male: 289 (73.9%)
	Female: 101 (26.1%)
Current Smoker (n, %)	116 (29.7)
Alcohol Consumption (n, %)	67 (17.2%)
Comorbidities (n, %)	
Hypertension	156 (40 %)
Diabetes mellitus	76 (19.5 %)
Coronary artery disease	31 (7.9 %)
BMI (kg/m^2)*	30.8 ± 5.5
Neck Circumference (cm)*	40.9 ± 4.2
Waist Circumference (cm)*	106.1 ± 14.6
Hip Circumference (cm)*	110.1 ± 11.2
Epworth Sleepiness Score*	9.8 ± 6.0
Apnea-hypopnea index (/hour)*	33.2 ± 30.3

BMI: Body mass index, NC: Neck circumference, WC: Waist circumference, HC: Hip circumference, SpO$_2$: Oxygen saturation, FVC: Forced vital capacity, FEV1%: Forced expiratory volume ratio in one second, ESS: Epworth Sleepiness Scale's score, TS: Tonsil size. *Values are expressed as mean (SD).

TABLE 2: Variables identified to be related to AHI in Spearman's rho test and their correlation coefficients.

Variable	Correlation coefficient	Variable	Correlation coefficient
BMI	0.491	FVC	−0.149
NC	0.358	FEV1%	−0.101
WC	0.371	FEV1/FVC	−0.085
HC	0.112	PaO$_2$	−0.203
Smoking	0.190	PaCO$_2$	0.161
ESS	0.103	SpO$_2$	−0.242
		TS	0.431

regression analysis. Each variable was integrated into the regression in order to identify how these variables as a whole affected the AHI via a step-by-step, multiple linear regression analysis. When the P value was <0.05, it was regarded as statistically significant.

3. Results

The demographic data (age, gender, smoking history, and alcohol and psychotropic drug use), anthropometric measurements (height, weight, body mass index, and circumferences of the neck, waist, and hips), and medical history variables are shown in Table 1.

Variables that were integrated into the regression analysis after we found that they were correlated with the AHI in Spearman's rho test were the BMI, NC, WC, hip circumference (HC), smoking rate in packages/year, force vital capacity (FVC), forced expiratory volume ratio in one second (FEV1%), FEV1/FVC ratio, Pao2, PaCO2, ESS score, oxygen saturation level via a pulse oximeter, the Epworth Scale score, and tonsil size. Correlation coefficients of these variables in

TABLE 3: Parameters used to identify independent predictors of apnea-hypopnea index.

Parameter	Beta	T	P value
Body mass index	0.797	2.132	0.034
Neck circumference	2.286	6.696	<0.0001
Oxygen saturation	−1.272	−9.094	<0.0001
Waist circumference	0.314	2.274	0.24
Tonsil size	5.114	2.261	0.024

nonparametric Spearman's rank order correlation analysis are shown in Table 2.

Thereafter, each variable was integrated into the regression analysis in order to identify how these variables as a whole affected the AHI via a step-by-step multiple linear regression analysis. In the seventh phase, the explanatory power of the model reached its peak: R^2 = 0.682. Therefore, the following model was developed to predict the AHI: AHI prediction = (0.797 × BMI) + (2.286 × NC) − (1.272 × SpO$_2$) + (5.114 × TS) + (0.314 × WC). The most significant variables in the regression model developed to the AHI prediction via a step-by-step multilinear regression analysis are shown in Table 3.

We found this model to be statistically significant (F = 155.348, P < 0.05). According to this formula, 68.2% of the variation in the AHI could be explained via these variables, while 32.8% could be attributed to other variables. Bland Altman plot comparing real AHI values obtained from PSG and the predicted AHI values obtained from the prediction formula is shown in Figure 1.

4. Discussion

Some studies have shown that data based on medical history and the findings of the physical examination may be useful to detect OSAS in patients. Hoffstein and Szalai obtained a sensitivity of 60% and a specificity of 63% in the detection of OSAS in patients in a study that included 594 patients and aimed to analyze the statistical relevance of data related to medical history and physical examinations [7]. In our study to predict the AHI, a clinical formula with 0.682 explanatory power was found including these parameters: body mass index, neck circumference, waist circumference, peripheral oxygen saturation, and tonsil size.

Sleep apnea, despite being the most common reason for EDS, was not considered to be a useful clinical feature for detecting OSAS in patients because 30 to 50% of the society claim moderate to sleepiness [1, 2]. In addition, other sleep disorders and diseases may cause EDS. Bausmer et al. did not find a significant correlation between the ESS score and the AHI [8]. In a study analyzing the relation between clinical parameters and OSAS on a group of 80 people, similar to our present study, no significant correlation was found between subjective sleepiness measured via the ESS and the AHI [9].

Obesity is an important risk factor for OSAS, and 70% of OSAS patients suffer from it. The most commonly used measurements in the diagnosis of obesity are BMI, WC, and HC. Bouloukaki et al. stated that BMI was a better indicator

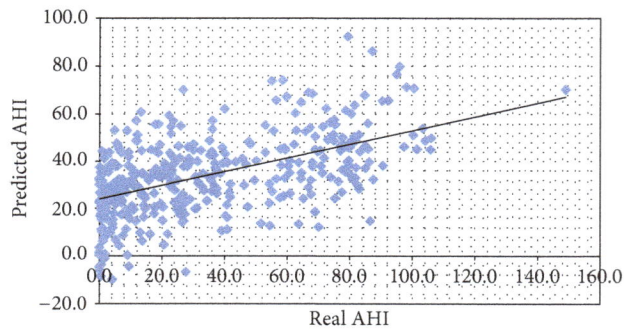

FIGURE 1: Distribution of predicted AHI values regarding real AHI values.

than other obesity indicators, such as waist-to-hip ratio, in OSAS predictability [10]. In many studies, NC, which is related to fat deposition around the upper airway, was defined as an important predictor factor for OSAS [3]. The value of NC in predicting OSAS is still controversial. In a study of 2,690 patients, Bouloukaki et al. reported that NC was the most significant correlate with the AHI [10]. In this study, similar to the findings in previous studies, NC and BMI were found to be significant parameters for the AHI prediction.

It is a challenging issue for otolaryngologists to identify and to improve the location of obstruction level(s) in the upper airway (UAW) in patients suspected of OSAS. The UAW is assumed to be narrower and/or more prone to collapse multilevelly in OSAS patients. The relationship between anatomic abnormalities and the severity of OSAS has not been well established in previous studies because UAW abnormalities are not the only causative factors [11]. In this study just TS was found significant in predicting the AHI among the physical examination findings of UAW, we only found TS to be significant in predicting the AHI. It is generally acknowledged that tonsillar hypertrophy causes airway obstruction. TS has been related to the AHI in a few different studies. Friedman revealed a relation between the increase in TS and the AHI through grading tonsil sizes in OSAS patients [4]. Enlarged tonsils are associated with OSAS, and surgical removal is thought to be an important part of the treatment. Cahali et al. reported that the tonsil grade has a strong correlation with the AHI in OSAS patients [12].

There is no consensus regarding the effect of nasal airway blockage on OSAS pathogenesis and the severity of the disease. While some authors argued that the nasal passage affects OSAS development and is related to AHI, other authors claimed the converse [13]. In this study, no statistically significant correlation between nasal obstruction and the AHI was detected.

The Mallampati index, which was defined by anesthesiologists in 1985 to identify difficult intubation, was later suggested as an MMI to be used in predicting OSAS [4]. This index is used to evaluate oropharyngeal structures and relative tongue size. Some studies reported that relative tongue size may be related to AHI. Liistro et al. [14] and Schellenberg et al. [15] concluded that MMI and tongue-base hypertrophy were related to AHI. However, in this study,

similar to Dreher et al.'s findings, we found no significant relationship between tongue-base hypertrophy, MMI, and the AHI [16].

In many studies, pulmonary function tests were not included in the data to detect OSAS predictors. Herer et al. evaluated 102 obese patients by clinical features, pulmonary function tests, arterial blood gas tensions, and oximetry for prediction of OSAS prior to PSG and stated that none of these data is sufficient to prove the existence of OSAS [17]. In a study which attempted to develop a predictive index for OSAS based on pulmonary function parameters, conducted with obese snorers suspected of OSAS, it is found out that daytime oxygen saturation contributed to the model significantly. It was argued that this model could help decrease redundant PSG applications by 38% [18]. In our study, among spirometric parameters, the FVC, FEV1%, and FEV1/FVC ratios were found to be correlated with the AHI, but these parameters were eliminated in the regression analysis and did not come out in the AHI predictive model as independent variables. The relationship between the levels of AHI and desaturation were also argued, and no strong significance was identified about this issue. Since it is easier to apply and it is more cost-effective, transcutaneous pulse oximetry has become more and more widely used in initial screenings of OSAS. Mulgrew et al. stated that PSG applied to patients suspected of OSAS is by no means superior to ambulatory methods based on oximeter readings combined with clinical data [19]. In their study of 275 patients, Chiner et al. found that a preliminary pulse oximeter may decrease redundant PGS ratios by 38% in a group of patients where the AHI is more than 15 [20]. On the other hand, no desaturation can be seen among hypopnea period and in cases where upper airway resistance has increased even when oxygen desaturation is prevalent in obstructive apnea. Therefore, an oximeter may be useful on its own, particularly as far as higher average levels of OSAS are concerned and where they cannot rule out the diagnosis [21]. Because putting all patients through overnight oximeters conflicts with the practicability of our study, we analyzed the pulse oximeters and oxygen saturations in peripheral blood in policlinic environment and found that evaluation was one of the most significant parameters in the AHI prediction model.

However, such formulas include different variables within different populations, whose differences may be a significant limitation of this study. Therefore, this method may not be sufficient since a screening technique and its validity need to be further tested in other series and would need to include more patients. It is our next aim to design a prospective study to evaluate the predictability of the formula obtained from this study.

As a result, a mathematical model created via data obtained through simple office procedures to predict OSAS may reduce redundant PSG and result in more rapid diagnoses and treatment processes. The potential advantage of this approach is its ease of use, its cost effectiveness, its applicable nature in office environments, and its contribution to more rapid decisions. Validity of this prediction formula needs to be further tested in other prospective researches. It is not possible to make a clear clinical statement about this formula yet. Validated prediction models, which will be created via collective studies by more sleep centers and with more groups of patients, are needed because no single, sufficient model has yet been described.

Conflict of Interests

The authors declare that there is no conflict of interests regarding the publication of this paper.

References

[1] T. Young, M. Palta, J. Dempsey, J. Skatrud, S. Weber, and S. Badr, "The occurrence of sleep-disordered breathing among middle-aged adults," *The New England Journal of Medicine*, vol. 328, no. 17, pp. 1230–1235, 1993.

[2] C. Bucca, L. Brussino, M. M. Maule et al., "Clinical and functional prediction of moderate to severe obstructive sleep apnoea," *Clinical Respiratory Journal*, vol. 5, no. 4, pp. 219–226, 2011.

[3] J. A. Rowley, L. S. Aboussouan, and M. S. Badr, "The use of clinical prediction formulas in the evaluation of obstructive sleep apnea," *Sleep*, vol. 23, no. 7, pp. 929–936, 2000.

[4] M. Friedman, H. Tanyeri, M. La Rosa et al., "Clinical predictors of obstructive sleep apnea," *Laryngoscope*, vol. 109, no. 12, pp. 1901–1907, 1999.

[5] C. Iber, S. Ancoli-Israel, A. L. Chesson, and S. F. Quan, *The AASMmanual 2007 for the Scoring of Sleep and Associated Events: Rules, Terminology and Technical Specifications*, American Academy of Sleep Medicine, Westchester, Ill, USA, 2007.

[6] American Academy of Sleep Medicine, *International Classification of Sleep Disorders: Diagnostic and Coding Manual*, American Academy of Sleep Medicine, Westchester, Ill, USA, 2005.

[7] V. Hoffstein and J. P. Szalai, "Predictive value of clinical features in diagnosing obstructive sleep apnea," *Sleep*, vol. 16, no. 2, pp. 118–122, 1993.

[8] U. Bausmer, H. Gouveris, O. Selivanova, B. Goepel, and W. Mann, "Correlation of the Epworth Sleepiness Scale with respiratory sleep parameters in patients with sleep-related breathing disorders and upper airway pathology," *European Archives of Oto-Rhino-Laryngology*, vol. 267, no. 10, pp. 1645–1648, 2010.

[9] J. F. Thong and K. P. Pang, "Clinical parameters in obstructive sleep apnea: are there any correlations?" *Journal of Otolaryngology—Head and Neck Surgery*, vol. 37, no. 6, pp. 894–900, 2008.

[10] I. Bouloukaki, F. Kapsimalis, C. Mermigkis et al., "Prediction of obstructive sleep apnea syndrome in a large Greek population," *Sleep and Breathing*, vol. 15, no. 4, pp. 657–664, 2011.

[11] A. I. Zonato, L. R. Bittencourt, F. L. Martinho, J. Ferreira Santos Jr., L. C. Gregório, and S. Tufik, "Association of systematic head and neck physical examination with severity of obstructive sleep apnea-hypopnea syndrome," *Laryngoscope*, vol. 113, no. 6, pp. 973–980, 2003.

[12] M. B. Cahali, C. F. de Paula Soares, D. A. da Silva Dantas, and G. G. S. Formigoni, "Tonsil volume, tonsil grade and obstructive sleep apnea: is there any meaningful correlation?" *Clinics*, vol. 66, no. 8, pp. 1347–1351, 2011.

[13] F. Lofaso, A. Coste, M. P. D'Ortho et al., "Nasal obstruction as a risk factor for sleep apnoea syndrome," *European Respiratory Journal*, vol. 16, no. 4, pp. 639–643, 2000.

[14] G. Liistro, P. Rombaux, C. Belge, M. Dury, G. Aubert, and D. O. Rodenstein, "High Mallampati score and nasal obstruction are associated risk factors for obstructive sleep apnoea," *European Respiratory Journal*, vol. 21, no. 2, pp. 248–252, 2003.

[15] J. B. Schellenberg, G. Maislin, and R. J. Schwab, "Physical findings and the risk for obstructive sleep apnea: the importance of oropharyngeal structures," *The American Journal of Respiratory and Critical Care Medicine*, vol. 162, no. 2, pp. 740–748, 2000.

[16] A. Dreher, R. De La Chaux, C. Klemens et al., "Correlation between otorhinolaryngologic evaluation and severity of obstructive sleep apnea syndrome in snorers," *Archives of Otolaryngology—Head and Neck Surgery*, vol. 131, no. 2, pp. 95–98, 2005.

[17] B. Herer, N. Roche, M. Carton, C. Roig, V. Poujol, and G. Huchon, "Value of clinical, functional, and oximetric data for the prediction of obstructive sleep apnea in obese patients," *Chest*, vol. 116, no. 6, pp. 1537–1544, 1999.

[18] F. Zerah-Lancner, F. Lofaso, M. P. D'Ortho et al., "Predictive value of pulmonary function parameters for sleep apnea syndrome," *The American Journal of Respiratory and Critical Care Medicine*, vol. 162, no. 6, pp. 2208–2212, 2000.

[19] A. T. Mulgrew, N. Fox, N. T. Ayas, and C. F. Ryan, "Diagnosis and initial management of obstructive sleep apnea without polysomnography: a randomized validation study," *Annals of Internal Medicine*, vol. 146, no. 3, pp. 157–166, 2007.

[20] E. Chiner, J. Signes-Costa, J. M. Arriero, J. Marco, I. Fuentes, and A. Sergado, "Nocturnal oximetry for the diagnosis of the sleep apnoea hypopnoea syndrome: a method to reduce the number of polysomnographics?" *Thorax*, vol. 54, no. 11, pp. 968–971, 1999.

[21] N. Netzer, A. H. Eliasson, C. Netzer, and D. A. Kristo, "Overnight pulse oximetry for sleep-disordered breathing in adults: a review," *Chest*, vol. 120, no. 2, pp. 625–633, 2001.

23

Prevalence of K-RAS Codons 12 and 13 Mutations in Locally Advanced Head and Neck Squamous Cell Carcinoma and Impact on Clinical Outcomes

Eric Bissada,[1] Olivier Abboud,[1] Zahi Abou Chacra,[1] Louis Guertin,[1] Xiaoduan Weng,[2] Phuc Félix Nguyen-Tan,[3] Jean-Claude Tabet,[1] Ève Thibaudeau,[1] Louise Lambert,[3] Marie-Lise Audet,[2] Bernard Fortin,[3] and Denis Soulières[2]

[1] *Department of Head and Neck Surgery, Centre Hospitalier de l'Université de Montréal (CHUM), Montreal, QC, Canada*
[2] *Department of Hematology and Medical Oncology, CHUM, Montreal, QC, Canada*
[3] *Department of Radiation Oncology, CHUM, Montreal, QC, Canada*

Correspondence should be addressed to Denis Soulières; denis.soulieres.chum@ssss.gouv.qc.ca

Academic Editor: David W. Eisele

Background. RAS gene mutations have an impact on treatment response and overall prognosis for certain types of cancer. *Objectives*. To determine the prevalence and impact of K-RAS codons 12 and 13 mutations in patients with locally advanced HNSCC treated with primary or adjuvant chemo-radiation. *Methods*. 428 consecutive patients were treated with chemo-radiation therapy and followed for a median of 37 months. From these, 199 paraffin embedded biopsy or surgical specimens were retrieved. DNA was isolated and analyzed for K-RAS mutational status. *Results*. DNA extraction was successful in 197 samples. Of the 197 specimens, 3.5% presented K-RAS codon 12 mutations. For mutated cases and non-mutated cases, complete initial response to chemoradiation therapy was 71 and 73% ($P = 0.32$). LRC was respectively 32 and 83% ($P = 0.03$), DFS was 27 and 68% ($P = 0.12$), distant metastasis-free survival was 100 and 81% ($P = 0.30$) and OS was 57 and 65% ($P = 0.14$) at three years. K-Ras codon 13 analysis revealed no mutation. *Conclusion*. K-RAS codon 12 mutational status, although not associated with a difference in response rate, may influence the failure pattern and the type of therapy offered to patients with HNSCC. Our study did not reveal any mutation of K-RAS codon 13.

1. Introduction

Head and neck squamous cell carcinoma (HNSCC) accounts for 47 000 new malignancies diagnosed each year in the USA and is the sixth most common human neoplasm, representing about 3% of all cancers [1]. Despite efforts to improve conventional treatment, survival rates for these cancers have not changed significantly over the past decade.

Initial evaluation of patients includes clinical assessment, study of tumor histological characteristics and tumor grading, as well as local-regional and distant metastasis status. Traditional clinical, radiological, and histopathological characteristics are however limited in their ability to accurately predict response to treatment. This has motivated many researchers to identify molecular characteristics that may influence overall prognosis.

A recent interest in molecular biology and genetics is motivated by the belief that understanding the origins of cancer can lead to more logical means of treating malignancies [2]. Identification of molecular events that lead to HNSCC may represent a key to predicting biological behaviour and may consequently lead to new treatment modalities that could lead to increases in survival rates. [3, 4]. Despite the recent progress in the field of molecular biology, clinicians need more tools to predict response to therapy or to identify patients at high risk of poor outcome. Identification of biological markers predictive of treatment failure would potentially permit the use of more targeted therapies or adaptation of current protocols to these patient groups in order to improve results.

Oncogenes of the *RAS* family are strongly implicated in the pathogenesis of cancer. *K-RAS* gene mutations have been reported in approximately 15–30% of human solid tumours [5–7]. This mutation is the most common abnormality of dominant oncogenes in human tumors and is a common event in the development and progression of adenocarcinomas of the pancreas (90%), colon (50%), thyroid (50%), bladder (50%), and lung (30%). The *RAS* family of genes is of particular interest in HNSCC because a mechanism for mutation (activation) of K-RAS by tobacco carcinogens has been suggested [8]. Furthermore, *RAS* mutations have been observed in other tobacco-related cancers, namely, pancreatic carcinoma and non-small cell lung carcinoma [4].

The *RAS* gene is known to encode for a family of related proteins, termed p21s, which are associated with the plasma membrane and participate in the transduction of signals involved in cellular growth and differentiation. The conversion of normal *RAS* proto-oncogenes, specifically K-RAS, to activated oncogenes is usually accomplished by point mutations involving the 12th and occasionally the 13th and 61st codons on chromosome 12. Several carcinogens preferentially bind codon 12 to create DNA adducts [9]. This results in the expression of abnormal p21 proteins harboring a single amino acid substitution favoring an active, GTP-bound state. This activates the RAS-RAF pathway and culminates in a pathologic activation of cellular mitosis.

K-RAS mutations are known to be associated with resistance to chemotherapy and radiation therapy, particularly in non-small cell lung and colorectal cancers [10, 11]. For metastatic cancer, the response rate to classical regimens of chemotherapy or to tyrosine kinase inhibitors is much lower in patients with the mutation. Hence, survival is lower and *K-RAS* mutations are considered a negative prognostic factor. These results have not been reproduced in HNSCC.

A limited number of publications have examined the frequency of these mutations in the development of HNSCC. In a 1990 study published in 1990, Howell et al. [12] first described an activated RAS oncogene specific to HNSCC. Following that report, others have attempted, through different techniques, to quantify the presence of this specific mutation in head and neck cancers. While some suggested that mutational activation of RAS was not associated with the occurrence of HNSCC [2, 4, 5, 13–20], others found that *K-RAS* mutations had a direct causal role in the development of these cancers [21–23].

Current literature describes a low frequency of these mutations in the western hemisphere. Investigations of *RAS* mutations in the Western World have estimated the incidence of these mutations to be less than 5% [4, 13, 15–18, 20, 24]. The prevalence of this mutation increases to 18% in countries such as Spain and Taiwan [21, 25] and may be even higher in India [23, 26]. Whereas *H-RAS* mutation was detected in as much as 35% of Indian oral cancer specimens [27] and has been associated with betel nut chewing, *K-RAS* mutation prevalences vary considerably [23, 27]. Some investigators have looked at the possible association between *K-RAS* mutations and clinical correlates. The existing literature is however scarce and derived from studies with small patient numbers and wide inclusion criteria, rendering cohorts too heterogeneous for results to be interpreted.

From these data, some authors have concluded that HNSCC with or without RAS mutations do not seem to differ clinically from each other [25].

Overexpression of the of the *RAS* gene product p21 in HNSCC has been reported by a number of groups, despite the low incidence of RAS mutations in head and neck cancers [28]. Abnormal expression of *RAS* genes may be attributed to mutation in the gene promoters and not to the coding region itself. Expression of this protein seems to be increased in well differentiated cancers, while its expression is low in severely dysplastic lesions and poorly differentiated cancers [29]. Authors have found a correlation between increased p21 and a more malignant and invasive biological behavior [3, 17, 28, 30–33], whereas others have correlated increased p21 expression with a favorable clinical prognosis [20, 29, 34]. In contrast, increased RAS p21 was found in poorly differentiated cancers, correlating with increased disease-free survival [34]. Oral cancers positive for *H-RAS* mutations may actually fare better than those who do not harbor, the mutation as suggested by Anderson et al. [5]. This finding, however, was not shown to be statistically significant due to the small number of positive tumors. No reference to prognosis was made by Saranath et al., whose group determined that 20 out of 57 oral tumor specimens tested positive for the mutation [27, 35].

The objectives of our study were to determine the prevalence of K-RAS codon 12 and 13 mutations, in patients with locally advanced HNSCC treated with chemoradiation therapy with or without surgery, and to evaluate the impact of these mutations on loco-regional control as well as overall, disease-free and distant metastasis-free survival at three years.

2. Patients and Methods

2.1. Patient Population. Four hundred and twenty-eight patients with stage III and IV HNSCC treated with chemoradiation therapy at Centre Hospitalier de l'Université de Montréal—Hôpital Notre-Dame and followed for a minimum of 24 months were included in this study.

2.2. Data Collection. Data were collected prospectively from a regular assessment of outcome variables such as response rates, local or regional recurrences, and survival rates by means of regular clinical and radiological evaluations. All patients had histological confirmation of SCC based on histological features in hematoxylin and eosin-stained tissue sections diagnosed by a pathologist experienced in head and neck pathology.

2.3. Sample Preparation. Three to eight sections of 10 μm were obtained from each tumor. To avoid cross-contamination during sectioning, disposable microtome blades were used, and the microtome was cleaned after cutting each specimen. The paraffin was removed by xylene and ethanol, and the tissue was then incubated in $200\,\mu L$ lysis buffer (10 mM Tris-HCl, pH 8.0, 1 mM EDTA, pH 8.0, 20 mM NaCl) containing 0.2 mg/mL proteinase K for 2 hours at 55°C. The mixture was then heated at 96°C for 5 minutes in order to inactivate proteinase K. Optic density was calculated for the supernatant after centrifugation of the mixture at 12000 G for 20 minutes. Four hundred nanograms of the prepared DNA were used as the template for K-RAS gene amplification and the remaining mixture was stored at −80°C for repeat analysis using the nested PCR technique.

2.4. PCR Amplification of K-RAS of Codons 12 and 13. PCR was performed in $100\,\mu L$ of reaction mixture containing a 400 to 500 ng of DNA, following a technique described by Hatzaki et al. [36]. Forward primer incorporated a C residue mismatch at the first position of codon 11. This created a BstNI restriction enzyme cleaving site in the amplified normal allele after PCR amplification. This cleaving site was absent in the amplified mutated DNA strand when any of the known point mutations were found on codon 12. Reverse primer incorporated a G residue mismatch at the first intron as a positive control for BstNI digestion. For codon 13, a mismatched downstream primer was used, creating a HaeIII restriction site in the wild-type allele.

2.5. Digestion of PCR End Products. For codon 12, digestion was carried out with BstN1. HaeIII digestion was carried out for codon 13. Samples were then analyzed with 6% polyacrylamide gel electrophoresis. Mutated K-RAS codon 12 resulted in a 143-bp strand, whereas wild-type resulted in two strands of 114 bp and 29 bp. Mutated K-RAS codon 13 showed two strands of 85 bp and 74 bp, whereas wild-type resulted in three strands measuring 85 bp, 48 bp, and 26 bp. Positive controls for all mutations (derived from cell lines) were run with each PCR. Cell line SW480 (ATCC inc., Manassas, VA, USA) has a homozygous mutation of K-RAS codon 12. Cell line HCT116 (ATCC inc., Manassas, VA, USA) has a heterozygous mutation of codon 13.

2.6. Statistical Analysis. Statistical analysis was performed using Fisher's test for categorical data and Kaplan-Meier's curves and log-rank statistics for disease-free survival, overall survival, and loco-regional control.

2.7. Ethical Aspects. This study was approved by our institution's ethics board (reference number 09.254).

3. Results

All available tissue samples from 428 consecutive patients treated with chemoradiation therapy in our institution were retrieved. In total, 199 paraffin embedded biopsy or surgical specimens were recovered. DNA extraction was accomplished successfully in 197 of these. Patient characteristics did not differ statistically. Seventy-seven percent of specimens were from male subjects. Primary tumor site is listed in Table 1. Seventy-nine percent of patients initially

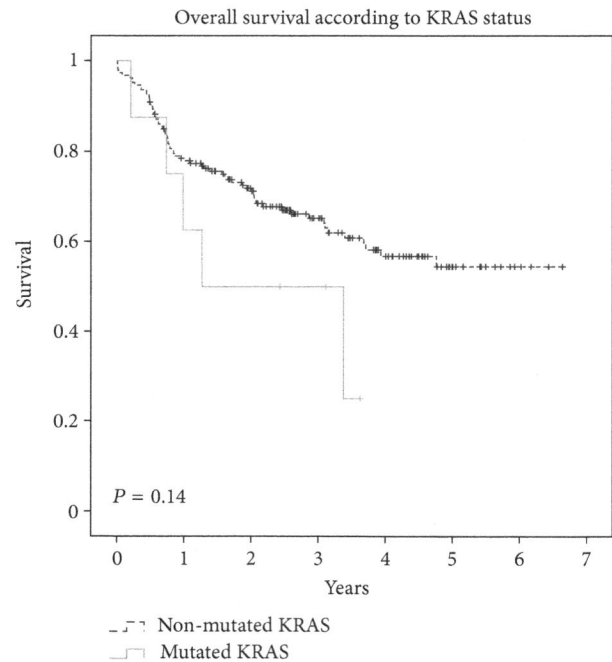

FIGURE 1: Kaplan Meier projected overall survival of wild-type K-RAS compared to mutated K-RAS.

presented with stage IV HNSCC. Chemotherapy regimens consisted of combined carboplatin and 5FU in the majority of patients (55%), and of single agent platinum salts-based drugs for the remainder of patients. K-RAS codon 12 mutations were detected in 7 of 197 DNA samples (3.5%). This value increased to 8 (4%) with the use of nested PCR techniques, suggesting an adequate sensitivity in detecting K-RAS mutations with simple PCR-RFLP. Results were reproducible, which confirmed test accuracy (data not shown). None of the samples showed mutations involving codon 13.

No statistically significant correlation could be made between degree of histological differentiation and presence or absence of K-RAS codon 12 mutations, nor could a correlation be made between this mutation and disease stage, recurrence, or second primary tumor formation. Mutations involving K-RAS codon 12 were not more prevalent according to gender. Four of the mutations were from oropharyngeal cancers, with an even distribution between base of tongue and tonsilar lesions. The remaining three mutations were from laryngeal specimens, consisting of two supraglottic and one glottic carcinomas.

Complete initial response to chemoradiation therapy was not influenced by mutational status. For mutated cases and nonmutated cases, complete initial response to chemoradiation therapy was 71 and 73%, respectively ($P = 0.32$). At three years, a statistically significant difference was observed for local-regional control between mutated and nonmutated cases, with respective values of 32% and 83% ($P = 0.03$). Disease-free survival was 27% and 68% ($P = 0.12$), distant metastasis-free survival was 100% and 81% ($P = 0.30$), and overall survival (see Figure 1) was 57% and 65% ($P = 0.14$)

TABLE 1: Patient characteristics and treatment intentions.

Characteristic	K-RAS codon 12 (no mutation)	K-RAS codon 12 (mutation)	K-RAS codon 13	All
Sex—M/F	144/44	6/1	—	150/45
Age—yr	56	62	—	56
Stage				
II	2	0	0	2
III	31	0	0	31
IV	148	6	0	154
Relapse	7	1	0	8
Site of primary tumor				
Mouth	21	0	0	21
Oropharynx	119	4	0	123
Larynx	26	3	0	29
Hypopharynx	11	0	0	11
Other	11	0	0	11
Tumor stage				
T1	21	1	0	22
T2	39	1	0	40
T3	60	1	0	61
T4	61	3	0	64
Nodal stage				
N0	21	0	0	21
N1	31	0	0	31
N2	103	5	0	108
N3	25	1	0	26
Radiotherapy				
Conventional	170	6	0	176
Adjuvant	18	0	0	18
Chemotherapy				
Cisplatin	61	1	0	62
Carboplatin	126	6	0	132

at three years. Lifetime results were not different when using the nested technique (data not shown).

4. Discussion

The prevalence of K-RAS codon 12 mutations in our study population is in agreement with previously published data from the western world. The PCR technique used here to detect codon 12 and 13 mutations has previously been validated in the clinical setting with a demonstration of high specificity (100%) and a detection at a low level of presence (1%) [37]. Contrary to one report, which could only identify K-RAS codon 12 mutations using a nested technique, our results indicate that simple PCR-RFLP was able to clearly identify 7 of the 8 mutated specimens studied. However, K-RAS codon 13 mutation is a very rare event in HNSCC. In a study on sinonasal carcinoma, 1% of squamous cell carcinomas harbored a K-RAS codon 12 mutations, and there were no mutations in codon 13 [9]. Furthermore, no codon 13 mutations were found in 22 SCC of the larynx in a study by Rizos et al. [18]. Also, in the study conducted by Weber et

al., only one case of HNSCC out of 89 harboured a codon 13 mutation [38].

Our study does not include analysis of the two other well-known RAS oncogenes. Our estimate may therefore be conservative in that RAS gene mutations other than K-RAS may be present in our population. K-RAS gene mutations may only represent 50% of RAS mutations in head and neck cancer specimens [25]. Furthermore, K-RAS mutations themselves may have been underestimated since codon 59 and 61 were not evaluated in our study; however, mutations of these codons are even less frequent.

On the other hand, K-RAS mutations found in head and neck specimens may possibly represent mutations in the lymphocytic infiltration of the carcinoma and not the malignant epithelium itself, as was previously described by Chang et al. [39]. Blood sampling verifying this possibility was not carried out in our population. Tissue samples showing K-RAS codon 12 mutations did not show a more aggressive pattern on histology than those without the mutation.

Our study failed to determine the chronological occurrence of these mutations since all tissue specimens studied were from advanced stage III and IV cancers. All mutations were found in advanced stage IV disease and recurrences.

The role of K-RAS mutations in early stages of carcinogenesis could thus not be ascertained. Whether or not K-RAS activation plays a part in early carcinogenesis remains unknown [19, 22]. Inducible activation of K-RAS in the oral cavity of mice has been objectified by Caulin et al. [22]. These tumors represent early stages of tumor progression, and their differentiation characteristics resemble those observed in benign human oral lesions.

In our population, tumors demonstrating K-RAS codon 12 mutations did not show an increased metastatic potential compared to their nonmutated counterparts. Thyroid cancer, on the other hand, demonstrates a substantial difference in occurrence of RAS gene activation between papillary (20%) and follicular (80%) cancers, suggesting a relation between this pattern and the marked difference in metastatic potential of these cancers [40]. RAS gene activation, usually by point mutation, may be an important event in the transformation of glandular tissue to adenocarcinoma, but seems to play a lesser role in SCC formation [15].

Treatment of HNSCC has evolved over the last two decades to incorporate modalities that have resulted in decreased patient morbidity. Unfortunately, there has been little improvement in mortality rates over the same period.

5. Conclusion

Although the prevalence of K-RAS codon 12 mutations is below 5% in the western hemisphere, the benefit of searching for such a mutation is considerable. Just as sarcomas represent only a fraction of laryngeal tumors and are treated surgically, HNSCC with K-RAS codon 12 mutations may represent a subset of tumors requiring special treatment considerations in order to improve outcomes. Though histology has long been accepted as the gold standard to classify tumors and orient treatment of HNSCC, molecular biology and the search for specific markers must be considered as an added tool to distinguish tumors with similar histological appearance but different behaviors. The use of biological markers may thus help overcome limitations inherent to histological classification and improve treatment outcomes by allowing the use of more specific treatment modalities.

Conflict of Interests

There is no conflict of interests to declare. None of the coauthors have direct financial relations with any of the trademarks mentioned in this paper.

Authors' Contribution

The first two authors (E. Bissada and O. Abboud) participated equally in the creation of this paper.

References

[1] A. Jemal, R. Siegel, E. Ward et al., "Cancer statistics, 2008," *CA: A Cancer Journal for Clinicians*, vol. 58, no. 2, pp. 71–96, 2008.

[2] J. C. Irish and A. Bernstein, "Oncogenes in head and neck cancer," *Laryngoscope*, vol. 103, no. 1, part 1, pp. 42–52, 1993.

[3] J. S. McDonald, H. Jones, Z. P. Pavelic, L. J. Pavelic, P. J. Stambrook, and J. L. Gluckman, "Immunohistochemical detection of the H-ras, K-ras, and N-ras oncogenes in squamous cell carcinoma of the head and neck," *Journal of Oral Pathology and Medicine*, vol. 23, no. 8, pp. 342–346, 1994.

[4] W. G. Yarbrough, C. Shores, D. L. Witsell, M. C. Weissler, M. E. Fidler, and T. M. Gilmer, "ras mutations and expression in head and neck squamous cell carcinomas," *Laryngoscope*, vol. 104, no. 11, part 1, pp. 1337–1347, 1994.

[5] J. A. Anderson, J. C. Irish, and B. Y. Ngan, "Prevalence of RAS oncogene mutation in head and neck carcinomas," *Journal of Otolaryngology*, vol. 21, no. 5, pp. 321–326, 1992.

[6] J. M. Spencer, S. M. Kahn, W. Jiang, V. A. DeLeo, and I. B. Weinstein, "Activated ras genes occur in human actinic keratoses, premalignant precursors to squamous cell carcinomas," *Archives of Dermatology*, vol. 131, no. 7, pp. 796–800, 1995.

[7] M. Barbacid, "ras genes," *Annual Review of Biochemistry*, vol. 56, pp. 779–827, 1987.

[8] S. A. Belinsky, T. R. Devereux, R. R. Maronpot, G. D. Stoner, and M. W. Anderson, "Relationship between the formation of promutagenic adducts and the activation of the K-ras protooncogene in lung tumors from A/J mice treated with nitrosamines," *Cancer Research*, vol. 49, no. 19, pp. 5305–5311, 1989.

[9] J. Bornholdt, J. Hansen, T. Steiniche et al., "K-ras mutations in sinonasal cancers in relation to wood dust exposure," *BMC Cancer*, vol. 8, article 53, 2008.

[10] M. Huncharek, J. Muscat, and J. F. Geschwind, "K-ras oncogene mutation as a prognostic marker in non-small cell lung cancer: a combined analysis of 881 cases," *Carcinogenesis*, vol. 20, no. 8, pp. 1507–1510, 1999.

[11] C. S. Karapetis, S. Khambata-Ford, D. J. Jonker et al., "K-ras mutations and benefit from cetuximab in advanced colorectal cancer," *The New England Journal of Medicine*, vol. 359, no. 17, pp. 1757–1765, 2008.

[12] R. E. Howell, F. S. H. Wong, and R. G. Fenwick, "A transforming Kirsten ras oncogene in an oral squamous carcinoma," *Journal of Oral Pathology and Medicine*, vol. 19, no. 7, pp. 301–305, 1990.

[13] S. E. Chang, P. Bhatia, N. W. Johnson et al., "Ras mutations in United Kingdom examples of oral malignancies are infrequent," *International Journal of Cancer*, vol. 48, no. 3, pp. 409–412, 1991.

[14] D. Saranath, L. T. Bhoite, M. G. Deo et al., "Detection and cloning of potent transforming gene(s) from chewing tobacco-related human oral carcinomas," *European Journal of Cancer B*, vol. 30, no. 4, pp. 268–277, 1994.

[15] G. Rumsby, R. L. Carter, and B. A. Gusterson, "Low incidence of ras oncogene activation in human squamous cell carcinomas," *British Journal of Cancer*, vol. 61, no. 3, pp. 365–368, 1990.

[16] W. A. Yeudall, L. K. Torrance, K. A. Elsegood, P. Speight, C. Scully, and S. S. Prime, "ras gene point mutation is a rare event in premalignant tissues and malignant cells and tissues from oral mucosal lesions," *European Journal of Cancer B*, vol. 29, no. 1, pp. 63–67, 1993.

[17] R. L. M. Ruíz-Godoy, C. M. García-Cuellar, N. E. Herrera González et al., "Mutational analysis of K-ras and Ras protein expression in larynx squamous cell carcinoma," *Journal of Experimental and Clinical Cancer Research*, vol. 25, no. 1, pp. 73–78, 2006.

[18] E. Rizos, G. Sourvinos, D. A. Arvanitis, G. Velegrakis, and D. A. Spandidos, "Low incidence of H-, K- and N-ras oncogene mutations in cytological specimens of laryngeal tumours," *Oral Oncology*, vol. 35, no. 6, pp. 561–563, 1999.

[19] T. Hirano, P. E. Steele, and J. L. Gluckman, "Low incidence of point mutation at codon 12 of K-ras proto-oncogene in squamous cell carcinoma of the upper aerodigestive tract," *Annals of Otology, Rhinology and Laryngology*, vol. 100, no. 7, pp. 597–599, 1991.

[20] H. Kiaris, D. A. Spandidos, A. S. Jones, E. D. Vaughan, and J. K. Field, "Mutations, expression and genomic instability of the H-ras proto-oncogene in squamous cell carcinomas of the head and neck," *British Journal of Cancer*, vol. 72, no. 1, pp. 123–128, 1995.

[21] M. Y. P. Kuo, J. H. Jeng, C. P. Chiang, and L. J. Hahn, "Mutations of Ki-ras oncogene codon 12 in betel quid chewing-related human oral squamous cell carcinoma in Taiwan," *Journal of Oral Pathology and Medicine*, vol. 23, no. 2, pp. 70–74, 1994.

[22] C. Caulin, T. Nguyen, M. A. Longley, Z. Zhou, X. J. Wang, and D. R. Roop, "Inducible activation of oncogenic K-ras results in tumor formation in the oral cavity," *Cancer Research*, vol. 64, no. 15, pp. 5054–5058, 2004.

[23] N. Das, J. Majumder, and U. B. Dasgupta, "ras gene mutations in oral cancer in eastern India," *Oral Oncology*, vol. 36, no. 1, pp. 76–80, 2000.

[24] J. K. Field, "The role of oncogenes and tumour-suppressor genes in the aetiology of oral, head and neck squamous cell carcinoma," *Journal of the Royal Society of Medicine*, vol. 88, no. 1, pp. 35P–39P, 1995.

[25] F. Nunez, O. Dominguez, E. Coto, C. Suarez-Nieto, P. Perez, and C. Lopez-Larrea, "Analysis of ras oncogene mutations in human squamous cell carcinoma of the head and neck," *Surgical Oncology*, vol. 1, no. 6, pp. 405–411, 1992.

[26] D. Saranath, R. G. Panchal, R. Nair et al., "Oncogene amplification in squamous cell carcinoma of the oral cavity," *Japanese Journal of Cancer Research*, vol. 80, no. 5, pp. 430–437, 1989.

[27] D. Saranath, S. E. Chang, L. T. Bhoite et al., "High frequency mutation in codons 12 and 61 of H-ras oncogene in chewing tobacco-related human oral carcinoma in India," *British Journal of Cancer*, vol. 63, no. 4, pp. 573–578, 1991.

[28] M. Hoa, S. L. Davis, S. J. Ames, and R. A. Spanjaard, "Amplification of wild-type K-ras promotes growth of head and neck squamous cell carcinoma," *Cancer Research*, vol. 62, no. 24, pp. 7154–7156, 2002.

[29] E. Freer, N. W. Savage, G. J. Seymour, T. L. Dunn, M. F. Lavin, and R. A. Gardiner, "RAS oncogene product expression in normal and malignant oral mucosa," *Australian Dental Journal*, vol. 35, no. 2, pp. 141–146, 1990.

[30] M. Azuma, N. Furumoto, H. Kawamata et al., "The relation of ras oncogene product p21 expression to clinicopathological status criteria and clinical outcome in squamous cell head and neck cancer," *Cancer Journal*, vol. 1, no. 9, pp. 375–380, 1987.

[31] M. Y. Kuo, H. H. Chang, L. J. Hahn, J. T. Wang, and C. P. Chiang, "Elevated ras p21 expression in oral premalignant lesions and squamous cell carcinomas in Taiwan," *Journal of Oral Pathology and Medicine*, vol. 24, no. 6, pp. 255–260, 1995.

[32] A. Ruol, J. K. Stephens, F. Michelassi et al., "Expression of ras oncogene p21 protein in esophageal squamous cell carcinoma," *Journal of Surgical Oncology*, vol. 44, no. 3, pp. 142–145, 1990.

[33] M. Oft, R. J. Akhurst, and A. Balmain, "Metastasis is driven by sequential elevation of H-ras and Smad2 levels," *Nature Cell Biology*, vol. 4, no. 7, pp. 487–494, 2002.

[34] J. K. Field, M. Yiagnisis, T. D. A. Spandidos et al., "Low levels of ras p21 oncogene expression correlates with clinical outcome in head and neck squamous cell carcinoma," *European Journal of Surgical Oncology*, vol. 18, no. 2, pp. 168–176, 1992.

[35] D. Saranath, L. T. Bhoite, and M. G. Deo, "Molecular lesions in human oral cancer: the Indian scene," *European Journal of Cancer B*, vol. 29, no. 2, pp. 107–112, 1993.

[36] A. Hatzaki, E. Razi, K. Anagnostopoulou et al., "A modified mutagenic PCR-RFLP method for K-ras codon 12 and 13 mutations detection in NSCLC patients," *Molecular and Cellular Probes*, vol. 15, no. 5, pp. 243–247, 2001.

[37] D. Soulières, W. Greer, A. M. Magliocco et al., "KRAS mutation testing in the treatment of metastatic colorectal cancer with anti-EGFR therapies," *Current Oncology*, vol. 17, supplement 1, pp. S31–S40, 2010.

[38] A. Weber, L. Langhanki, F. Sommerer, A. Markwarth, C. Wittekind, and A. Tannapfel, "Mutations of the BRAF gene in squamous cell carcinoma of the head and neck," *Oncogene*, vol. 22, no. 30, pp. 4757–4759, 2003.

[39] S. E. Chang, W. E. Marnock, P. J. Shirlaw et al., "Novel KI-ras codon 61 mutation in infiltrating leucocytes of oral squamous cell carcinoma," *The Lancet*, vol. 1, no. 8645, p. 1014, 1989.

[40] N. R. Lemoine, E. S. Mayall, F. S. Wyllie et al., "Activated ras oncogenes in human thyroid cancers," *Cancer Research*, vol. 48, no. 16, pp. 4459–4463, 1988.

24

Hearing Benefit in Allograft Tympanoplasty Using Tutoplast Processed Malleus

Anja Lieder and Wolfgang Issing

Department of Otolaryngology, Freeman Hospital, Freeman Road, High Heaton, Newcastle upon Tyne NE7 7DN, UK

Correspondence should be addressed to Wolfgang Issing; wolfgang.issing@nuth.nhs.uk

Academic Editor: Leonard P. Rybak

Objectives. Tutoplast processed human cadaveric ossicular allografts are a safe alternative for ossicular reconstruction where there is insufficient material suitable for autograft ossiculoplasty. We present a series of 7 consecutive cases showing excellent air-bone gap closure following canal-wall-down mastoidectomy for cholesteatoma and reconstruction of the middle ear using Tutoplast processed malleus. *Patients and Methods.* Tympanoplasty with Tutoplast processed malleus was performed in seven patients to reconstruct the middle ear following canal-wall-down mastoidectomy in a tertiary ENT centre. *Main Outcome Measures.* Hearing improvement and recurrence-free period were assessed. Pre-and postoperative audiograms were performed. *Results.* The average pre operative hearing loss was 50 ± 13 dB, with an air-bone gap of 33 ± 7 dB. Post operative audiograms at 25 months demonstrated hearing thresholds of 29 ± 10 dB, with an air-bone gap of 14 ± 6 dB. No prosthesis extrusion was observed, which compares favourably to other commercially available prostheses. *Conclusions.* Tutoplast processed allografts restore conductive hearing loss in patients undergoing mastoidectomy and provide an excellent alternative when there is insufficient material suitable for autograft ossiculoplasty.

1. Introduction

Human cadaveric allografts have been used in middle ear reconstruction for half a century. They fully integrate into the middle ear and may be used to reconstruct the ossicular chain where there is insufficient autologous material. Tutoplast processed ossicular allografts (Tutoplast Ossicula auditus) consist of dehydrated human malleus or incus and provide a matrix for new bone formation through bone remodelling. They are derived from selected donors using the Tutoplast process. This process involves osmotic destruction of tissue cells, followed by denaturation using sodium hydroxide and hydrogen peroxide to inactivate all pathogens, and finally dehydration and sterilization by gamma irradiation. The Tutoplast process inactivates all living organisms and spores from donated tissue and achieves Sterility Assurance Level of 10^{-6}. Each transplant can be tracked back to the original donor [1, 2]. Tutoplast Ossicula auditus is licensed as a medical product in Germany and fulfils European Union and USA medical drug regulations.

We present a series of 7 consecutive cases demonstrating excellent long-term hearing improvements in tympanoplasty using Tutoplast processed malleus to reconstruct the middle ear following mastoidectomy.

2. Patients and Methods

Seven consecutive patients with cholesteatoma aged 11–69 years (four male, three female) underwent canal-wall-down mastoidectomy and tympanoplasty between May 2009 and January 2011. Two cases were revisions. All patients had canal-wall-down mastoidectomy for removal of cholesteatoma, followed by ype III tympanoplasty including myringoplasty with tragal perichondrium in a single-stage procedure. This would entail the placement of a Tutoplast processed malleus (Tutoplast Ossicula auditus, Tutogen Medical GmbH, Neunkirchen, Germany) onto the stapes if the patient's own ossicles were found to be either absent, eroded or unsuitable for an autograft. One patient had additional

TABLE 1: Comparison between pre- and postoperative audiograms and assessment of air-bone gap.

TABLE 1: Comparison between pre- and postoperative audiograms and assessment of air-bone gap.

	Patient								
	1	2	3	4	5	6	7	Mean	SD
Operated ear									
Preoperative hearing (air conduction; 500–4000 Hz)	50	41	55	73	54	38	36	**49.5**	*12.7*
Preoperative air-bone gap (500–4000 Hz)	30	23	28	43	38	34	35	**32.7**	*6.6*
Follow-up (months)	34	26	29	29	20	22	15	25	6
Postoperative hearing (air conduction; 500–4000 Hz)	28	28	39	45	28	19	19	**29.1**[a]	*9.7*
Postoperative air-bone gap (500–4000 Hz)	18	5	24	14	15	9	13	**13.8**[b]	*6.0*
Air-bone gap closure achieved	13	18	4	29	23	25	23	18.9	8.5

[a]$P = 0.0061$; [b]$P = 0.00012$. Bold: Mean values. Italic: Standard deviation.

reconstruction of posterior canal wall using tragal cartilage. All patients had their ear dressed with 2 silastic sheets, one being placed in the mastoid cavity to facilitate epithelialisation of the cavity and the other to cover the tympanic membrane. Bismuth iodine paste gauze dressing was applied into the external auditory meatus for 2-3 weeks. Once sufficient healing was ascertained, patients were instructed in the Valsalva manoeuvre and were encouraged to perform it 20–30 times per day.

Hearing assessment was by pure tone audiograms in accordance with the British Society of Audiology recommended procedure (2004). Values are given in Decibel Hearing Level (dB HL) for testing frequencies of 250, 500, 1000, 2000, 4000, and 8000 Hertz (Hz). Air-bone gaps were calculated in accordance with the American Academy of Otolaryngology-Head and Neck Surgery (AAO-HNS) 1995 guideline. The testing frequency of 3000 Hz was substituted with 4000 Hz. Audiograms were read by two observers independently. Average hearing levels are given in dB HL and standard deviations are applied where appropriate. Where applicable, Student's t-test (equal sample size, unequal variance) was performed and P values were given.

3. Ethical Considerations

Written consent, including the use of Tutoplast Ossicula auditus, was obtained. All investigations and procedures were performed according to best clinical practice and the medical principles of the Declaration of Helsinki. The National Research Ethics Service of the United Kingdom has confirmed that formal ethics approval procedure is not required (NRES Ref 04/26/31) as this is a retrospective study using a fully licensed product.

4. Results

Postoperative complications were not observed. The stapes suprastructure was fully intact in six patients. There was partial destruction of the stapes suprastructure in one patient, with one crus being present, and, in this case, the prosthesis was placed on the preserved crus.

The average preoperative hearing loss (air conduction) was 49.5 ± 12.7 dB (36–73 dB). The average preoperative air-bone gap was 32.7 ± 6.6 dB (23–43 dB) (Table 1). Patients

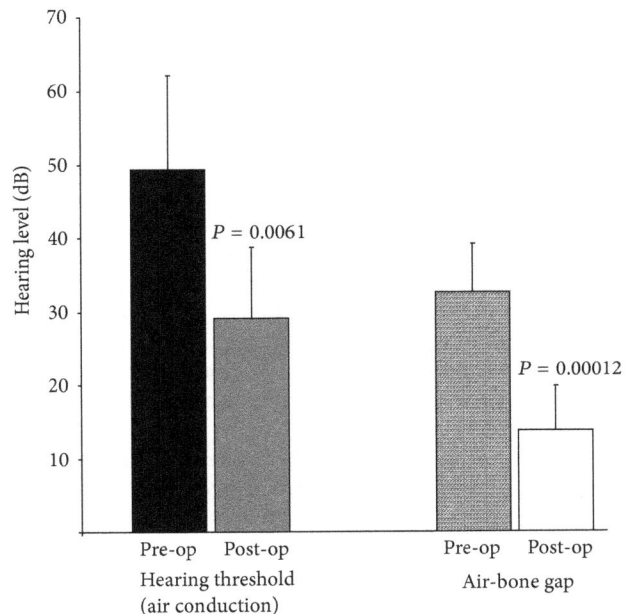

FIGURE 1: Hearing thresholds before and after surgery. Preoperative (pre-op) and postoperative (post-op) hearing thresholds in db Hearing Level including standard deviation are shown. The first group of two columns (black and grey column, resp.) denotes the hearing threshold on air conduction preoperatively and postoperatively. The second group of two columns denotes the air-bone gap preoperatively and postoperatively (patterned and white column, resp.).

were followed up between 15 and 34 months after surgery, on average 25 ± 6 months. Recurrence or prosthesis extrusion was not observed. All patients had a safe dry ear upon clinical examination and reported substantial improvement to their hearing.

Postoperative hearing thresholds (air conduction) in the operated ear had improved to 29.1 ± 9.7 dB ($P = 0.006$). The air-bone gap had narrowed to 13.8 ± 6.0 dB after surgery (4–24 dB) ($P = 0.0001$). Six patients (86%) had a postoperative air-bone gap of less than 20 dB. The air-bone gap closure achieved was on average 18.9 ± 8.5 dB (4–29 dB, Table 1 and

Figure 1). Representative pre- and postoperative pure tone audiograms are shown in Figure 2.

5. Discussion

Middle ear reconstruction following cholesteatoma surgery can be challenging. Auditory ossicles are often eroded, making them insufficient for ossiculoplasty, and they can also harbour remnants of cholesteatoma matrix which can facilitate disease recurrence. Surgical options in these cases include the use of ossicular replacement prostheses or ossicular allografts. Apprehension in using such allografts over a fear of infection transmission has not made them widely known surgical options in recent years and many surgeons have no experience in using them. Tutoplast processed malleus is safe. Since the inception of Tutoplast processed human cadaveric allografts in the 1970s and, there have been no reported cases of graft rejection or disease transmission [2].

Tutoplast processed malleus acts as a collagen matrix for bone regeneration and remodelling. Studies on allograft ossiculoplasty dating back to the 1970s demonstrate that allograft ossicles (notched incus homograft) achieve excellent integration and restoration of hearing [3]. Tutoplast processed bone grafts achieve the highest mesenchymal stem cell adherence in vitro, hence making it an ideal environment for bone regeneration [4]. A study on a postmortem temporal bone confirms minimal resorption of allograft ossicles [5] and longevity of these grafts is excellent, as no osteoclastic bone resorption occurs [6].

Ossicular replacement prostheses are used in middle ear reconstruction with extensively published evidence. A series of 465 cases reported closure of air-bone gap to ≤ 15 dB in 63% of cases and to ≤ 20 dB in 73% of cases with partial ossicular replacement prostheses (PORP) [7]. A series of 650 cases, also using Plastipore PORP, reported postoperative air-bone gaps of ≤ 20 dB in 68%, although the average air-bone gap was 18 ± 11 dB after 12 months [8]. Another group reported postoperative air-bone gap closure (≤20 dB) in tympanoplasty following mastoidectomy for 46% and 33% for titanium and hydroxyapatite prostheses, respectively. Average postoperative air-bone gap was 26.5 dB, with 23.8 dB for titanium group and 29.8 dB for hydroxyapatite group after 1 year [9]. Closure of the air-bone gap fourteen years following mastoidectomy and tympanoplasty using Plastipore PORP was reported to be 60% in a group of 5 patients [10].

Tympanoplasty with allogeneic ossicles can restore hearing to levels comparable to autograft, and hearing benefit is often favourable to prostheses. Early reports by Wehrs report a graft take rate between 92 and 96% and a satisfactory hearing outcome between 77 and 89% [11]. In a case series on using homologous or autologous incus interposition grafts, there was no significant difference in hearing gain between allografts and autografts. Postoperative air-bone gap was 19 dB, with 66% of patients achieving an air-bone gap closure of 20 dB or better after 15 months [12]. Another study on malleus allograft ossiculoplasties reported air-bone gap closure of ≤ 20 dB in 81% of cases one year postoperatively, but, in all cases, stapes suprastructure was missing and ossiculoplasty was performed as a secondary procedure, making these outcomes less straightforward to compare [13].

Others report less favourable hearing outcomes compared to autografts or glass ionomer cement. In a study of 293 patients comparing different means of ossicular reconstruction, cholesteatoma removal was the primary cause for surgery in 62 cases (21%), with a mean postoperative air-bone gap of 15 ± 8 dB. Allograft ossicles were used in 39 out of 293 cases (13%), resulting in a postoperative air-bone gap of 13 ± 9 dB (mean air-bone gap closure 17 ± 9 dB). There is no distinct group undergoing canal-wall-down mastoidectomy for cholesteatoma using allograft ossicles in this study, which again makes this difficult to compare with other studies [14].

Our postoperative air-bone gap is 13.8 dB. The average closure of the air-bone gap is 18.9 dB, and 86% of patients had a postoperative air-bone gap of 20 dB or less. Our outcomes gained from a single-stage procedure exceed the air-bone gap closures reported for PORP in some of the larger studies of tympanoplasty [7, 8]. They also compare favourably to results achieved in canal-wall-down mastoidectomy [9, 10, 13]. Moreover, the majority of operations in these studies were performed for chronic suppurative otitis media or were secondary procedures, and canal-wall-down mastoidectomy was either performed as a separate stage or not at all.

In addition to potentially advantageous hearing benefit, allogeneic ossicular grafts integrate into the middle ear and rarely extrude, with historic failure rates between 4 and 8% [11] and more recent extrusion rates of 0% [13]. Extrusion rates between 4-5% [8, 10] and 7% [7] have been reported in studies using prostheses. No extrusion was observed in our series but, due to its low group size, a conclusion on graft extrusion rates is not possible.

6. Conclusion

(i) We demonstrate that Tutoplast processed malleus restores hearing in 7 patients undergoing canal-wall-down mastoidectomy and tympanoplasty for cholesteatoma.

(ii) We recommend consideration of Tutoplast processed malleus in cases of cholesteatoma where autologous material cannot be used and where a single-step operative procedure to eradicate cholesteatoma with concomitant reconstruction of the middle ear is desired.

(iii) In this small study with a 25-month follow-up, no graft extrusion or other complications were observed, and we are encouraged to offer allograft ossicular reconstruction as an alternative to ossicular prostheses to our patients undergoing mastoid exploration for cholesteatoma who wish to have ossiculoplasty but who have insufficient autologous ossicles.

Conflict of Interests

The authors declare that there is no conflict of interests regarding the publication of this paper.

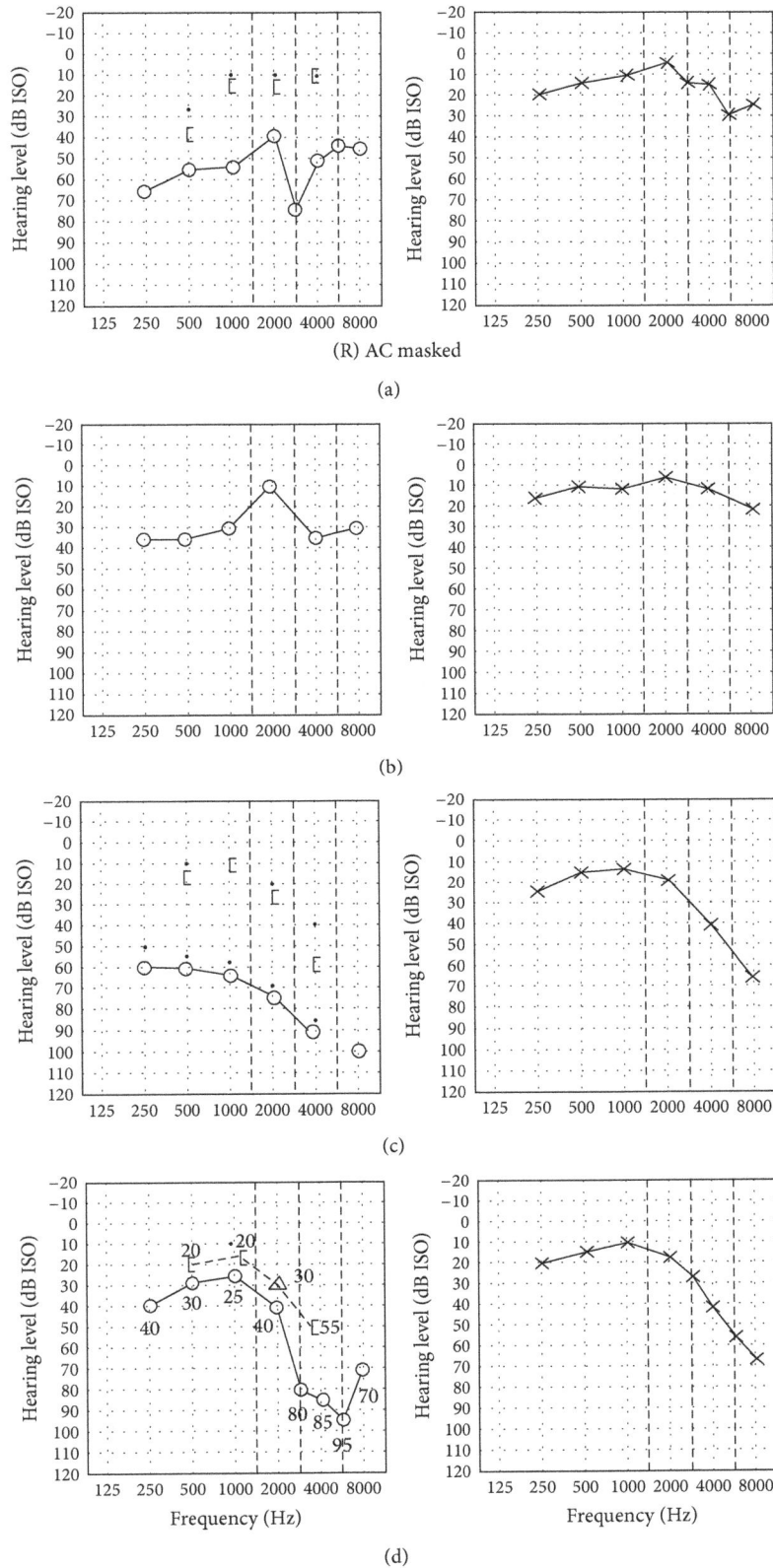

FIGURE 2: Representative pre- and postoperative original PTA from two patients. Two representative preoperative and postoperative PTA of two patients. Patient 1 (rows (a) and (b)) showed good closure of his operated right ear ABG from 30 dB to 18 dB postoperatively. Patient 4 (rows (c) and (d)) showed excellent ABG closure over 29 dB with a residual ABG of 14 dB in the operated right ear.

Acknowledgments

The authors declare that they have received no funding to support this study. Mr. Wolfgang Issing has received speaker fees from Tutogen Medical GmbH.

References

[1] C. Schoepf, "Allograft safety: efficacy of the Tutoplast process," *Implants-International Magazine of Oral Implantology*, vol. 7, no. 1, pp. 10–15, 2006.

[2] Tutogen GmbH, "Der Tutoplast prozess—weltweit einzigartig," http://www.tutogen.de/de/unternehmen/herstellung -tutoplast-prozess.html.

[3] R. E. Wehrs, "Homograft ossicles in tympanoplasty," *The Laryngoscope*, vol. 92, no. 5, pp. 540–546, 1982.

[4] C. Seebach, J. Schultheiss, K. Wilhelm, J. Frank, and D. Henrich, "Comparison of six bone-graft substitutes regarding to cell seeding efficiency, metabolism and growth behaviour of human mesenchymal stem cells (MSC) *in vitro*," *Injury*, vol. 41, no. 7, pp. 731–738, 2010.

[5] V. Goodhill and R. Gussen, "The fate of an ossicular allograft in tympanoplasty," *The Laryngoscope*, vol. 93, no. 5, pp. 578–582, 1983.

[6] J. Lang, A. G. Kerr, and G. D. Smyth, "Long-term viability of transplanted ossicles," *The Journal of Laryngology & Otology*, vol. 100, no. 7, pp. 741–747, 1986.

[7] D. E. Brackmann, J. L. Sheehy, and W. M. Luxford, "TORPs and PORPs in tympanoplasty: a review of 1042 operations," *Otolaryngology*, vol. 92, no. 1, pp. 32–37, 1984.

[8] J. W. House and K. B. Teufert, "Extrusion rates and hearing results in ossicular reconstruction," *Otolaryngology*, vol. 125, no. 3, pp. 135–141, 2001.

[9] L. O. Redaelli de Zinis, "Titanium vs hydroxyapatite ossiculoplasty in canal wall down mastoidectomy," *Archives of Otolaryngology*, vol. 134, no. 12, pp. 1283–1287, 2008.

[10] A. Eleftheriadou, T. Chalastras, S. Georgopoulos et al., "Long-term results of plastipore prostheses in reconstruction of the middle ear ossicular chain," *Journal for Oto-Rhino-Laryngology and its Related Specialties*, vol. 71, no. 5, pp. 284–288, 2009.

[11] R. E. Wehrs, "Results of homografts in middle ear surgery," *The Laryngoscope*, vol. 88, no. 5, pp. 808–815, 1978.

[12] R. C. O'Reilly, S. P. Cass, B. E. Hirsch, D. B. Kamerer, R. A. Bernat, and S. P. Poznanovic, "Ossiculoplasty using incus interposition: hearing results and analysis of the middle ear risk index," *Otology & Neurotology*, vol. 26, no. 5, pp. 853–858, 2005.

[13] J.-P. Vercruysse, F. E. Offeciers, T. Somers, I. Schatteman, and P. J. Govaerts, "The use of malleus allografts in ossiculoplasty," *The Laryngoscope*, vol. 112, no. 10, pp. 1782–1784, 2002.

[14] S. A. Felek, H. Celik, A. Islam, A. H. Elhan, M. Demirci, and E. Samim, "Type 2 ossiculoplasty: prognostic determination of hearing results by middle ear risk index," *American Journal of Otolaryngology*, vol. 31, no. 5, pp. 325–331, 2010.

25

Demography and Histologic Pattern of Laryngeal Squamous Cell Carcinoma in Kenya

Owen Pyeko Menach,[1,2] **Asmeeta Patel,**[2] **and Herbert Ouma Oburra**[1,2]

[1] *Department of Surgery, ENT Division, University of Nairobi, P.O. Box 330-00202, Nairobi, Kenya*
[2] *ENT Head & Neck Department, Kenyatta National Hospital, P.O. Box 20723-00202, Nairobi, Kenya*

Correspondence should be addressed to Owen Pyeko Menach; menachpyeko@yahoo.com

Academic Editor: David W. Eisele

Background. Laryngeal squamous cell carcinoma is a common head and neck cancer worldwide. *Objective.* To determine the demographic characteristics of patients with laryngeal cancer, establish their tumor characteristics and relate it to their smoking and alcohol ingestion habits. *Methods.* Fifty cases and fifty controls were recruited of matching age, sex, and region of residence. History and pattern of cigarette smoking and alcohol ingestion was taken and analyzed. *Results.* 33 (66%) of the cases and 3 (6%) among controls were current cigarette smokers. 74% had smoked for more than 30 years, $P < 0.0001$ OR 21.3 (95% CI: 2.6–176.1). There was a male predominance (96%) and most cases (62%) were from the ethnic communities in the highland areas of Kenya predominantly in Central and Eastern provinces. Very heavy drinkers had increased risk of $P < 0.0001$ OR, 6.0 (95% CI: 1.957–18.398) and those who smoked cigarettes and drank alcohol had poorly differentiated tumors G3, $P < 0.001$, OR 11.652 (95% CI 2.305–58.895), and G4, $P = 0.52$ OR 7.286 (95% CI 0.726–73.075). They also presented with advanced disease (73.6%). *Conclusion.* Cigarette smoking and alcohol ingestion are strong risk factors for development of late stage and poorly differentiated laryngeal squamous cell carcinoma in Kenya.

1. Background

The commonest causes of death in Kenya are infectious diseases followed closely by cardiovascular illnesses and cancer in that order [1]. Cancer cases in Kenya have however been steadily rising due to the increasing prevalence of cigarette smoking which is a known cause of various neoplasias, more so the upper aerodigestive tract and lung tumors [1, 2]. This rise has been documented and published by the Nairobi Cancer Registry [3], but it is not thought to depict the accurate situation on the ground because cancer diagnosis and notification from health institutions are not as meticulous as desirable. This increase has not been captured in local studies especially with regard to head and neck cancer in general and laryngeal carcinoma in particular.

From previous published work, cigarette smoking and alcohol ingestion have been shown to be major risk factors for laryngeal squamous cell carcinoma in this locality as seen in other populations [4]. The incidence of this cancer may increase considering the rising prevalence of smoking in Kenya especially among men in the 45–49 years of age bracket [1, 2]. Moreover, it is also quite worrying that 13% of schooling children smoke cigarettes and, just like in adults, males smoke more than females [5, 6]. If not checked, there is likelihood of increased cancer burden corresponding to the shifting trends and rising prevalence of cigarette smoking in this population.

Globally, about a fifth of the world's population smoke cigarettes and these figures are increasing exponentially due to extensive and aggressive marketing done by cigarette manufacturing companies [7]. The smoking pattern in the world seems to vary in the various continents with Russia and China leading to the prevalence of the disease. This trend seems to be reducing in the West while it is increasing in the developing world though the prevalence is still higher in the Western countries, Europe, and Asia [7, 8].

Concurrent cigarette smoking and ingestion of ethanol have been shown to increase mucosal penetration of tobacco carcinogens as well as production of carcinogenic metabolites in the upper aerodigestive tract [9, 10]. The risk imparted by both factors has been shown to be synergistic thus increasing the risk of squamous cell carcinoma by many fold [4, 9, 10]. However, alcohol as an independent risk factor for laryngeal cancer remains controversial [10]. The relation between histologic differentiation of squamous cell carcinoma with cigarette smoking and alcohol ingestion has been documented [11]. These risk factors have been shown to predispose to poorly differentiated forms and therefore have a poorer outcome than more differentiated ones though other authors dispute this finding [11, 12]. Overall, the prevalence of cigarette smoking and alcohol ingestion is increasing, but its relation to cancer has not been clearly elucidated with regard to laryngeal squamous cell carcinoma in this population.

2. Objective

The objective of this study was to determine the demographic characteristics of patients with laryngeal squamous cell carcinoma, establish their tumor characteristics, and relate it to their cigarette smoking and alcohol ingestion habits.

3. Study Design

This was a hospital based case-control study.

4. Sample Size Calculation

The sample size was calculated using the Hennekens and Buring [13] formula for comparing two proportions.

5. Methodology

The study was conducted between March and May, 2011, at the Kenyatta National Hospital.

5.1. Recruitment of Study Patients. A total of 50 cases whose histology had been confirmed to be squamous cell carcinoma were recruited for the study. 78% were recruited from the Otorhinolaryngology Head and Neck Department whereas 22% were recruited from the Radiation-Oncology Department. All the cases were staged clinically, endoscopically, and radiologically by computerized tomography scanning and finally discussed in the Otorhinolaryngology Head and Neck Tumor Board. Six cases that had nonsquamous cell histologies were excluded from the study whereas two others were declined.

5.2. Recruitment of Controls. A total of 50 controls were recruited. 72% were recruited from the Orthopedic Wards whereas 28% were recruited from the Orthopedic Clinic. Among the controls, three patients were found to have dysphonia whereas one had a neck swelling and was referred to the otorhinolaryngology clinic for detailed assessment. 62% had been admitted with fractures and dislocations, 25% with benign spinal ailments, and the rest had inflammatory and infectious ailments. Controls were matched by age with the cases within a range of five years.

5.3. Establishment of Demographic Data, Presence and Nature of Smoking Habit and Alcohol Ingestion. The patient's demographic data including age, sex, and region of origin, occupation as well as smoking and alcohol intake habits were documented. Symptomatology and nasolaryngoscopy data were obtained from the control subjects with a focus to rule out laryngeal cancer. The controls that did not have symptoms and nasolaryngoscopy evidence of laryngeal cancer were included in the study. Their alcohol intake habits, including the type, were categorized as per NIAAA [14] guidelines while cigarette smoking habits were classified in pack-years in both groups.

6. Data Management and Analysis

All the information was recorded in a data collection questionnaire. This data was then entered into a password protected Microsoft Access database. Quality control was performed by comparing the data entered into the Microsoft Access database with the hard copy forms, identifying inconsistent ones and making appropriate corrections. The data was thereafter exported to SPSS 17.0 statistical package which was used for subsequent data analysis. Results were presented in tables, graphs, and pie charts. Mean, median, and standard deviation were computed and used to summarize continuous variables while simple counts, frequencies, and proportions were used to summarize nominal variables. Chi-squared and Fisher's exact tests were used to detect associations between nominal variables whereas ANOVA and t-tests were used to detect associations between continuous and nominal variables. Multivariate logistic regression methods were used to detect associations between continuous variables.

7. Results

7.1. Age Distribution. The youngest age for the cases was 42 years while the oldest was 84 years with a mean age of 63 years. There was no statistically significant difference between the case and control group whose mean age was 61 years ($P = 0.297$).

7.2. Sex Distribution. Out of the 50 cases, only 2 were female (4%) whereas the rest were male (96%) suggesting that this is predominantly a male disease.

7.3. Region of Origin. The highland areas of Central province (46%) and Eastern province (16%) were the most affected geographical areas. The lowlands of Rift Valley, Nyanza and Western followed suit with 16%, 8%, and 6%, respectively (Figure 1). The least number of cases was seen in Nairobi province ($P = 0.281$). Some cases from Nyanza and coast province were controlled against controls recruited from other regions due to unavailability of the suitable age and sex. This study did not determine to what extent ethnicity contributed to regional biases.

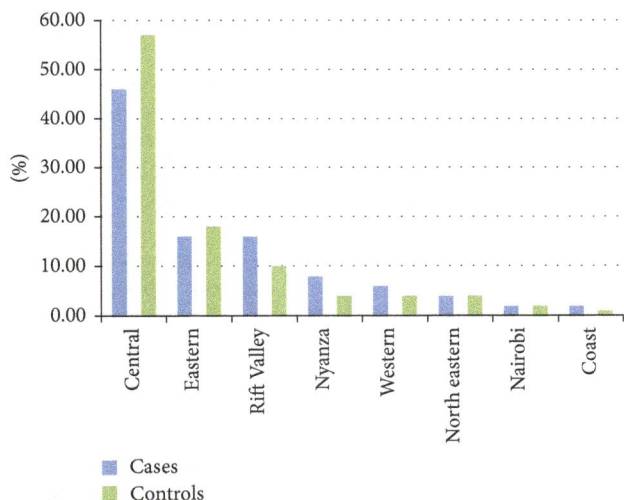

FIGURE 1: Distribution of cases and controls by region.

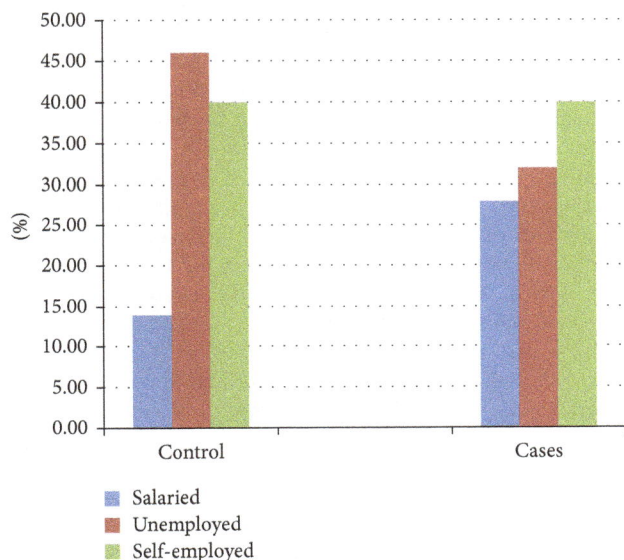

FIGURE 3: Levels of education among cases and controls.

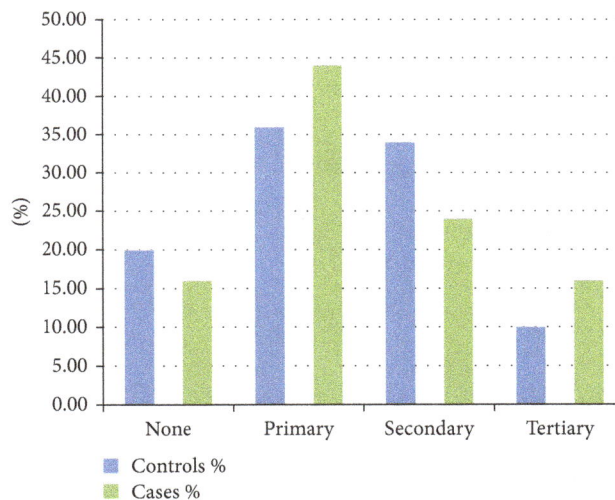

FIGURE 2: Occupation among cases and controls.

TABLE 1: Smoking history and habits.

	Controls	Cases	P value
Smoker			
No	94.00%	34.00%	<0.0001
Yes	6.00%	66.00%	
Cigarette type smoked			
Filtered	86.70%	69.80%	0.198
Nonfiltered	13.30%	30.20%	
Lives with smoker			
No	98.00%	96.00%	0.558
Yes	2.00%	4.00%	
Smokes in the house			
No	98.00%	94.00%	0.307
Yes	2.00%	6.00%	

7.4. Occupation. An equal proportion of cases and controls were self-employed whereas more of the controls were unemployed compared to the cases. Twice as much of the cases were salaried compared to the controls although these findings were not statistically significant ($P = 0.166$) (Figure 2).

7.5. Education. Majority of the cases had attained primary education compared to controls whereas other levels of education were comparable ($P = 0.57$) (Figure 3).

In general, the characteristics of the cases in terms of sex, age, region of origin, occupation, and level of education were similar with the distribution among controls.

7.6. Smoking History. The prevalence of the respondents who lived with someone who smoked in the house was comparable between cases and controls at 3% and 2%, respectively.

The P values for living with a smoker and smoking in the house were 0.558 and 0.307, respectively (Table 1).

Similarly, the mean age of starting cigarette smoking among the cases was 20.18 whereas it was 25 among the controls ($P = 0.044$). Those who started smoking below the age of 20 years had $P < 0.0001$, OR of 31.733 (95% CI: 8.74–115.04) whereas those who started smoking between 21 and 40 years of age had $P < 0.001$, OR of 7.727 (95% CI: 2.409–24.787). P value for those who began smoking after 40 years was 1.00. Those who smoked more than 30 pack-years among the cases had higher risks compared to controls, OR of 21.3 ($P < 0.0001$, 95% CI 2.6–176.1). This confirms the fact that longer duration and greater intensity of cigarette smoking portend a great risk for laryngeal SCC.

7.7. Alcohol Consumption. 38 (76%) cases consumed alcohol compared to 29 (58%) controls. This was statistically significant, $P = 0.05$, OR of 2.3 (95% CI: 1.0–5.4), though it was more pronounced among those who were very heavy drinkers $P = 0.002$ OR 6.0 (95% CI: 11.957–18.398).

TABLE 2: Tumor characteristics and stage of disease.

	Count	Column N%
Differentiation		
Well differentiated (G1)	19	38.00%
Moderately differentiated (G2)	17	34.00%
Poorly differentiated (G3)	10	20.00%
Undifferentiated (G4)	4	8.00%
Stage		
1	3	6.40%
2	10	20%
3	24	46%
4	13	27.60%

7.8. Tumor Characteristics and Stage of Tumor. In this study, majority of the cases had histological diagnosis of well differentiated (G1) squamous cell carcinoma followed by moderately differentiated (G2), and poorly differentiated (G3) and the least was undifferentiated carcinoma (G4).

Majority of the cases presented in stages 3 and 4 of the disease (Table 2).

7.9. Risk Factors in relation to Histological Grade. On analyzing the histological grades against the risk exposures being studied, 4 cases smoked but did not drink alcohol and developed G1 carcinoma. Of note is that none of those who smoked without ingesting alcohol developed poorly differentiated cancer and none of those who drank alcohol without smoking cigarettes developed G1 carcinoma. This relation was of statistical significance, P value < 0.0001, OR of 21.333 (95% CI 2.227–204.364), when compared to controls.

7.10. Cigarette Smoking and Alcohol Ingestion. There was a statistically significant increased risk for laryngeal squamous cell carcinoma on all histological grades except for G1 tumors among those who smoked cigarettes and consumed alcohol concurrently, but, notably, they were more predisposed to develop poorly differentiated tumors G3 and G4 (Table 3).

Multivariate logistic regression was performed on variables that had significant P values. The variables included were being a current smoker ($P \leq 0.0001$), duration since stopping smoking ($P = 0.029$), age of smoking debut ($P = 0.044$), cumulative pack-years ($P < 0.0001$), duration of smoking ($P < 0.0001$), prevalence of alcohol intake ($P = 0.05$), drinks taken per week ($P = 0.028$), G1 tumors ($P < 0.001$) and G2 tumors (P 0.022). Only being a current smoker OR of 14.576 (95% CI 2.624–80.979), and long duration of smoking, OR of 7.312 (95% CI 1.619–33.024), were independently associated with increased risk for laryngeal squamous cell carcinoma in this population.

8. Discussion

According to the results of this study, majority of the cases of laryngeal squamous cell carcinoma were elderly males. This is comparable to studies done elsewhere since men tend to consume more alcohol and smoke more cigarettes than females as is found in Kenyan surveys [1, 2, 7]. In these surveys, about 2% of women used tobacco in its various forms whereas 1% smoked cigarettes which translate to the low prevalence of laryngeal squamous cell carcinoma among females. Studies in other populations show male prevalence of laryngeal squamous cell carcinoma as high as 100% [15]. Gallus et al. [16] carried a study among female patients and found that cigarette smoking was still the most important risk factor for laryngeal squamous cell carcinoma. With this in mind, it would be prudent to formulate policies that will reduce the prevalence and incidence of cigarette smoking among males to reduce cancer burden in this population.

Of the cases recruited, majority of them came from highland areas of Kenya's Central, Eastern, and Rift Valley provinces. This distribution is in keeping with work published by Onyango and Macharia [17] and mirrors the higher prevalence of cigarette smoking in these provinces [1, 2]. The proximity of these regions to Kenyatta National Hospital which hosts the only comprehensive public cancer treatment centre may also be a contributing factor. We can therefore postulate that the higher rates of cigarette smoking in Central and Eastern provinces, which are nearly ethnically homogenous, are responsible for the higher prevalence of laryngeal squamous cell carcinoma encountered. The contribution of genetic predisposition was not captured in this research since other regions like Coast province had high prevalence of cigarette smoking but did not have correspondingly high laryngeal cancer cases. This is an area for further research since only 62% cases of laryngeal squamous cell carcinoma have been shown to be directly linked to these two risk factors in Kenya [4].

On the other hand, there was no relation between occupation, level of education, and laryngeal cancer as opposed to findings in previous published work by Onyango and Macharia [17]. That study may not be comparable to the present one since the former had a larger sample size and included head and neck cancers in general. In other populations, low levels of education have been associated with low socioeconomic status which has been shown to confer a higher risk for laryngeal squamous cell carcinoma [18–20]. This has been attributed to higher prevalence of cigarette smoking among patients of low socioeconomic status who smoke cheaper hand rolled nonfilter cigarettes which have higher levels of carcinogens [21].

Patients who were current smokers had a significant risk for laryngeal squamous cell carcinoma in general compared to controls and there was no significant risk for laryngeal squamous cell carcinoma from environmental tobacco smoke. It should be pointed out that the respondents were few in both categories.

Earlier age of commencement of cigarette smoking has been shown at molecular level to increase risk for cancer in the aerodigestive tract [22]. This has a significant bearing in this population since it has been shown that majority of them start smoking in primary and secondary school levels [23]. Measures to reduce cigarette smoking in this age group should therefore be formulated so as to reduce cancer burden in the coming generations. On the other hand, majority

TABLE 3: Histological grade for concurrent smoking and alcohol intake.

Grade	Yes	No	P value	OR	Lower CI	Upper CI
G1	8	11				
G2	10	7	0.006	4.218	1.425	12.285
G3	8	2	<0.001	11.652	2.305	58.895
G4	3	1	0.052	7.286	0.726	73.075

of cases had smoked more than 30 pack-years increasing their risk for laryngeal cancer more than 21 times compared to controls. These facts confirm that longer duration and greater intensity of cigarette smoking portend a great risk for laryngeal SCC as shown in studies performed worldwide [24].

Alcohol consumption has been positively associated with laryngeal SCC mostly as a cofactor and also as an independent factor [10, 25]. In this study, there was an overall increased risk for laryngeal squamous cell carcinoma though the risk was significantly higher among very heavy drinkers. This finding seems to be significantly higher compared to other studies [26]. Alcohol ingestion is therefore an independent risk factor for laryngeal squamous cell carcinoma in Kenya. Such variance with other populations may be linked to the fact that majority of the alcohol consumed among the cases was traditional brew and unregulated beer.

With regard to histologic findings, majority of the patients who smoked cigarettes but did not drink alcohol developed G1 carcinoma which is not in keeping with published data [11]. The numbers involved in this study were small and therefore we may not make statistical inference based on this. Moreover, confounding factors such as GERD and human papilloma virus (HPV) may have contributed to cancer causation despite this being a controlled study as they are now acknowledged risks for head and neck squamous cell carcinoma in general including laryngeal ones. In this study, alcohol consumption predisposed to G2 carcinoma while those who were alcohol drinkers and cigarette smokers as well developed the less differentiated G3 and G4 SCC. This is in keeping with various studies done globally [11, 12, 27]. Many molecular epidemiologic studies have shown that alcohol intake and cigarette smoking cause mutation of p53 and p16 genes as well as overexpression of cyclin D1 [11, 28]. P53 gene mutation and cyclin D1 over expression among others predispose to less differentiated squamous cell carcinoma in the head and neck region [28, 29]. These may explain the histologic pattern encountered in this study. The scope of this study did not capture whether host factors influenced the histologic type and is therefore an avenue for further research.

Lastly, majority of the patients presented stage, 3 and 4 of laryngeal cancer (73.6%). From published data, tumors that are causally linked to cigarette smoking and alcohol ingestion have been shown to progress rapidly and present late [30]. These tumors are aggressive and have high recurrence rate although various other factors come into play in this region as regards late presentation as shown earlier by Oburra [31] and later by Onyango and Macharia [17]. These include their health seeking behaviour, ignorance and poverty, and lack of adequate health facilities and personnel as well as high cost of health care.

In conclusion, cigarette smoking and alcohol ingestion are important risk factors for laryngeal SCC in this population, more so in Central and Eastern provinces. Cigarette smoking without ingestion of alcohol had higher associations with well differentiated carcinoma whereas concurrent cigarette smoking and alcohol intake predisposed more to the less differentiated SCC of the larynx. The results of this study provide epidemiologic evidence that cigarette smoking and alcohol ingestion are strongly associated with poorly differentiated laryngeal squamous cell carcinoma. These tumors generally have a poorer outcome especially in the study population where cancer diagnosis, assessment, referral, management, and followup are not optimum [17].

More emphasis should be put in place to strengthen the existing tobacco control bill [32] including improved budgetary allocation for the relevant bodies to help reduce the prevalence of cigarette smoking as well as improve cancer diagnosis, treatment, and followup. A specific effort should be put to reduce cigarette smoking among school going children and college students as this will go a long way in reducing new cancer cases in future.

There were some limitations in this study. A few cases were controlled by age and sex but not geographical region of origin. This was also a hospital based study and therefore it may not reflect the true picture of the general population. Being a case-control study, recall bias may have impacted on the responses we got from the research subjects. The orthopedic trauma patients, some of whom were used in this study, may have had alcohol related accidents thus may have not been ideal controls.

Declaration

This paper was presented during the Kenya Ear Nose and Throat Society (KENTS) Scientific Conference in May 2013 and at the 20th International Federation of Otorhinolaryngological Societies (IFOS 2013) Congress in June 2013. A summarized version was also submitted by the corresponding author to the IFOS 2013 Congress Scientific Secretariat where he won the Young Scientist of the Year Award.

Ethical Approval

This study was reviewed and approved by the Kenyatta National Hospital and University of Nairobi Ethics & Research Committee (P8/01/2011).

Conflict of Interests

The authors declare that there is no conflict of interests regarding the publication of this paper.

Acknowledgments

The authors would like to acknowledge the cooperation of Kenyatta National Hospital who allowed this research to be performed in their premises. The authors wish to declare that this study was funded by the principal researcher.

References

[1] Central Bureau of Statistics (CBS) [Kenya], Ministry of Health (MOH) [Kenya] and ORC Macro, *Kenya Demographic and Health Survey 2003: Key Findings*, CBS, MOH and ORC Macro, Calverton, Md, USA, 2004.

[2] Kenya National Bureau of Statistics (KNBS) and ICF Macro, *Kenya Demographic and Health Survey 2008-2009*, KNBS and ICF Macro, Calverton, Md, USA, 2010.

[3] G. Z. Mutuma and A. Rugutt-Korir, "Cancer Incidence Report NAIROBI 2000-2002," Nairobi Cancer Registry Kenya Medical Research Institute, Nairobi, Kenya, http://www.healthresearch-web.org/files/CancerIncidenceReportKEMRI.pdf.

[4] P. Menach, H. O. Oburra, and A. Patel, "Cigarette Smoking and Alcohol Ingestion as Risk Factors for Laryngeal Squamous Cell Carcinoma at Kenyatta National Hospital, Kenya," *Clinical Medicine Insights: Ear, Nose and Throat*, vol. 5, pp. 17–24, 2012.

[5] "Kenya Global School-based Student Health Survey 2003 Fact Sheet," http://www.who.int/chp/gshs/kenya/en/index.html.

[6] J. N. Nato, "Report on the results of the Global Youth Tobacco Survey in Kenya (GYTSKenya 2001)," http://www.afro.who.int/index.php?option=com_docman&task=doc_download&gid=5496.

[7] World Health Organization International Agency for Research on Cancer, *IARC Monographs on the Evaluation of Carcinogenic Risks to Humans. Volume 83. Tobacco Smoke and Involuntary Smoking*.

[8] J. Mackay and J. Crofton, "Tobacco and the developing world," *British Medical Bulletin*, vol. 52, no. 1, pp. 206–221, 1996.

[9] C. A. Squier, P. Cox, and B. K. Hall, "Enhanced penetration of nitrosonornicotine across oral mucosa in the presence of ethanol," *Journal of Oral Pathology*, vol. 15, no. 5, pp. 276–279, 1986.

[10] A. Zeka, R. Gore, and D. Kriebel, "Effects of alcohol and tobacco on aerodigestive cancer risks: a meta-regression analysis," *Cancer Causes and Control*, vol. 14, no. 9, pp. 897–906, 2003.

[11] M. Bodnar, H. Rekwirowicz, P. Burduk, R. Bilewicz, W. Kaźmierczak, and A. Marszałek, "Impact of tobacco smoking on biologic background of laryngeal squamous cell carcinoma," *Przegląd Lekarski*, vol. 66, no. 10, pp. 598–602, 2009 (Polish).

[12] L. Mao, W. K. Hong, and V. A. Papadimitrakopoulou, "Focus on head and neck cancer," *Cancer Cell*, vol. 5, no. 4, pp. 311–316, 2004.

[13] C. H. Hennekens and J. E. Buring, *Epidemiology in Medicine*, Little Brown, Boston, Mass, USA, 1987.

[14] National Institute on Alcohol Abuse and Alcoholism, "Helping Patients Who Drink Too Much: A Clinician's Guide," http://www.niaaa.nih.gov/guide.

[15] F. Islami, I. Tramacere, M. Rota et al., "Alcohol drinking and laryngeal cancer: overall and dose-risk relation—a systematic review and meta-analysis," *Oral Oncology*, vol. 46, no. 11, pp. 802–810, 2010.

[16] S. Gallus, C. Bosetti, S. Franceschi, F. Levi, E. Negri, and C. La Vecchia, "Laryngeal cancer in women: tobacco, alcohol, nutritional, and hormonal factors," *Cancer Epidemiology Biomarkers & Prevention*, vol. 12, no. 6, pp. 514–517, 2003.

[17] J. F. Onyango and I. M. Macharia, "Delays in diagnosis, referral and management of head and neck cancer presenting at Kenyatta National Hospital, Nairobi," *East African Medical Journal*, vol. 83, no. 4, pp. 85–91, 2006.

[18] M. S. Cattaruzza, P. Maisonneuve, and P. Boyle, "Epidemiology of laryngeal cancer," *European Journal of Cancer Part B*, vol. 32, no. 5, pp. 293–305, 1996.

[19] U. Kapil, P. Singh, S. Bahadur, S. N. Dwivedi, R. Singh, and N. Shukla, "Assessment of risk factors in laryngeal cancer in India: a case-control study," *Asian Pacific Journal of Cancer Prevention*, vol. 6, no. 2, pp. 202–207, 2005.

[20] H. S. Raitiola and J. S. Pukander, "Etiological factors of laryngeal cancer," *Acta Oto-Laryngologica, Supplement*, no. 529, pp. 215–217, 1997.

[21] E. De Stefani, F. Oreggia, S. Rivero, and L. Fierro, "Hand-rolled cigarette smoking and risk of cancer of the mouth, pharynx and larynx," *Cancer*, vol. 70, no. 3, pp. 679–682, 1992.

[22] J. K. Wiencke, S. W. Thurston, K. T. Kelsey et al., "Early age at smoking initiation and tobacco carcinogen DNA damage in the lung," *Journal of the National Cancer Institute*, vol. 91, no. 7, pp. 614–619, 1999.

[23] E. M. Nturibi, A. A. Kolawole, and S. A. McCurdy, "Smoking prevalence and tobacco control measures in Kenya, Uganda, the Gambia and Liberia: a review," *International Journal of Tuberculosis and Lung Disease*, vol. 13, no. 2, pp. 165–170, 2009.

[24] C. Bosetti, S. Gallus, R. Peto et al., "Tobacco smoking, smoking cessation, and cumulative risk of upper aerodigestive tract cancers," *American Journal of Epidemiology*, vol. 167, no. 4, pp. 468–473, 2008.

[25] G. Pöschl and H. K. Seitz, "Alcohol and cancer," *Alcohol and Alcoholism*, vol. 39, no. 3, pp. 155–165, 2004.

[26] M. Dosemeci, I. Gokmen, M. Unsal, R. B. Hayes, and A. Blair, "Tobacco, alcohol use, and risks of laryngeal and lung cancer by subsite and histologic type in Turkey," *Cancer Causes and Control*, vol. 8, no. 5, pp. 729–737, 1997.

[27] T. Bundgaard, S. M. Bentzen, and H. Sogaard, "Histological differentiation of oral squamous cell cancer in relation to tobacco smoking," *European Journal of Cancer Part B*, vol. 31, no. 2, pp. 118–121, 1995.

[28] D. J. Slamon, J. B. DeKernion, I. M. Verma, and M. J. Cline, "Expression of cellular oncogenes in human malignancies," *Science*, vol. 224, no. 4646, pp. 256–262, 1984.

[29] D. Chin, G. M. Boyle, D. R. Theile, P. G. Parsons, and W. B. Coman, "Molecular introduction to head and neck cancer (HNSCC) carcinogenesis," *The British Journal of Plastic Surgery*, vol. 57, no. 7, pp. 595–602, 2004.

[30] D. J. Trigg, M. Lait, and B. L. Wenig, "Influence of tobacco and alcohol on the stage of laryngeal cancer at diagnosis," *Laryngoscope*, vol. 110, no. 3 I, pp. 408–411, 2000.

[31] H. O. Oburra, "Late presentation of laryngeal and nasopharyngeal cancer in Kenyatta National Hospital," *East African Medical Journal*, vol. 75, no. 4, pp. 223–226, 1998.

[32] Republic of Kenya, "Kenya Law reports. Tobacco control bill 2007," *Kenya Gazette Supplement*, no. 95, pp. 133–176.

26

The Relationship between the Efficacy of Tonsillectomy and Renal Pathology in the Patients with IgA Nephropathy

Tsutomu Nomura, Yoshimi Makizumi, Tsuyoshi Yoshida, and Tatsuya Yamasoba

Department of Otolaryngology and Head and Neck Surgery, Faculty of Medicine, University of Tokyo, 7-3-1 Hongo, Bunkyo-ku, Tokyo 113-8655, Japan

Correspondence should be addressed to Tsutomu Nomura; t-nomura@bc5.so-net.ne.jp

Academic Editor: David W. Eisele

Objective. The aim of this study was to evaluate the effects of tonsillectomy as a treatment for IgA nephropathy in relation to renal pathological findings. *Methods.* This is a retrospective analysis of 13 patients having IgA nephropathy treated by tonsillectomy. *Results.* UP/UCre levels decreased from 820.8 to 585.4 one month postsurgery and then showed slight worsening to 637.3 at the most recent follow-up. There was no significant difference in the improvement rate between pathological grades I–III and IV. There was positive correlation between Pre-UP/UCre level and the reduction rate of UP/UCre, which was statistically significant ($R = 0.667$, $R^2 = 0.445$, and $P = 0.01$). *Conclusions.* Reduction of UP/UCre at one month postsurgery is considered to be an overall prognostic factor, and tonsillectomy is considered to be an effective therapy for IgA patients regardless of the grade of renal pathology.

1. Introduction

IgA nephropathy (IgAN) is the most common form of chronic glomerulonephritis with IgA deposits present mainly in the mesangial areas in Japan. Several retrospective studies have investigated the effect of tonsillectomy on IgA nephropathy [1–3]. A great deal of data regarding the effect of tonsillectomy on patients with IgA nephropathy has been reported, although few reports have examined the relationship between the efficacy of tonsillectomy and renal pathology.

In terms of renal pathology, Akagi and Nishizaki [4] recommended tonsillectomy for IgA patients with grade I to III renal pathology. Xie et al. [5] reported that tonsillectomy was not effective in IgA patients with marked renal damage.

The purpose of this study is to evaluate the effects of tonsillectomy as a treatment for IgAN in relation to renal pathological findings.

2. Materials and Methods

We performed a retrospective review of 13 patients, 4 males and 9 females, with IgAN referred from the nephrology department of our university hospital. All patients underwent tonsillectomy (Table 1). The age at tonsillectomy was 30.3 years on average (range: 13 to 65 years). Mean follow-up interval was 186 months from the first visit and 19 months from tonsillectomy. Three patients had steroid pulse therapy after tonsillectomy. Almost all patients had medication of angiotensin converting enzyme inhibitor (ACEI), angiotensin II receptor blocker (ARB), and diuretics.

Renal biopsy findings were classified in terms of prognosis as good (grade I), relatively good (grade II), relatively poor (grade III), and poor (grade IV) using the criteria of the Committee of IgA Nephropathy—the Special Study Group of Progressive Glomerular Disease, the Ministry of Health, Labor and Welfare of Japan [6]. Through renal biopsy, 4, 3, 1, and 5 patients were classified as grades I, II, III, and IV, respectively.

Criteria of IgA pathology are as follows.

Grade I: slight mesangial proliferation and increased matrix were observed. No glomerulosclerosis, crescent formation, or adhesion to Bowman's capsules was observed. No prominent changes were seen in the interstitium, renal tubuli, or blood vessels.

TABLE 1: Baseline characteristic of 13 patients with IgA nephropathy.

Gender (male/female)	4/9
Age at tonsillectomy	30.3 (13–65) years
Follow-up interval	
After the first visit	186 m
After tonsillectomy	19 m

TABLE 2: Overall examined data.

	Presurgery	One month PS*	Recent
Cre	0.8 ± 0.3	0.8 ± 0.3	0.8 ± 0.3
IgA	242.2 ± 67.5	212.7 ± 64.0	222.3 ± 77
eGFR	90.1 ± 29.6	89.3 ± 30.7	86.4 ± 30.5
UP/UCre	820.8 ± 813.5	585.4 ± 427.2	637.3 ± 832.1
Hematuria	10/13	10/13	10/13

*PS: postsurgery.

Grade II: slight mesangial cell proliferation and increased matrix were observed. Glomerulosclerosis, crescent formation, or adhesion to Bowman's capsules was observed in less than 10% of all biopsied glomeruli. Interstitial and vascular findings were the same as in Group I.

Grade III: moderate, diffuse mesangial proliferation and increased matrix were observed. Glomerulosclerosis, crescent formation, or adhesion to Bowman's capsules was observed in less than 10–30% of all biopsied glomeruli.

Cellar infiltration was slight in the interstitium except around some sclerosed glomeruli. Tubular atrophy was slight, and mild vascular sclerosis was observed.

Grade IV: severe, diffuse mesangial proliferation and increased matrix were observed. Glomerulosclerosis, crescent formation, or adhesion to Bowman's capsules was observed in more than 30% of all biopsied glomeruli. When sites of sclerosis are totaled and converted to global sclerosis, the sclerosis rate was more than 50% of all glomeruli. Some glomeruli also showed compensatory hypertrophy.

Presurgery, one month postsurgery, and most recent serous IgA level, serous creatinine, and extent of hematuria were reviewed. The rate of urine protein/urine creatinine (UP/UCre) and estimated glomerular filtration rate (eGFR) were calculated. The reduction rate of UP/UCre was calculated with the following formula.

2.1. (Pre-UP/UCre-Post-UP/UCre)/Pre-UP/UCre. For statistical analysis, Mann-Whitney U test was performed to compare the two means, χ^2 test was used for rate analysis, and regression analysis to determine correlation was carried out with SPSS ver.10.0.

3. Results

The data obtained before surgery, one month after surgery, and at most recent visit are presented in Table 2. Creatinine, IgA, eGFR, and hematuria levels exhibited virtually no change when compared to presurgery. UP/UCre levels decreased from 820.8 (presurgery) to 585.4 one month postsurgery and then showed slight increase to 637.3 at the most recent visit, but the difference was not statistically significant (Figure 1). The change was not related to the presence of postoperative steroid pulse therapy.

TABLE 3: The improvement rate one month postsurgery compared to presurgery in terms of renal pathology.

	UP/UCre	Hematuria	IgA
Grade			
I	2/4	2/4 (3/4)	3/3
II	2/3	1/3	2/3
III	1/1	0/1	1/1
IV	2/5	1/5 (2/5)	2/4

*( ): data at most recent.

The improvement rate one month postsurgery compared to presurgery in terms of renal pathology is shown in Table 3. The UP/UCre level was reduced in 2, 2, 1, and 2 patients classified as grades I, II, III, and IV, respectively. Hematuria was improved in 2, 1, 1, and 1 patients in grades I, II, III, and IV, respectively. Serous IgA was improved in 3, 2, and 2 patients in grades I, II, and IV, respectively.

The improvement rate at the most recent visit compared to presurgery is presented also in Table 3. Hematuria showed slight improvement in all grades, but levels of other factors remained almost the same. There was no significant difference in the improvement rate between pathological grades I–III and IV.

The correlation between UP/UCre and the reduction rate of UP/UCre is plotted in Figure 2. The Pre-UP/UCr had a positive correlation with the reduction rate of UP/UCre, with a statistical significance ($R = 0.667$, $R^2 = 0.445$, and $P = 0.01$).

4. Discussion

IgA nephropathy (IgAN) is the most common form of chronic glomerulonephritis with IgA deposits present mainly in the mesangial areas in Japan [6]. Tonsillitis is believed to play an important role in the pathogenesis in IgAN. Several retrospective studies have investigated the effect of tonsillectomy on IgA nephropathy [1–3]. Although tonsillectomy has been recommended for patients exhibiting grade I to III renal pathology, not those exhibiting grade IV [5], the current study suggested that an improvement in the extent of urine protein, IgA, and hematuria can be achieved also in patients with grade IV renal pathology.

The UP/UCre level is presumed to reflect daily protein excretion dose and therefore state of renal function. The UP/UCre level was decreased one month postsurgery, and

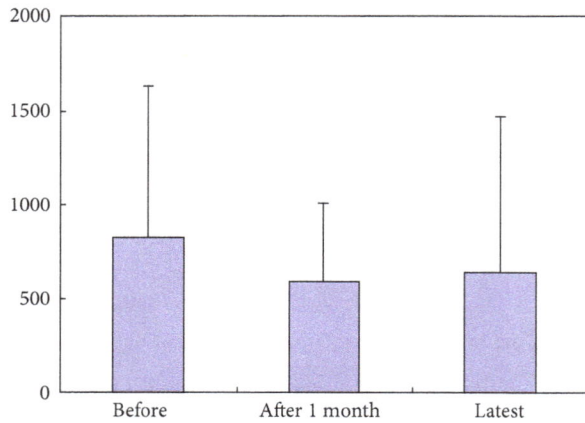

FIGURE 1: UP/UCre levels.

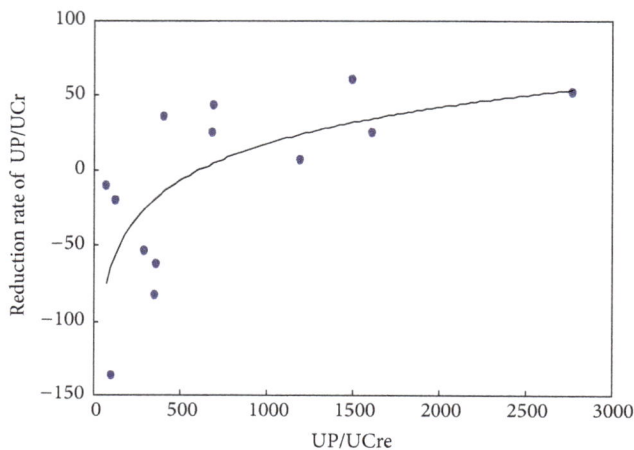

FIGURE 2: The correlation between UP/UCre and the reduction rate of UP/UCre.

Conflict of Interests

The authors declare that there is no conflict of interests regarding the publication of this paper.

References

[1] H. Akagi, M. Kosaka, K. Hattori et al., "Long-term results of tonsillectomy as a treatment for IgA nephropathy," *Acta Oto-Laryngologica Supplement*, vol. 124, no. 555, pp. 38–42, 2004.

[2] C. Ponticelli, "Tonsillectomy and IgA nephritis," *Nephrology Dialysis Transplantation*, vol. 27, no. 7, pp. 2610–2613, 2012.

[3] I. Maeda, T. Hayashi, K. K. Sato et al., "Tonsillectomy has beneficial effects on remission and progression of IgA nephropathy independent of steroid therapy," *Nephrology Dialysis Transplantation*, vol. 27, no. 7, pp. 2806–2813, 2012.

[4] H. Akagi and K. Nishizaki, "Indication criteria for tonsillectomy in patients with IgA nephropathy," *Japan Society for Stomato-Phalingology*, vol. 17, no. 2, pp. 197–204, 2005.

[5] Y. Xie, X. Chen, S. Nishi, I. Narita, and F. Gejyo, "Relationship between tonsils and IgA nephropathy as well as indications of tonsillectomy," *Kidney International*, vol. 65, no. 4, pp. 1135–1144, 2004.

[6] Y. Tomino and H. Sakai, "Clinical guidelines for immunoglobulin a (IgA) nephropathy in Japan, second version," *Journal of Clinical and Experimental Nephrology*, vol. 7, no. 2, pp. 93–97, 2003.

although it showed slight worsening at the most recent visit, it remained to be improved when compared to presurgery.

In terms of the correlation between the UP/UCre level and the reduction rate of UP/UCre, the Pre-UP/UCre level had positive correlation with the reduction rate of UP/UCre. This suggests that the effect of tonsillectomy is not related to the clinical stage of IgAN. Thus, the reduction of UP/UCre level at one month postsurgery is considered to be an overall prognostic factor, and tonsillectomy is considered to be an effective therapy for IgA patients regardless of the grades of renal pathology.

5. Conclusion

Reduction of UP/UCre level one month after tonsillectomy is considered to be an overall prognostic factor, and tonsillectomy is considered to be an effective therapy for IgA regardless of renal pathological grades.

27

Management of Globus Pharyngeus

S. Kortequee,[1] P. D. Karkos,[1] H. Atkinson,[1] N. Sethi,[2] D. C. Sylvester,[1] R. S. Harar,[2] S. Sood,[1] and W. J. Issing[3]

[1] *Department of Otolaryngology, Bradford Royal Infirmary, Bradford BD9 6RJ, UK*
[2] *Department of Otolaryngology, Pinderfields Hospital, Wakefield WF1 4DG, UK*
[3] *Department of Otolaryngology, The Freeman Hospital, Newcastle upon Tyne NE7 7DN, UK*

Correspondence should be addressed to S. Kortequee; sahrkortequee@mac.com

Academic Editor: David W. Eisele

Globus pharyngeus is a common ENT condition. This paper reviews the current evidence on globus and gives a rational guide to the management of patients with globus. The aetiology of globus is still unclear though most ENT surgeons believe that reflux whether acidic or not plays a significant role. Though proton pump inhibitors are used extensively in practice, there is little evidence to support their efficacy. Most patients with globus can be discharged after simple office investigations. The role of pepsin-induced laryngeal injury is an exciting concept that needs further study. Given the benign nature of globus pharyngeus, in most cases, reassurance rather than treatment or extensive investigation with rigid oesophagoscopy or contrast swallows is all that is needed. We need more research into the aetiology of globus.

1. Introduction

Globus pharyngeus, the sensation of something stuck in the throat, has been noted since the time of Hippocrates. Purcell first used the term globus hystericus in the early 18th century [1]. In 1968, Malcomson [2] suggested the term globus pharyngeus as a more accurate description since not all patients with globus were either hysterical or female.

Typically, globus is relieved by ingestion of solids or liquids and tends to be worse on dry swallows. Globus may be associated with throat irritation, soreness, dryness, catarrh, or constant throat clearing. It forms a large part of ENT practice and may account for about 4% of referrals to our outpatient clinics [3]. The prevalence is much higher in the general population as most people may not present to hospital with it. A recent study by Ali and Wilson [4] found that up to 78% of patients presenting to non-ENT clinics had had globus-type symptoms.

2. Aetiology

Despite the high prevalence in the community, the aetiology of globus remains unclear and highly controversial. It is slowly being accepted that it may be multifactorial and that when it occurs in isolation it rarely hides any sinister pathology [5]. Most of the recent work has suggested several mechanisms in isolation or not uncommonly in combination are to blame for the manifestation of globus pharyngeus; these include psychological factors, gastro-esophageal reflux (GOR), pharyngeal dysmotility, hypertonic upper oeso-phageal sphincter (UOS), and local anatomic abnormalities [6–11].

2.1. Psychological Factors. As its earlier name, globus hystericus, suggests, there has been a long history of links between globus and psychological factors. It is the fourth most discriminating symptom of a somatisation disorder after vomiting, aphonia, and painful extremities [12]. As most of the globus patients are quite rightly referred to ENT surgeons rather than to psychiatrists, a psychogenic basis must always be borne in mind. Gale et al. [13] in a detailed medical and psychological examinations including assessment with the Minnesota Multiphasic Personality Inventory (MMPI) of 4240 US male veterans demonstrated a 6.4% incidence of globus. This globus group scored higher in nine out of ten of the MMPI clinical scales. They concluded that in men there is a significant link to depression and somatization disorder and as a result other related treatable psychopathology should be investigated.

Harris et al. [14] when comparing globus patients with other ENT patients (as a control group) found that globus patients had had more severe life events in the year and less confiding relationships than controls. Social stress may thus play a role in either initiating or maintaining globus.

2.2. Reflux. The link between GOR and globus has been a matter of controversy for over forty years. Chevalier et al. [6] looked at globus patients with and without typical GOR symptoms. They found that 66.6% of the nonreflux globus group and 80% of the GOR globus group had significant episodes of reflux (based on pH monitoring). In direct contrast, Chen et al. in a similar study found no evidence of reflux in globus patients based on ambulatory pH monitoring [7].

Reflux is, however, best detected by impedance. Anandasabapathy and Jaffin [15] using multichannel intraluminal impedance and pH monitoring (MII-pH) have suggested that globus may also be due to nonacid (NAR) reflux. As MII-pH can detect reflux episodes independent of acid changes, it is allegedly more accurate at picking up proximal reflux. This latter study found NAR and proximal reflux to be significant predictors of globus.

Based on porcine models, pepsin has been shown to increase the levels of laryngeal protective proteins and thus explain the NAR link. Even though low pH is needed to activate pepsin, its stability means that it may be activated intracellularly or when the larynx is later exposed to acid [16].

2.3. Pharyngeal and Upper Oesophageal Sphincter Function (UOS). Hypertonicity of the UOS has been suggested as a cause of globus, but several studies have yielded conflicting results. This has largely been due to possible technical difficulties in assessing UOS pressure profiles. It has long been recognised that the UOS pressure profile is asymmetrical, especially when using multilumen catheters. Therefore, earlier studies that have not taken this into account must be viewed with caution. Also, oral movement during swallowing and compression from surrounding structures complicates pressure readings.

UOS pressure measurements obtained using circumferential transducers are regarded as being more reflective of true intraluminal pressure. Sun et al. [17] looked at twenty-four healthy volunteers and thirty-two patients with globus and found UOS pressure to be normal in most of the globus patients and could not suggest it as a possible aetiological factor. Interestingly they found that videofluoroscopic evidence of pharyngeal dysfunction especially laryngeal penetration had a strong association with globus.

Tokashiki et al. [18], however, showed that perfusion of HCl into the distal oesophagus was related to a sensation of globus associated with a rise in UOS pressure. This rise in pressure was independent of the detection of a rise in pH in the hypopharynx.

2.4. Local Mechanical Abnormalities. Recently there have been reports of very subtle changes in anatomy that when rectified have given relief of globus.

Agada et al. [9] published a small series of patients with globus having "abnormally" retroverted epiglottises. The definition of a retroverted epiglottis is if the tip touches the tongue base when the tongue is protruded.

Ulug and Ulubil [10] have presented a case of corniculate cartilage subluxation presenting with globus. Other postulated causes include Eagles syndrome (calcified stylohyoid ligament), impalpable thyroid nodules [11], cervical osteophytes, lingual tonsils, or prominent greater cornu of the hyoid.

Gastric inlet patches have also been aetiologically linked to globus [19, 20]. These are congenital islands of ectopic gastric mucosa found in the cervical oesophagus. With the incidence of gastric inlet patch being quite common (3.6%), it is hard to establish a causal relationship. Alagozlu et al. [21] have gone further to suggest that it is *H. pylori* infection of the inlet patch that causes altered cervical perception and hence globus. What is worrying about this is that these patches have been associated with both squamous cell carcinomas and adenocarcinomas of the upper oesophagus [19, 22].

More interestingly though Shiomi et al. [12] looked at the mucus in the epipharynx of patients with globus and compared it with that from healthy volunteers, they found that there were significantly increased concentrations of fucose and sialic acid (the main determinants of mucus viscosity) in the mucus of those with globus as compared to normal subjects.

Lastly, though there is no evidence to suggest this, some ENT surgeons believe that globus may "simply" be a local sensory abnormality just like tinnitus.

3. Investigation

As with all our patients, the key is in taking a proper history. Pointers that would suggest sinister underlying pathology would include dysphagia, aspiration, regurgitation, weight loss, voice change, and pain. The presence of overt symptoms of GOR should be noted.

The head and neck should be thoroughly examined. This should include transnasal fibre-optic laryngoscopy (FOL) or if available transnasal flexible laryngooesophagoscopy (TNO). Any further investigation should be based on the findings at history and examination.

3.1. Radiology. In ENT departments in the UK, contrast swallows are the most popular radiological investigations used to investigate globus, with some departments historically using them to screen patients for upper aerodigestive tract malignancy [23, 24]. They have been favoured because they are safe (compared to rigid endoscopy), quick, and believed to increase diagnostic yield.

Unfortunately there is particular concern that this modality may miss a malignancy. One of the authors (RPH) retrospectively reviewed a series of 1275 patients that had barium swallows [24]. Six hundred and ninety-nine patients had globus and 451 of these patients had globus without sinister symptoms. In these patients, barium swallows did not show any sinister pathology. Another review of barium swallows by Hajioff and Lowe [25] looked at 2854 barium swallows from two centres, and of the 2011 patients that presented with globus, none had a worrying abnormality on barium swallow. Only one retrospective case series [26] has found an association between isolated globus and hypopharyngeal cancer. Two cases out of twenty-three cases were retrospectively found to have malignancies (a piriform fossa and postcricoid tumour). More recent and larger studies have failed to make a similar association.

In the light of the previously mentioned we do not recommend barium swallows routinely for globus. The diagnostic yield for malignancy is poor though it may reassure the patient [27].

3.2. Endoscopy. Direct visualisation of the upper digestive tract is another means of investigating globus. The main drawback of this is that flexible oesophagoscopy often requires sedation, while rigid endoscopy requires a general anaesthetic and carries a small but significant risk of perforation.

Lorenz et al. [28] carried out flexible endoscopies on patients that had been referred by ENT for further investigation of globus, and all of the patients had had a normal outpatient ENT examination and barium swallow. 62.7% of the patients were found to have pathology that could possibly have caused their globus though no sinister pathology was noted. Similarly, Nagano et al. [29] in their study found a 36.5% incidence of benign oesophageal pathology in patients with globus on flexible endoscopy, but again no malignancies were identified.

Takwoingi et al. [30] retrospectively reviewed 250 patients that had undergone rigid endoscopy for globus. The most common recorded anomalies were cricopharyngeal spasm (4.8%) and reflux (4.4%). No tumours were found, and they concluded that rigid endoscopy played a limited role in the investigation of globus. One patient had a perforation that was successfully treated conservatively.

The most recent major advance in endoscopy is transnasal oesophagoscopy (TNO). It combines the main advantages of both conventional flexible and rigid oesophagoscopy with none of the major disadvantages. It can be done with just topical anaesthesia and vasoconstriction. There is total examination of the upper digestive tract down to the stomach with the ability to take biopsies at the same time. It has been shown to be safe with a high patient satisfaction rate [31].

Though TNO is not yet routinely available in the UK, we think that it is the ideal investigation for those ENT surgeons who want a relatively safe, cheap, and quick way of visualising the upper digestive tract especially the hypopharynx and postcricoid regions. Where TNO is available, almost 90% patients with globus can be discharged after their first visit [32]. We eagerly await studies comparing the diagnostic yield of TNO to that of rigid oesophagoscopy.

3.3. Symptom Scores and Indices. Despite the controversies, a large number of UK ENT surgeons believe that reflux plays a role in globus. Many of us do not use any scores or indices in our assessment of patients with globus [33]. The reflux symptom index and the reflux finding score are not particularly valid diagnostic tools when used in globus

patients [34]. The Glasgow Edinburgh Throat Score (GETS) has been validated for use in globus but is not widely used [4].

3.4. Impedance and pH Studies. Because of the benign nature of globus, we rarely ever ask for pH or impedance studies in our patients. They often require referrals to the gastroenterologists and rarely contribute to our management plan. They are used mainly as a research tool. However, this may change in the future.

4. Treatment

Where there is uncertainty about the aetiology there will be uncertainty about the management. If patients have overt signs or symptoms suggestive of reflux in addition to globus, we would treat them aggressively with a proton pump inhibitor (PPi) twice daily and a reflux suppressant for at least 4 months [35]. We do not routinely use H2 receptor antagonists. A study from the Cleveland Clinic using a regimen similar to ours has been found to be effective in controlling the symptoms of laryngopharyngeal reflux (LPR). Most of the ENT surgeons in the UK seem to be prescribing suboptimal doses of PPis [33].

In cases where there is globus but with no evidence of GOR, there is little merit in treating them with PPis. Two recent meta-analyses of the role of PPis in reflux related laryngeal disease have shown little or no benefit over placebo [36, 37]. They both recommend that more studies are required to define the subgroup of patients that will benefit from PPis.

PPis are useful in controlling symptoms secondary to gastric inlet mucosa. Where this fails, then argon plasma ablation has been useful in controlling symptoms [20]. *H. pylori* eradication therapy should also be performed if there was evidence of infection.

Speech and language therapists may have a role to play in managing globus patients. A few trials have shown that globus symptom scores do improve after a course of speech therapy [38, 39]. What is not clear from these studies is whether there is a specific effect from speech therapy or if improvement is due to increased reassurance. Hypnotically Assisted Relaxation (HAR) therapy has also been reported in a recent case series [40] to improve globus sensation regardless of the cause. Manometric UOS readings in the patients showed no change before and after HAR.

In cases where there are anatomical anomalies, the trend seems to be excision of the offending local structure, most often some part of the cartilaginous framework of the larynx [9, 10]. There have been surprisingly no issues with aspiration or voice change following these procedures. These results have to be viewed with caution as the numbers are small with short follow-up intervals.

We must also remember to assess the whole patient and make referrals to the psychiatrists where it is indicated. Therefore in most cases of globus, if the history and examination of the patient suggest no sinister pathology, then reassurance is often enough. Rowley showed that at 7 years about 55% of patients were asymptomatic and none had developed an upper aerodigestive tract malignancy [5]. At the present, we do not recommend any further radiologic or endoscopic examination for the patient with isolated globus.

5. Conclusion

Globus is a clinical diagnosis and not a diagnosis of exclusion. A complete head and neck examination including fibreoptic laryngoscopy is more than adequate to confidently discharge the classic globus pharyngeus patients. The introduction of TNO in one stop globus clinics has meant that with appropriate training otolaryngologists can nowadays and in selected cases complete a thorough upper aerodigestive tract examination, thus avoiding the need for any other investigations such as barium swallows or oesophagoscopies under general anaesthesia. Overinvestigating these patients can often add unnecessary stress to a group of patients who already seem to have higher levels of depression, anxiety, and other somatic concerns. In fact the authors believe that both barium swallow and panendoscopy under GA are things of the past and should not form part of the standard globus assessment.

More research needs to be carried out into the aetiology, treatment, and long-term prognosis of persistent globus.

References

[1] J. Purcell, *A Treatise of Vapours or Hysterick Fits*, Edward Place, London, UK, 2nd edition, 1707.

[2] K. G. Malcomson, "Globus vel pharynges (a reconnaissance of proximal vagalmodalities)," *The Journal of Laryngology & Otology*, vol. 82, pp. 219–230, 1968.

[3] P. J. Moloy and R. Charter, "The globus symptom. Incidence, therapeutic response, and age and sex relationships," *Archives of Otolaryngology*, vol. 108, no. 11, pp. 740–744, 1982.

[4] K. H. M. Ali and J. A. Wilson, "What is the severity of globus sensation in individuals who have never sought health care for it?" *Journal of Laryngology and Otology*, vol. 121, no. 9, pp. 865–868, 2007.

[5] H. Rowley, T. P. O'Dwyer, A. S. Jones, and C. I. Timon, "The natural history of globus pharyngeus," *Laryngoscope*, vol. 105, no. 10, pp. 1118–1121, 1995.

[6] J. M. Chevalier, E. Brossard, and P. Monnier, "Globus sensation and gastroesophageal reflux," *European Archives of Oto-Rhino-Laryngology*, vol. 260, no. 5, pp. 273–276, 2003.

[7] C. Chen, C. Tsai, A. S. Chou, and J. Chiou, "Utility of ambulatory pH monitoring and videofluoroscopy for the evaluation of patients with globus pharyngeus," *Dysphagia*, vol. 22, no. 1, pp. 16–19, 2007.

[8] M. J. Corso, K. G. Pursnani, M. A. Mohiuddin et al., "Globus sensation is associated with hypertensive upper esophageal sphincter but not with gastroesophageal reflux," *Digestive Diseases & Sciences*, vol. 43, no. 7, pp. 1513–1517, 1998.

[9] F. O. Agada, A. P. Coatesworth, and A. R. H. Grace, "Retroverted epiglottis presenting as a variant of globus pharyngeus," *Journal of Laryngology and Otology*, vol. 121, no. 4, pp. 390–392, 2007.

[10] T. Ulug and S. A. Ulubil, "An unusual cause of foreign-body sensation in the throat: corniculate cartilage subluxation," *American Journal of Otolaryngology*, vol. 24, no. 2, pp. 118–120, 2003.

[11] J. N. Marshall, G. McGann, J. A. Cook, and N. Taub, "A prospective controlled study of high-resolution thyroid ultrasound in patients with globus pharyngeus," *Clinical Otolaryngology and Allied Sciences*, vol. 21, no. 3, pp. 228–231, 1996.

[12] Y. Shiomi, N. Oda, Y. Shiomi, and S. Hosoda, "Hyperviscoelasticity of epipharyngeal mucus may induce globus pharyngis," *Annals of Otology, Rhinology and Laryngology*, vol. 111, no. 12, pp. 1116–1119, 2002.

[13] C. R. Gale, J. A. Wilson, and I. J. Deary, "Globus sensation and psychopathology in men: the vietnam experience study," *Psychosomatic Medicine*, vol. 71, no. 9, pp. 1026–1031, 2009.

[14] M. B. Harris, I. J. Deary, and J. A. Wilson, "Life events and difficulties in relation to the onset of globus pharyngis," *Journal of Psychosomatic Research*, vol. 40, no. 6, pp. 603–615, 1996.

[15] S. Anandasabapathy and B. W. Jaffin, "Multichannel intraluminal impedance in the evaluation of patients with persistent globus on proton pump inhibitor therapy," *Annals of Otology, Rhinology and Laryngology*, vol. 115, no. 8, pp. 563–570, 2006.

[16] N. Johnston, P. W. Dettmar, B. Bishwokarma, M. O. Lively, and J. A. Koufman, "Activity/stability of human pepsin: implications for reflux attributed laryngeal disease," *Laryngoscope*, vol. 117, no. 6, pp. 1036–1039, 2007.

[17] J. Sun, B. Xu, Y. Yuan, and J. Xu, "Study on the function of pharynx & upper esophageal sphincter in globus hystericus," *World Journal of Gastroenterology*, vol. 8, no. 5, pp. 952–955, 2002.

[18] R. Tokashiki, N. Funato, and M. Suzuki, "Globus sensation and increased upper esophageal sphincter pressure with distal esophageal acid perfusion," *European Archives of Oto-Rhino-Laryngology*, vol. 267, no. 5, pp. 737–741, 2010.

[19] A. Alaani, P. Jassar, A. T. Warfield, D. R. Gouldesbrough, and I. Smith, "Heterotopic gastric mucosa in the cervical oesophagus (inlet patch) and globus pharyngeus—an under-recognised association," *Journal of Laryngology and Otology*, vol. 121, no. 9, pp. 885–888, 2007.

[20] A. Meining, M. Bajbouj, M. Preeg et al., "Argon plasma ablation of gastric inlet patches in the cervical esophagus may alleviate globus sensation: a pilot trial," *Endoscopy*, vol. 38, no. 6, pp. 566–570, 2006.

[21] H. Alagozlu, Z. Simsek, S. Unal, M. Cindoruk, S. Dumlu, and A. Dursun, "Is there an association between Helicobacter pylori in the inlet patch and globus sensation?" *World Journal of Gastroenterology*, vol. 16, no. 1, pp. 42–47, 2010.

[22] S. Satoh, T. Nakashima, K. Watanabe et al., "Hypopharyngeal squamous cell carcinoma bordering ectopic gastric mucosa "inlet patch" of the cervical esophagus," *Auris Nasus Larynx*, vol. 34, no. 1, pp. 135–139, 2007.

[23] G. W. Back, P. Leong, R. Kumar, and R. Corbridge, "Value of barium swallow in investigation of globus pharyngeus," *Journal of Laryngology and Otology*, vol. 114, no. 12, pp. 951–954, 2000.

[24] R. P. S. Harar, S. Kumar, M. A. Saeed, and D. J. Gatland, "Management of globus pharyngeus: review of 699 cases," *Journal of Laryngology and Otology*, vol. 118, no. 7, pp. 522–527, 2004.

[25] D. Hajioff and D. Lowe, "The diagnostic value of barium swallow in globus syndrome," *International Journal of Clinical Practice*, vol. 58, no. 1, pp. 86–89, 2004.

[26] A. Tsikoudas, N. Ghuman, and M. A. Riad, "Globus sensation as early presentation of hypopharyngeal cancer," *Clinical Otolaryngology*, vol. 32, no. 6, pp. 452–456, 2007.

[27] A. K. Mahrous, C. Kaoutzanis, K. Amin, and P. Gluckman, "Positive findings on barium swallow in patients presenting with a "sensation of a lump in the throat"," *European Archives of Oto-Rhino-Laryngology*, vol. 269, no. 3, pp. 1047–1050, 2012.

[28] R. Lorenz, G. Jorysz, and M. Clasen, "The globus syndrome: value of flexible endoscopy of the upper gastrointestinal tract," *Journal of Laryngology and Otology*, vol. 107, no. 6, pp. 535–537, 1993.

[29] H. Nagano, K. Yoshifuku, and Y. Kurono, "Association of a globus sensation with esophageal diseases," *Auris Nasus Larynx*, vol. 37, no. 2, pp. 195–198, 2010.

[30] Y. M. Takwoingi, U. S. Kale, and D. W. Morgan, "Rigid endoscopy in globus pharyngeus: how valuable is it?" *Journal of Laryngology and Otology*, vol. 120, no. 1, pp. 42–46, 2006.

[31] M. R. Amin, G. N. Postma, M. Setzen, and J. A. Koufman, "Transnasal esophagoscopy: a position statement from the American Bronchoesophagological Association (ABEA)," *Otolaryngology—Head and Neck Surgery*, vol. 138, no. 4, pp. 411–414, 2008.

[32] G. N. Postma, J. T. Cohen, P. C. Belafsky et al., "Transnasal esophagoscopy: revisited (over 700 consecutive cases)," *Laryngoscope*, vol. 115, no. 2, pp. 321–323, 2005.

[33] P. D. Karkos, J. Benton, S. C. Leong et al., "Trends in laryngopharyngeal reflux: a British ENT survey," *European Archives of Oto-Rhino-Laryngology*, vol. 264, no. 5, pp. 513–517, 2007.

[34] K. H. Park, S. M. Choi, S. U. K. Kwon, S. W. Yoon, and S. U. K. Kim, "Diagnosis of laryngopharyngeal reflux among globus patients," *Otolaryngology—Head and Neck Surgery*, vol. 134, no. 1, pp. 81–85, 2006.

[35] J. A. McGlashan, L. M. Johnstone, J. Sykes, V. Strugala, and P. W. Dettmar, "The value of a liquid alginate suspension (Gaviscon Advance) in the management of laryngopharyngeal reflux," *European Archives of Oto-Rhino-Laryngology*, vol. 266, no. 2, pp. 243–251, 2009.

[36] M. A. Qadeer, C. O. Phillips, A. R. Lopez et al., "Proton pump inhibitor therapy for suspected GERD-related chronic laryngitis: a meta-analysis of randomized controlled trials," *American Journal of Gastroenterology*, vol. 101, no. 11, pp. 2646–2654, 2006.

[37] L. Gatta, D. Vaira, G. Sorrenti, S. Zucchini, C. Sama, and N. Vakil, "Meta-analysis: the efficacy of proton pump inhibitors for laryngeal symptoms attributed to gastro-oesophageal reflux disease," *Alimentary Pharmacology and Therapeutics*, vol. 25, no. 4, pp. 385–392, 2007.

[38] F. Millichap, M. Lee, and T. Pring, "A lump in the throat: should speech and language therapists treat globus pharyngeus?" *Disability and Rehabilitation*, vol. 27, no. 3, pp. 124–130, 2005.

[39] H. S. Khalil, M. W. Bridger, M. Hilton-Pierce, and J. Vincent, "The use of speech therapy in the treatment of globus pharyngeus patients. A randomised controlled trial," *Revue de Laryngologie Otologie Rhinologie*, vol. 124, no. 3, pp. 187–190, 2003.

[40] J. L. Kiebles, M. A. Kwiatek, J. E. Pandolfino, P. J. Kahrilas, and L. Keefer, "Do patients with globus sensation respond to hypnotically assisted relaxation therapy? A case series report," *Diseases of the Esophagus*, vol. 23, no. 7, pp. 545–553, 2010.

28

Nasal Involvement in Obstructive Sleep Apnea Syndrome

Daniel de Sousa Michels,[1] **Amanda da Mota Silveira Rodrigues,**[2] **Márcio Nakanishi,**[1] **André Luiz Lopes Sampaio,**[1,2] **and Alessandra Ramos Venosa**[1,2]

[1] *Department of Otorhinolaryngology and Head and Neck Surgery, Brasília University Hospital, HUB, SGAN 605, Avenida L2 Norte, 70830-200 Brasília, DF, Brazil*
[2] *Universidade de Brasília (UnB), Campus Universitário Darcy Ribeiro, 70910-900 Brasília, DF, Brazil*

Correspondence should be addressed to Daniel de Sousa Michels; dsmichels@gmail.com

Academic Editor: David W. Eisele

Numerous studies have reported an association between nasal obstruction and obstructive sleep apnea syndrome (OSAS), but the precise nature of this relationship remains to be clarified. This paper aimed to summarize data and theories on the role of the nose in the pathophysiology of sleep apnea as well as to discuss the benefits of surgical and medical nasal treatments. A number of pathophysiological mechanisms can potentially explain the role of nasal pathology in OSAS. These include the Starling resistor model, the unstable oral airway, the nasal ventilatory reflex, and the role of nitric oxide (NO). Pharmacological treatment presents some beneficial effects on the frequency of respiratory events and sleep architecture. Nonetheless, objective data assessing snoring and daytime sleepiness are still necessary. Nasal surgery can improve the quality of life and snoring in a select group of patients with mild OSAS and septal deviation but is not an effective treatment for OSA as such. Despite the conflicting results in the literature, it is important that patients who are not perfectly adapted to CPAP are evaluated in detail, in order to identify whether there are obstructive factors that could be surgically corrected.

1. Introduction

In "Morbis Popularibis," Hippocrates observed that nasal polyps were associated with restless sleep [1]. In practice, most people experience difficulty sleeping during episodes of nasal congestion associated with upper airways infections. Thus, a link between nasal breathing and sleep, as well as an improvement in sleep quality after a relief of the nasal obstruction, appears to be intuitive [2].

Many nose and pharynx abnormalities may cause or worsen snoring and sleep apnea, such as septal deviation, nasal polyps, turbinate hypertrophy, and rhinitis. Adenoid hypertrophy, nasopharyngitis, and nasopharyngeal tumors can also cause narrowing of the airways in the nasopharyngeal region [3].

Epidemiological studies have demonstrated a relationship between the measure of nasal airflow and snoring [4], but attempts to find a linear correlation between nasal obstruction and sleep apnea have been less successful [5]. A weak correlation between nasal resistance measured by posterior rhinomanometry and severity of sleep apnea has been recently reported [6].

This paper aimed to summarize data and theories on the role of the nose in the pathophysiology of sleep apnea as well as to discuss the benefits of surgical and medical nasal treatments.

2. Nasal Involvement in the Pathophysiology of Obstructive Sleep Apnea Syndrome (OSAS)

The nose accounts for over 50% of the total upper airway resistance and plays an important role in the establishment of physiological functions such as humidification, heating, and air filtration [7].

Among the places of greatest resistance to nasal airflow are the vestibule and nasal valve area, determined by the alar cartilages, septum, and inferior turbinates [8].

The nasal mucosa is a dynamic organ controlled by the autonomic nervous system. Periodic nasal congestion and decongestion have been termed the "nasal cycle" by Heetderks [9]. This cycle occurs in approximately 80% of the adult population. In patients with permanent unilateral nasal obstruction, the nasal cycle may contribute to a significant increase in total airway resistance [10].

In healthy individuals, the lateral decubitus increases congestion in the ipsilateral nasal cavity and reduces airflow resistance in the contralateral nasal cavity. This does not occur due to a hydrostatic effect, but rather as a reflex response caused by asymmetric pressure on the body [11, 12]. This reflex interrupts the nasal cycle [13]. However, in the assessment of both nasal cavities, no significant changes were observed in the cross-sectional area when comparing supine and lateral decubitus [14].

To fully explain the relationship between airflow, nasal obstruction, and sleep apnea, it is necessary to understand some dynamic theories of physics.

Among the physiological mechanisms that elucidate the relationship between nasal airflow and breathing during sleep are the Starling resistor model, the unstable oral airway proposition, the nasal respiratory reflex, and the role of nitric oxide (NO) [2].

According to the Starling resistor model (Figure 1), the upper airways function as a hollow tube with a constriction near the entrance hole, which corresponds to the nostrils, and a posterior collapsible segment, which corresponds to the oropharynx. This model predicts that the presence of a further upstream obstructive factor (nose) will generate a suction force, that is, a negative intraluminal pressure downstream (oropharynx), resulting in pharyngeal collapse in predisposed individuals [15, 16].

A closed jaw and proper dental occlusion stabilize the flow in the upper airways [17]. When nasal resistance exceeds a certain level, an air bypass occurs and leads to mouth breathing, resulting in a decrease in the retroglossal dimension, due to the subsequent retraction of the tongue, narrowing of the pharyngeal lumen, and increased oscillation and vibration of the soft palate and redundant tissue of the pharynx [14]. This shift from nasal to oral breathing is physiologically disadvantageous to the individual, leading to an unstable breathing pattern [2].

Central respiratory events have also been increasingly associated with oral breathing during sleep. Tanaka and Honda [18] proposed that, after a switch to oral breathing during sleep, there is greater CO_2 elimination during expiration, caused by an increase in respiratory stimulus. The increase in central apneas suggests that the nose plays an important role in the regulation of respiration and not only in the maintenance of airway patency.

A third factor is the nasal ventilatory reflex. An experimental application of local anesthetics in the nasal mucosa of healthy patients led to a significant increase of obstructive and central apnea episodes, of the same magnitude as those reported with complete nasal obstruction [19]. Similar results from other experiments [20] confirmed that the activation of nasal receptors during nasal breathing had a direct positive effect on spontaneous ventilation, leading to a higher resting

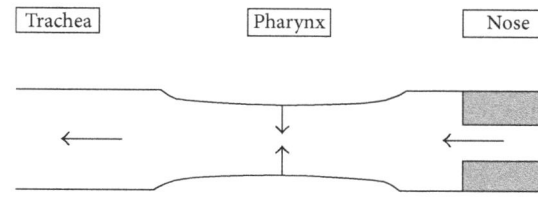

FIGURE 1: Starling resistor model.

breathing frequency and minute ventilation. Mouth breathing reduces the activation of these nasal receptors, leading to deactivation of the nasal-respiratory reflex and reduction of spontaneous ventilation, which can trigger respiratory events in susceptible individuals with subclinical OSAS [21] or exacerbate apnea episodes [22].

Finally, NO appears to play a role in maintaining the patency of the upper airways, as a transmitter between the nose, pharyngeal muscles, and lungs [23]. NO is produced in significant quantities in the nose and in the paranasal sinuses and has been proven (including in clinical practice) to be a potent pulmonary vasodilator, improving oxygenation and ventilation-perfusion ratio [24]. As the total amount of inspired NO varies according to the nasal flow [25], it appears logical that a decrease in nasal breathing would result in reduction of NO delivery to the lungs and a reduction in blood oxygenation. NO also plays a role in the maintenance of muscle tone, regulation of neuromuscular pathways in the pharyngeal muscles, spontaneous respiration, and sleep regulation. In general, the role of NO in the regulation of nasal OSAS, although probably significant, is still not completely understood [26].

The nasal pathophysiology in the pathogenesis of OSAS is summarized in Table 1.

3. Clinical and Experimental Evidence

Evidence suggests that experimental reduction of nasal patency and flow has a significant effect on breathing during sleep.

Suratt et al. [27] induced obstructive apneas in healthy subjects through nasal occlusion with gauze. Lavie et al. [28] investigated the influence of partial and complete obstruction of the nose in healthy subjects and observed a significant increase in the number of apneas during sleep.

Evidence from several observational and cross-sectional studies demonstrates that the objective increase in measures of nasal resistance and the presence of allergic rhinitis (AR) are associated with OSAS. Lofaso et al. [6] performed posterior rhinomanometry in 528 patients and observed an increased nasal resistance in OSAS patients compared to the control group. In a large population study, Young et al. [29] identified chronic nasal congestion as a risk factor for OSAS.

Data from an electromyographic study in healthy men performed by Basner et al. [30] demonstrated that the upper airway tone is lower during oral breathing than during nasal breathing, suggesting that the activity of the dilator muscles of the upper airway can be modulated by receptors in the

TABLE 1: Nasal pathophysiology in the pathogenesis of OSAS.

Starling resistor model	Increased nasal resistance results in negative oropharyngeal pressure (suction force).
Instability of mouth breathing	Significant increase in nasal resistance generates higher fraction of oral breathing, leading to unstable airway.
Nasal ventilatory reflex	Decrease in nasal airflow results in less activation of nasal receptors and, consequently, inhibition of muscle tone, respiratory rate, and minute ventilation.
Nitric oxide (NO)	Decrease in nasal flow generates lower concentration of pulmonary NO with reduced ventilation-perfusion ratio.

nasal mucosa, sensitive to airflow or pressure. However, two other studies demonstrated that the airway did not affect the electromyographic activity of the genioglossus muscle in normal individuals, but other pharyngeal dilator muscles have not been studied [31, 32].

Epidemiological studies [33] demonstrated that AR affects 9% to 42% of the population. The mechanism through which allergic rhinitis causes poor quality of sleep and daytime fatigue is not entirely clear, but it is believed that several factors are involved. Inflammatory mediators such as interferon- (IFN-) gamma, tumor necrosis factor- (TNF-) alpha, interleukin- (IL-) 1b, IL-4, IL-10 [34], postural changes, and certain therapeutic agents, such as antihistamines, may have a direct impact on sleep regulation. One study described a direct association between nasal resistance and the severity of OSAS in patients with AR [35], as well as between nasal obstruction and subjective sleep quality and daytime sleepiness [36]. A recent study observed that both the AR and nonallergic rhinitis (NAR) are associated with impaired sleep quality and demonstrated complaints in up to 83% of patients with NAR [37].

In a recent review, McNicholas [38] attempted to synthesize these apparently conflicting results, indicating that reversible nasal obstruction is perhaps more closely associated with OSAS than with permanent nasal obstruction. This finding was observed in studies of patients with temporary obstruction (including AR and iatrogenic causes), which demonstrated a more consistent association with OSAS than studies of patients with structural abnormalities, such as a deviated nasal septum.

Thus, it appears that nasal obstruction, especially the reversible type (whether artificial or disease-induced), is associated with snoring and mild OSAS. Nonetheless, a direct correlation between the degree of nasal obstruction and the severity of OSAS has not been observed; nasal obstruction does not appear to be the main contributing factor in the majority of patients with moderate to severe OSAS.

These are some lines of evidence that, even with limited methodology, show how the nasal respiratory dysfunction influences sleep apnea.

4. Nasal Treatment in OSAS

Treatment options for cases with nasal obstruction include nasal dilators, medical treatment, and surgical intervention. Some clinical trials have been performed, aiming to analyze the therapeutic possibilities; however, the evaluation of the results was not uniformly objective. Many of the studies are not randomized, do not include a control group, and have a small sample size and relatively short follow-up period [39].

5. Conservative Treatment

In patients with nasal obstruction secondary to chronic rhinitis, the main cause of increased nasal resistance is edema and turbinate hypertrophy. Among the options for drug treatment are topical corticosteroids and sympathomimetic decongestants. These medications reduce the levels of inflammatory mediators, or even directly cause vasoconstriction, thereby leading to a decrease in nasal resistance and improved sleep [39].

There is only one randomized controlled trial assessing the effect of topical nasal corticosteroids in adult OSAS (Table 1) [40]. In that study, Kiely et al. evaluated the effect of topical nasal fluticasone for four weeks in 23 patients with chronic rhinitis: 13 had moderate to severe OSAS (mean apnea-hypopnea index [AHI]: 26.5) and ten patients were snorers without OSAS (mean AHI: 3). A reduction in AHI (mean: −6.5) and in nasal resistance was observed in the OSAS group after treatment with fluticasone when compared to placebo. However, there was no improvement in subjective sleep quality (reported by the patient, or improvement in the snoring intensity reported by the partner), in sleep architecture (no change in the duration of REM sleep), or in oxyhemoglobin desaturation index (desaturation between average and minimum levels) in either group.

These findings suggest that nasal obstruction due to allergic rhinitis favors worsening of sleep apnea and that treatment with topical corticosteroids can be somewhat beneficial in cases of mild to moderate OSAS.

Studies on nasal decongestants, such as oxymetazoline [28, 41], were limited and were inconclusive (Table 2). The results demonstrate that nasal decongestants, whether or not associated with nasal dilators, are not effective in the management of OSA, as no improvement was observed in the degree of daytime sleepiness or AHI [42–45]. As their clinical use is limited to only a few days, nasal decongestants cannot be used for OSAS management.

It can be concluded that pharmacological improvement in nasal patency in patients with OSAS and chronic nasal obstruction presents some beneficial effects on the frequency of respiratory events and sleep architecture. Nonetheless, objective data assessing snoring and daytime sleepiness are still necessary.

The use of nasal dilators is an option for increasing nasal patency in the narrowest part of the airway, the nasal

TABLE 2: Studies on topical medication for the treatment of sleep disorders.

Study	Study design	Patients	Nasal pathology	Intervention	Results
Kiely et al., 2004 [40]	Double-blinded, controlled, randomized	10 snorers (mean AHI: 3), 13 OSAS (mean AHI: 26.5)	Allergic rhinitis without septal deviation	Fluticasone 100 mcg BD for four weeks versus placebo	Reduction in AHI and subjective nasal resistance. No difference in sleep architecture, snoring, or O_2 saturation.
McLean et al., 2005 [44]	Cross-sectional, blinded	10 moderate to severe OSAS	Chronic nasal obstruction	Topical oxymetazoline (0.2 mg BD) and external nasal dilator versus placebo	Reduction in AHI, improved sleep architecture, and reduced oral breathing. No alterations in sleepiness.
Kerr et al., 1992 [43]	Cross-sectional, blinded	10 moderate to severe OSAS	Chronic nasal obstruction	Topical oxymetazoline and nasal dilator versus placebo	Mild improvement in arousal index. No alterations in AHI, O_2 saturation, or sleepiness.

AHI: apnea-hypopnea index; OSAS: obstructive sleep apnea syndrome.

valve. Two of the nasal dilators available in the market are an external device, Breathe Right (CNS Inc.; Bloomington, MN, USA), and an internal device, Nozovent (Prevancure AB; Frölunda, Sweden). Five studies with small sample were retrieved, three using Breathe Right and two using Nozovent (Table 3) [46–48, 50].

Nasal dilators are generally not recommended in patients with OSAS, but they may be beneficial for those with simple snoring associated with rhinitis and/or nasal valve stenosis. Since they are affordable devices with few side effects, they can be useful in some selected cases, especially as a conservative option for patients with indication for surgical correction of the nasal valve.

6. Surgical Treatment

Nasal obstruction in patients with OSAS may be caused by septal deviation, nasal polyps, and turbinate hypertrophy, among several other abnormalities. In this context, surgical interventions, such as septoplasty, rhinoseptoplasty, functional endoscopic sinus surgery, turbinectomy, and nasal valve surgery, appear to be a good therapeutic option [51].

There is also a group of patients who may benefit from surgical intervention not for curative purposes, but as an adjuvant treatment to improve the effectiveness of the main therapeutic option, continuous positive airway pressure (CPAP).

Li et al. [52, 53] recently addressed the role of nasal surgery in patients with snoring and OSAS from two different perspectives. Initially [52], the efficacy of nasal surgery for relief of snoring and OSAS in patients with septal deviation was assessed. The authors concluded that complete relief of snoring was achieved in only 12% of patients. Secondly, the improvement in quality of life after nasal surgery alone in patients with OSAS and nasal obstruction was assessed [53]. This parameter was evaluated through generic and disease-specific questionnaires. Li et al. concluded that it is possible to significantly improve the quality of life by correcting an obstructed nasal airway and thus substantiated the role of

nasal surgery in treating these patients. Notwithstanding, despite the significant improvement observed in the quality of life parameters, there was no statistically significant improvement in the objective polysomnographic data. This discrepancy between objective and subjective outcomes was also observed in several other similar studies after nasal surgery alone for OSAS treatment. Verse et al. [54] studied a cohort of 26 patients, 19 of whom had OSAS and seven of whom were simple snorers. A variety of nasal surgical procedures, including rhinoplasty, septoplasty, endoscopic sinus surgery, and nasal valve surgery, were performed. They concluded that although nasal surgery significantly improved subjective sleep quality and daytime sleepiness, the surgical response rate in the apnea group was only 15%, based on objective parameters (AHI). Four patients presented worsening of sleep apnea, despite the reduction in arousal index. This paradoxical effect can be explained by the "first night effect," which occurs when the patient has the initial, preoperative, sleep study for the first time, he does not sleep well and as a result the study it may not reflect the true severity of the sleep apnea. In the postoperative evaluation, when the patient has already adapted to the methodology of the examination, the severity of the problem becomes more evident.

Morinaga et al. [55] evaluated how the pharyngeal morphology affects the outcomes of nasal surgery in patients with OSAS and nasal obstruction. The morphological characteristics analyzed included degree of tonsillar hypertrophy, Mallampati grade, and retroglossal space. They concluded that the most favorable surgical outcomes were observed in subjects whose soft palate was positioned higher and/or had larger retroglossal dimensions. Conversely, Li et al. [52] found a relationship between the degree of tonsillar hypertrophy and surgical outcomes. The most important (and only) randomized study was conducted in 2007, by Koutsourelakis et al., in Athens [56], who divided 49 patients with septal deviation and OSAS into two groups; one group underwent septoplasty and the other, a sham surgery. Despite the subjective improvement in nasal patency, no objective changes

TABLE 3: Studies on nasal dilators for treatment of sleep disorders.

Study	Patients	Study design, intervention	Results	Commentaries
Bahammam et al., 1999 [46]	18 snorers, mean AHI: 8.9	Cross-sectional, Breathe Right versus placebo	Improvement on desaturation time and sleep architecture. No difference in AHI or arousal index.	Nasal dilation increased nasal cross-section area. No information regarding snoring.
Pevernagie et al., 2000 [47]	12 snorers, mean AHI: 6, chronic rhinitis and nasal obstruction	Cross-sectional, Breathe Right versus placebo	Reduction of snoring. No difference in AHI, sleep architecture, or arousal index.	Nasal dilation significantly decreased nasal resistance.
Djupesland et al., 2001 [48]	18 snorers, mean AHI: 9.3, nocturnal nasal obstruction	Cross-sectional, Breathe Right versus placebo	No difference in O_2 saturation, snoring, or sleep architecture. Increase of AHI.	Nasal dilation increased cross-sectional area and nasal volume.
Schönhofer et al., 2003 [49]	38 OSAS, in use of CPAP, mean AHI: 17.1	Cross-sectional, Nozovent versus placebo	CPAP pressure reduction. No difference in AHI or O_2 saturation.	Nasal dilation was not controlled by objective or subjective measures.
Hoijer et al., 1992 [50]	10 OSAS, mean AHI: 18	Cross-sectional, Nozovent versus placebo	Reduction of snoring and O_2 saturation. No improvement on hypersomnolence.	Nasal dilation increased nasal airflow.

AHI: apnea-hypopnea index; OSAS: obstructive sleep apnea syndrome; CPAP: continuous positive airway pressure.

were observed on AHI or daytime sleepiness, assessed by the Epworth sleepiness scale. However, in the septoplasty group, four patients (14.8%) responded to surgery, according to the Sher criteria (AHI reduction by 50% or more), and only one patient was disease-free (AHI < 5). It was concluded that nasal surgery can improve the quality of life and snoring in a select group of patients with mild OSAS and septal deviation. Nasal surgery is certainly not the most effective treatment for all patients with OSAS, but further studies can better define subgroups of patients who can benefit from the surgical procedure.

7. Nasal Obstruction and CPAP

CPAP is the treatment of choice for moderate or severe OSAS; however, the rate of adherence to this form of therapy is less than 70% [57]. Over 50% of CPAP users complain of significant nasal symptoms, such as nasal congestion, rhinorrhea, nasal dryness, and sneezing [58], which may become more significant if the patient presents any structural abnormality of the nose.

Since the CPAP mask is in contact with the nose, it is reasonable to assume that nasal alterations constitute a limitation to its use. The presence of functional or anatomical abnormalities in the nasal cavity may require greater CPAP pressure titration for the elimination of respiratory events, causing patient discomfort and hindering adaptation to the device. Nonetheless, attributing the low adherence to CPAP to a condition of increased nasal resistance is a controversial hypothesis.

Tárrega et al. [59] evaluated, through rhinomanometry, 125 patients with indication for CPAP therapy and observed no correlation between nasal resistance and CPAP adherence. Haddad et al. [60] investigated the contribution of nasal factors on CPAP adherence and observed that the highest values of body mass index (BMI), neck circumference, and AHI were found in the group of patients with good CPAP adherence, while nasal parameters such as rhinoscopy, nasofibroscopy, and acoustic rhinometry showed no differences between the groups with good or poor adherence.

Conversely, Morris et al. [61] observed a greater minimum cross-sectional area in the interior turbinate of patients with good CPAP adherence. These results were corroborated by Sugiura et al. [62], who observed that nasal resistance was lower in patients who used CPAP during titration polysomnography. These data demonstrate the need of good nasal patency during the patient's initial adaptation to the device. So et al. [63] also investigated 36 patients using acoustic rhinometry and observed that the sum of the nasal area was greater in the group of patients with good CPAP adherence, but only in those with AHI < 60/hour.

Despite the conflicting results in the literature, it is important that patients who are not perfectly adapted to CPAP are evaluated in detail, in order to identify whether there are obstructive factors that could be surgically corrected. In a group of patients who underwent radiofrequency turbinectomy, Powell et al. [64] demonstrated a subjective improvement of nasal obstruction, which, in turn, increased

CPAP adherence. Similarly, Friedman et al. [65] showed a significant decrease in the levels of CPAP titration after nasal surgery alone. In that study, a reduction in pressure required for the cessation of obstructive events was observed in patients with mild, moderate, and severe OSAS. The average reduction in CPAP titration pressure was 9.3 cm H_2O preoperatively to 6.7 cm H_2O postoperatively. Nakata et al. [66] assessed 12 patients with nasal obstruction and severe OSAS who did not respond to treatment with CPAP. After nasal surgery, a significant decrease in nasal resistance and a significant increase in minimum O_2 saturation during sleep were observed. However, no change was evidenced in AHI, despite the decrease in CPAP titration pressure from 16.8 cm H_2O to 12 cm H_2O in five patients.

8. Final Considerations

Despite the recent progress in the study of the relation between OSAS and nasal obstruction, there are still areas of doubt. Many of the studies investigating this relationship had an inappropriate sample size, poorly defined patient populations, inadequate control groups, and inappropriate techniques to objectively evaluate nasal resistance.

It is established that an improvement in nasal resistance, whether through surgery, medication, or use of nasal dilators, may improve self-reported sleep quality. However, these results are not always followed by improvement in polysomnographic parameters. Despite the lack of evidence demonstrating the success of nasal surgery as an isolated treatment for moderate and severe OSAS, surgical procedures that improve nasal patency have a role in relieving symptoms of simple snoring and as part of multiple-level surgery in patients with OSAS. Nasal surgery may help in OSA patients who do not tolerate CPAP therapy, when there is a local obstructive factor in the nose.

Conflict of Interests

The authors declare that there is no conflict of interests regarding the publication of this paper.

References

[1] L. Hippocrates, *De Morbus Popularibus*, Frien, Sheep, London, UK, 1717.

[2] C. Georgalas, "The role of the nose in snoring and obstructive sleep apnoea: an update," *European Archives of Oto-Rhino-Laryngology*, vol. 268, no. 9, pp. 1365–1373, 2011.

[3] D. N. F. Fairbanks, "Effect of nasal surgery on snoring," *Southern Medical Journal*, vol. 78, no. 3, pp. 268–270, 1985.

[4] T. J. Craig, S. Teets, E. B. Lehman, V. M. Chinchilli, and C. Zwillich, "Nasal congestion secondary to allergic rhinitis as a cause of sleep disturbance and daytime fatigue and the response to topical nasal corticosteroids," *Journal of Allergy and Clinical Immunology*, vol. 101, no. 5, pp. 633–637, 1998.

[5] M. Atkins, V. Taskar, N. Clayton, P. Stone, and A. Woodcock, "Nasal resistance in obstructive sleep apnea," *Chest*, vol. 105, no. 4, pp. 1133–1135, 1994.

[6] F. Lofaso, A. Coste, M. P. D'Ortho et al., "Nasal obstruction as a risk factor for sleep apnoea syndrome," *European Respiratory Journal*, vol. 16, no. 4, pp. 639–643, 2000.

[7] B. G. Ferris Jr., J. Mead, and L. H. Opie, "Partitioning of respiratory flow resistance in man," *Journal of Applied Physiology*, vol. 19, pp. 653–658, 1964.

[8] M. Kohler, R. Thurnheer, and K. E. Bloch, "Side-selective, unobtrusive monitoring of nasal airflow and conductance," *Journal of Applied Physiology*, vol. 101, no. 6, pp. 1760–1765, 2006.

[9] D. R. Heetderks, "Observations on the reactions of normal nasal mucosa membrane," *The American Journal of the Medical Sciences*, vol. 174, pp. 231–244, 1927.

[10] K. O. Olsen and E. B. Kern, "Nasal influences on snoring and obstructive sleep apnea," *Mayo Clinic Proceedings*, vol. 65, no. 8, pp. 1095–1105, 1990.

[11] D. W. Hudgel and D. W. Robertson, "Nasal resistance during wakefulness and sleep in normal man," *Acta Oto-Laryngologica*, vol. 98, no. 1-2, pp. 130–135, 1984.

[12] P. Cole and J. S. J. Haight, "Posture and nasal patency," *American Review of Respiratory Disease*, vol. 129, no. 3, pp. 351–354, 1984.

[13] P. Cole and J. S. J. Haight, "Mechanisms of nasal obstruction during sleep," *Laryngoscope*, vol. 94, no. 12, pp. 1557–1559, 1984.

[14] T. Verse and W. Pirsig, "Impact of impaired nasal breathing on sleep-disordered breathing," *Sleep and Breathing*, vol. 7, no. 2, pp. 63–76, 2003.

[15] P. L. Smith, R. A. Wise, A. R. Gold, A. R. Schwartz, and S. Permutt, "Upper airway pressure-flow relationships in obstructive sleep apnea," *Journal of Applied Physiology*, vol. 64, no. 2, pp. 789–795, 1988.

[16] S. S. Park, "Flow-regulatory function of upper airway in health and disease: a unified pathogenetic view of sleep-disordered breathing," *Lung*, vol. 171, no. 6, pp. 311–333, 1993.

[17] S. T. Kuna and J. E. Remmers, "Neural and anatomic factors related to upper airway occlusion during sleep," *Medical Clinics of North America*, vol. 69, no. 6, pp. 1221–1242, 1985.

[18] Y. Tanaka and Y. Honda, "Nasal obstruction as a cause of reduced PCO_2 and disordered breathing during sleep," *Journal of Applied Physiology*, vol. 67, no. 3, pp. 970–972, 1989.

[19] W. T. McNicholas, M. Coffey, and T. Boyle, "Effects of nasal airflow on breathing during sleep in normal humans," *American Review of Respiratory Disease*, vol. 147, no. 3, pp. 620–623, 1993.

[20] N. J. Douglas, D. P. White, J. V. Weil, and C. W. Zwillich, "Effect of breathing route on ventilation and ventilatory drive," *Respiration Physiology*, vol. 51, no. 2, pp. 209–218, 1983.

[21] D. P. White, R. J. Cadieux, R. M. Lombard, E. O. Bixler, A. Kales, and C. W. Zwillich, "The effects of nasal anesthesia on breathing during sleep," *American Review of Respiratory Disease*, vol. 132, no. 5, pp. 972–975, 1985.

[22] R. B. Berry, K. G. Kouchi, J. L. Bower, and R. W. Light, "Effect of upper airway anesthesia on obstructive sleep apnea," *American Journal of Respiratory and Critical Care Medicine*, vol. 151, no. 6, pp. 1857–1861, 1995.

[23] J. Lundberg, "Airborne nitric oxide: Inflammatory marker and aerocrine messenger in man," *Acta Physiologica Scandinavica*, vol. 157, no. 633, pp. 1–27, 1996.

[24] M. L. Blitzer, E. Loh, M. A. Roddy, J. S. Stamler, and M. A. Creager, "Endothelium-derived nitric oxide regulates systemic and pulmonary vascular resistance during acute hypoxia in humans," *Journal of the American College of Cardiology*, vol. 28, no. 3, pp. 591–596, 1996.

[25] P. G. Djupesland, J. M. Chatkin, W. Qian et al., "Aerodynamic influences on nasal nitric oxide output measurements," *Acta Oto-Laryngologica*, vol. 119, no. 4, pp. 479–485, 1999.

[26] J. S. J. Haight and P. G. Djupesland, "Nitric oxide (NO) and obstructive sleep apnea (OSA)," *Sleep and Breathing*, vol. 7, no. 2, pp. 53–61, 2003.

[27] P. M. Suratt, B. L. Turner, and S. C. Wilhoit, "Effect of intranasal obstruction on breathing during sleep," *Chest*, vol. 90, no. 3, pp. 324–329, 1986.

[28] P. Lavie, N. Fischel, J. Zomer, and I. Eliaschar, "The effects of partial and complete mechanical occlusion of the nasal passages on sleep structure and breathing in sleep," *Acta Oto-Laryngologica*, vol. 95, no. 1-2, pp. 161–166, 1983.

[29] T. Young, L. Finn, and H. Kim, "Nasal obstruction as a risk factor for sleep-disordered breathing. The University of Wisconsin Sleep and Respiratory Research Group," *Journal of Allergy and Clinical Immunology*, vol. 99, no. 2, pp. S757–S762, 1997.

[30] R. C. Basner, P. M. Simon, R. M. Schwartzstein, S. E. Weinberger, and J. Woodrow Weiss, "Breathing route influences upper airway muscle activity in awake normal adults," *Journal of Applied Physiology*, vol. 66, no. 4, pp. 1766–1771, 1989.

[31] Y.-X. Shi, M. Seto-Poon, and J. R. Wheatley, "Breathing route dependence of upper airway muscle activity during hyperpnea," *Journal of Applied Physiology*, vol. 84, no. 5, pp. 1701–1706, 1998.

[32] J. S. Williams, P. L. Janssen, D. D. Fuller, and R. F. Fregosi, "Influence of posture and breathing route on neural drive to upper airway dilator muscles during exercise," *Journal of Applied Physiology*, vol. 89, no. 2, pp. 590–598, 2000.

[33] R. A. Settipane and D. R. Charnock, "Epidemiology of rhinitis: allergic and nonallergic," *Clinical Allergy and Immunology*, vol. 19, pp. 23–34, 2007.

[34] B. J. Ferguson, "Influences of allergic rhinitis on sleep," *Otolaryngology: Head and Neck Surgery*, vol. 130, no. 5, pp. 617–629, 2004.

[35] W. T. McNicholas, S. Tarlo, P. Cole et al., "Obstructive apneas during sleep in patients with seasonal allergic rhinitis," *American Review of Respiratory Disease*, vol. 126, no. 4, pp. 625–628, 1982.

[36] B. A. Stuck, J. Czajkowski, A.-E. Hagner et al., "Changes in daytime sleepiness, quality of life, and objective sleep patterns in seasonal allergic rhinitis: a controlled clinical trial," *Journal of Allergy and Clinical Immunology*, vol. 113, no. 4, pp. 663–668, 2004.

[37] A. F. Kalpaklıoğlu, A. B. Kavut, and M. Ekici, "Allergic and nonallergic rhinitis: the threat for obstructive sleep apnea," *Annals of Allergy, Asthma & Immunology*, vol. 103, no. 1, pp. 20–25, 2009.

[38] W. T. McNicholas, "The nose and OSA: variable nasal obstruction may be more important in pathophysiology than fixed obstruction," *European Respiratory Journal*, vol. 32, no. 1, pp. 3–8, 2008.

[39] B. Kotecha, "The nose, snoring and obstructive sleep apnoea," *Rhinology*, vol. 49, no. 3, pp. 259–263, 2011.

[40] J. L. Kiely, P. Nolan, and W. T. McNicholas, "Intranasal corticosteroid therapy for obstructive sleep apnoea in patients with co-existing rhinitis," *Thorax*, vol. 59, no. 1, pp. 50–55, 2004.

[41] N. J. Cassisi, H. F. Biller, and J. H. Ogura, "Changes in arterial oxygen tension and pulmonary mechanics with the use of posterior packing in epistaxis: a preliminary report," *Laryngoscope*, vol. 81, no. 8, pp. 1261–1266, 1971.

[42] T. J. Craig, C. D. Hanks, and L. H. Fisher, "How do topical nasal corticosteroids improve sleep and daytime somnolence in allergic rhinitis?" *Journal of Allergy and Clinical Immunology*, vol. 116, no. 6, pp. 1264–1266, 2005.

[43] P. Kerr, T. Millar, P. Buckle, and M. Kryger, "The importance of nasal resistance in obstructive sleep apnea syndrome," *Journal of Otolaryngology*, vol. 21, no. 3, pp. 189–195, 1992.

[44] H. A. McLean, A. M. Urton, H. S. Driver et al., "Effect of treating severe nasal obstruction on the severity of obstructive sleep apnoea," *European Respiratory Journal*, vol. 25, no. 3, pp. 521–527, 2005.

[45] C. F. Clarenbach, M. Kohler, O. Senn, R. Thurnheer, and K. E. Bloch, "Does nasal decongestion improve obstructive sleep apnea?" *Journal of Sleep Research*, vol. 17, no. 4, pp. 444–449, 2008.

[46] A. S. Bahammam, R. Tate, J. Manfreda, and M. H. Kryger, "Upper airway resistance syndrome: effect of nasal dilation, sleep stage, and sleep position," *Sleep*, vol. 22, no. 5, pp. 592–598, 1999.

[47] D. Pevernagie, E. Hamans, P. Van Cauwenberge, and R. Pauwels, "External nasal dilation reduces snoring chronic rhinitis patients: a randomized controlled trial," *European Respiratory Journal*, vol. 15, no. 6, pp. 996–1000, 2000.

[48] P. G. Djupesland, O. Skatvedt, and A. K. Borgersen, "Dichotomous physiological effects of nocturnal external nasal dilation in heavy snorers: the answer to a rhinologic controversy?" *American Journal of Rhinology*, vol. 15, no. 2, pp. 95–103, 2001.

[49] B. Schönhofer, J. Kerl, S. Suchi, D. Köhler, and K. A. Franklin, "Effect of nasal valve dilation on effective CPAP level in obstructive sleep apnea," *Respiratory Medicine*, vol. 97, no. 9, pp. 1001–1005, 2003.

[50] U. Hoijer, H. Ejnell, J. Hedner, B. Petruson, and L. B. Eng, "The effects of nasal dilation on snoring and obstructive sleep apnea," *Archives of Otolaryngology—Head and Neck Surgery*, vol. 118, no. 3, pp. 281–284, 1992.

[51] M. Kohler, K. E. Bloch, and J. R. Stradling, "The role of the nose in the pathogenesis of obstructive sleep apnea," *Current Opinion in Otolaryngology & Head & Neck Surgery*, vol. 17, no. 1, pp. 33–37, 2009.

[52] H. Y. Li, L. A. Lee, P. C. Wang, N. H. Chen, Y. Lin, and T. J. Fang, "Nasal surgery for snoring in patients with obstructive sleep apnea," *Laryngoscope*, vol. 118, no. 2, pp. 354–359, 2008.

[53] H.-Y. Li, Y. Lin, N.-H. Chen, L.-A. Lee, T.-J. Fang, and P.-C. Wang, "Improvement in quality of life after nasal surgery alone for patients with obstructive sleep apnea and nasal obstruction," *Archives of Otolaryngology: Head and Neck Surgery*, vol. 134, no. 4, pp. 429–433, 2008.

[54] T. Verse, J. T. Maurer, and W. Pirsig, "Effect of nasal surgery on sleep-related breathing disorders," *Laryngoscope*, vol. 112, no. 1, pp. 64–68, 2002.

[55] M. Morinaga, S. Nakata, F. Yasuma et al., "Pharyngeal morphology: a determinant of successful nasal surgery for sleep apnea," *The Laryngoscope*, vol. 119, no. 5, pp. 1011–1016, 2009.

[56] I. Koutsourelakis, G. Georgoulopoulos, E. Perraki, E. Vagiakis, C. Roussos, and S. G. Zakynthinos, "Randomised trial of nasal surgery for fixed nasal obstruction in obstructive sleep apnoea," *European Respiratory Journal*, vol. 31, no. 1, pp. 110–117, 2008.

[57] N. McArdle, G. Devereux, H. Heidarnejad, H. M. Engleman, T. W. Mackay, and N. J. Douglas, "Long-term use of CPAP therapy for sleep apnea/hypopnea syndrome," *American Journal of Respiratory and Critical Care Medicine*, vol. 159, no. 4, pp. 1108–1114, 1999.

[58] V. Hoffstein, S. Viner, S. Mateika, and J. Conway, "Treatment of obstructive sleep apnea with nasal continuous positive airway pressure: patient compliance, perception of benefits, and side effects," *The American Review of Respiratory Disease*, vol. 145, no. 4, pp. 841–845, 1992.

[59] J. Tárrega, M. Mayos, J. R. Montserrat et al., "Nasal resistance and continuous positive airway pressure treatment for sleep apnea/hypopnea syndrome," *Archivos de Bronconeumologia*, vol. 39, no. 3, pp. 106–110, 2003.

[60] F. L. M. Haddad, T. D. A. Vidigal, L. Mello-Fujita et al., "The influence of nasal abnormalities in adherence to continuous positive airway pressure device therapy in obstructive sleep apnea patients," *Sleep and Breathing*, vol. 17, no. 4, pp. 1201–1207, 2013.

[61] L. G. Morris, J. Setlur, O. E. Burschtin, D. L. Steward, J. B. Jacobs, and K. C. Lee, "Acoustic rhinometry predicts tolerance of nasal continuous positive airway pressure: a pilot study," *American Journal of Rhinology*, vol. 20, no. 2, pp. 133–137, 2006.

[62] T. Sugiura, A. Noda, S. Nakata et al., "Influence of nasal resistance on initial acceptance of continuous positive airway pressure in treatment for obstructive sleep apnea syndrome," *Respiration*, vol. 74, no. 1, pp. 56–60, 2006.

[63] Y. K. So, H.-J. Dhong, H. Y. Kim, S.-K. Chung, and J.-Y. Jang, "Initial adherence to autotitrating positive airway pressure therapy: Influence of upper airway narrowing," *Clinical and Experimental Otorhinolaryngology*, vol. 2, no. 4, pp. 181–185, 2009.

[64] N. B. Powell, A. I. Zonato, E. M. Weaver et al., "Radiofrequency treatment of turbinate hypertrophy in subjects using continuous positive airway pressure: a randomized, double-blind, placebo-controlled clinical pilot trial," *Laryngoscope*, vol. 111, no. 10, pp. 1783–1790, 2001.

[65] M. Friedman, H. Tanyeri, J. W. Lim, R. Landsberg, K. Vaidyanathan, and D. Caldarelli, "Effect of improved nasal breathing on obstructive sleep apnea," *Otolaryngology: Head and Neck Surgery*, vol. 122, no. 1, pp. 71–74, 2000.

[66] S. Nakata, A. Noda, H. Yagi et al., "Nasal resistance for determinant factor of nasal surgery in CPAP failure patients with obstructive sleep apnea syndrome," *Rhinology*, vol. 43, no. 4, pp. 296–299, 2005.

29

Treatment of Vertigo: A Randomized, Double-Blind Trial Comparing Efficacy and Safety of *Ginkgo biloba* Extract EGb 761 and Betahistine

Larysa Sokolova,[1] Robert Hoerr,[2] and Tamara Mishchenko[3]

[1] *Faculty of Neurology, Bohomolets National Medical University, Shevchenko Avenue, 13, Kiev 01601, Ukraine*
[2] *Clinical Research Department, Dr. Willmar Schwabe GmbH & Co. KG, Willmar-Schwabe-Straße 4, 76227 Karlsruhe, Germany*
[3] *Institute of Neurology, Psychiatry and Narcology of the NAMS of Ukraine SI, 46, Akademika Pavlova Street, Kharkiv 61068, Ukraine*

Correspondence should be addressed to Robert Hoerr; robert.hoerr@schwabe.de

Academic Editor: Michael D. Seidman

A multicenter clinical trial was performed to compare the efficacy and safety of *Ginkgo biloba* extract EGb 761 and betahistine at recommended doses in patients with vertigo. One hundred and sixty patients (mean age 58 years) were randomly assigned to double-blind treatment with EGb 761 (240 mg per day) or betahistine (32 mg per day) for 12 weeks. An 11-point numeric analogue scale, the Vertigo Symptom Scale—short form, the Clinical Global Impression Scales and the Sheehan Disability Scale were used as outcome measures. Both treatment groups were comparable at baseline and improved in all outcome measures during the course of treatment. There was no significant intergroup difference with regard to changes in any outcome measure. Numerically, improvements of patients receiving EGb 761 were slightly more pronounced on all scales. Clinical global impression was rated "very much improved" or "much improved" in 79% of patients treated with EGb 761 and in 70% receiving betahistine. With 27 adverse events in 19 patients, EGb 761 showed better tolerability than betahistine with 39 adverse events in 31 patients. In conclusion, the two drugs were similarly effective in the treatment of vertigo, but EGb 761 was better tolerated. This trial is registered with controlledtrials.com ISRCTN02262139.

1. Introduction

Dizziness is a symptom reported frequently in primary care, more often by women than men. In a nationally representative sample of 4869 adults in Germany, aged 18 to 79 years, the one-year prevalence of moderate to severe dizziness (including vestibular and nonvestibular vertigo) was 22.9% and the one-year prevalence of moderate to severe vestibular vertigo was 4.9% [1]. The one-year incidence of moderate to severe dizziness was 3.1% and the one-year incidence of moderate to severe vestibular vertigo was 1.4%. The lifetime prevalence of dizziness-related medical consultations amounted to 17.1% [1]. In a cross-national survey of emergency department visits in the United States, 3.3% of cases presented with dizziness. Of these, 32.9% were of otological/vestibular origin and 4% were due to cerebrovascular disease [2]. Centralvestibular vertigo (12.4%), bilateral peripheral vestibulopathy

(5.1%), and paroxysmal dysfunction of the vestibular nerve or vestibular organs (3.9%) are among the frequent types of vertigo. In 3.3% of patients, the cause of vertigo remains unclear [3]. Vertigo is frequent in patients with cerebrovascular disease. Compromised blood supply in the vertebrobasilar region has been reported to manifest itself by isolated vertigo in 24% of patients [4] and 17% of patients with cerebral microangiopathy complained of vertigo [5].

In vertigo associated with cerebrovascular disorders, drugs that improve cerebral blood flow are often prescribed. The international survey found betahistine to be the most frequently prescribed drug for the treatment of various kinds of vertigo, including Ménière's disease, benign paroxysmal positional vertigo, other peripheral vertigo, and peripheral vertigo of unknown origin, followed by piracetam and *Ginkgo biloba* extract [6]. Betahistine is a histamine analogue with agonistic activity at the H_1 and antagonistic activity at the H_3 histamine receptors. Its efficacy in the treatment of Ménière's disease and other vertiginous syndromes has been demonstrated by randomized, placebo-controlled trials [7, 8].

Ginkgo biloba extract EGb 761 enhances cerebral and vestibular blood flow [9, 10] by decreasing blood viscosity [11]. It improves neuronal plasticity [12] as well as mitochondrial function and energy metabolism [13] and protects neurons from oxidative damage [14]. Its efficacy in the treatment of vestibular and nonvestibular vertigo has also been proven by randomized, placebo-controlled trials [15].

The present study was conducted to compare efficacy and safety of EGb 761 to that of the most frequently prescribed antivertigo agent, betahistine, in patients with vertiginous syndromes.

2. Patients and Methods

This randomized, placebo-controlled, double-blind, multi-center clinical trial was conducted by outpatient clinics (mostly associated with departments of neurology) at 10 hospitals in Ukraine in accordance with the Declaration of Helsinki, the Guideline for Good Clinical Practice (GCP) of the International Conference on Harmonization (ICH), and applicable local laws. The protocol was approved by the ethics committee of the Ministry of Healthcare of Ukraine and the local ethics committees of the participating sites; it was registered under number ISRCTN02262139 before enrollment of the patients started. Informed consent was obtained from all patients before any trial-related procedures were undertaken.

2.1. Patient Selection. Patients of either sex, at least 45 years old, were eligible if they were diagnosed with peripheral vertigo not otherwise specified (H81.3) or vertiginous syndrome not otherwise specified (H81.9) as classified by the International Classification of Diseases, 10th edition (ICD-10) [16], had symptoms of vertigo for at least 3 months, scored at least 3 on a one-to-ten numeric analogue scale (NAS) at screening, and had sufficient Russian or Ukrainian language skills to respond to interview questions and complete questionnaires. A negative pregnancy test and adequate contraception were required from female patients. Patients with specific vertiginous syndromes (e.g., Ménière's disease, Lermoyez syndrome, and benign paroxysmal positional vertigo), vertigo due to specified somatic diseases (except cerebrovascular disease), severe other disorders, contraindications to one of the drugs under study, need for drugs that might interfere with the efficacy assessments, or gastrointestinal disorders with uncertain absorption of the active agents were excluded from the study.

2.2. Randomization and Treatment. Randomization stratified by centers was carried out by the sponsor's biometrics department using a validated computer program that matched treatments to drug numbers in a 1:1 ratio. Blinding was achieved by a double-dummy technique: that is, all patients received the same number of film-coated tablets (EGb 761 or placebo) and capsules (betahistine or placebo) in a way that each patient received only one active drug. Drug and placebo tablets and drug and placebo capsules, respectively, were indistinguishable in appearance and taste; all packages and labels were identical except for the drug numbers. Each patient was handed the drug package with the lowest drug number still available at the recruiting site. This procedure guaranteed blinding of patients, investigators, and site staff, concealment of allocation, and balance of treatment group sizes.

The treatment period was 12 weeks, during which patients took either 240 mg per day (120 mg b.i.d.) Ginkgo biloba extract EGb 761 or 32 mg per day (16 mg b.i.d.) betahistine dihydrochloride. EGb 761 is a dry extract from Ginkgo biloba leaves (35–67 : 1), extraction solvent: acetone 60% (w/w) (manufacturer: Dr. Willmar Schwabe GmbH & Co. KG, Karlsruhe, Germany; EGb 761 is a trade mark of Dr. Willmar Schwabe GmbH & Co. KG). The extract is adjusted to 22.0–27.0% ginkgo flavonoids calculated as ginkgo flavone glycosides and 5.0–7.0% terpene lactones consisting of 2.8–3.4% ginkgolides A, B, and C and 2.6–3.2% bilobalide and contains less than 5 ppm ginkgolic acids. The doses of both drugs were chosen in accordance with available evidence of efficacy derived from systematic reviews [7, 8, 15].

2.3. Visits and Assessments. To verify the diagnosis for inclusion and the criteria for eligibility, the medical history was recorded and a general physical examination, laboratory tests, and a clinical neurootological examination, including the Romberg test, the Unterberger stepping test, and an evaluation of spontaneous nystagmus with the aid of Frenzel glasses were performed. Assessments of efficacy and safety of the drugs were scheduled 4, 8, and 12 weeks after the baseline visit. Efficacy was evaluated using an eleven-point numeric analogue scale (NAS) with 0 indicating the absence of vertigo and 10 representing extremely severe vertigo, the short form of the Vertigo Symptom Scale (VSS-SF) [17], the Sheehan Disability Scale (SDS) [18], and the Clinical Global Impressions (CGI) Scale [19]. The 15-item VSS-SF is a self-rating scale taking into account frequency and severity of vertigo within the last month. It consists of two subscales to assess two dimensions of vertigo: vertigo-balance (VSS-V) and autonomic-anxiety (VSS-A) symptoms. The maximum score of 60 indicates the most severe symptoms. The SDS is a 3-item self-rating inventory originally designed to assess to what extent psychological symptoms disrupt a patient's work, social life, and family life. It has been used successfully in somatic diseases with emotional distress. Higher scores (maximum: 10) indicate more severe impairment. Of the CGI, items 2 (change) and 3 (therapeutic index) were rated by the investigators following interviews with the patients. To monitor the safety of the treatments, vital signs were examined at all visits and physical examination, 12-lead ECG, and laboratory tests were performed at the screening and final visits. All adverse events experienced by patients during the treatment period and a subsequent two-day washout period were recorded and assessed for seriousness, severity, and causality.

2.4. Statistical Analyses. For each of the efficacy variables, the EGb 761 group was compared to the betahistine group with methods of descriptive data analysis. Standard summary statistics (arithmetic mean and standard deviation) were calculated for all quantitative variables. Categorical values are presented in frequency tables including absolute and relative frequencies. Descriptive *P* values were calculated using Wilcoxon tests and Fisher's exact tests for quantitative and categorical parameters, respectively. Efficacy analyses were based on the full analysis data set including all patients who received randomized study treatment at least once and having at least one measurement of any efficacy parameter during the randomized treatment period. Additionally prespecified subgroups (age, gender, clinical neurootological findings, and severity of symptoms) were analyzed. Safety variables were evaluated for the safety population which included all patients randomized to study treatment and who took study medication at least once. Adverse events were summarized by means of appropriate frequency tables based on coded items and taking into account severity and relationship to study drug. Overall incidence rates were compared between treatment groups. Due to the exploratory nature of the study, no formal sample size calculation was performed. The sample size of $2 \times 80 = 160$ patients was considered to be large enough to allow for a valid comparison of the EGb 761 and the betahistine group with respect to efficacy and safety.

3. Results and Discussion

Of 169 patients screened, 160 were eligible, received treatment as randomly allocated, and were included in the full analysis set (EGb 761, 80 patients; betahistine, 80 patients). Three patients in the EGb 761 group (unexpected improvement/remission, 1 patient; violation of inclusion/exclusion criteria, 2 patients) and two patients in the betahistine group (withdrawal of informed consent without giving the reason) terminated the study prematurely. Patient disposition and analysis sets are depicted in Figure 1. Demographic data, rating scale scores, and clinical neurootological findings at enrollment are presented in Table 1. There were no conspicuous differences between the treatment groups when treatment was started.

3.1. Efficacy. Patient-rated overall severity of vertigo (NAS) as well as symptoms of vertigo (VSS-SF) and disability due to vertigo (SDS) improved markedly in both treatment groups (Table 2, Figure 2). Similarly, clinician-rated global impression of change and neurootological findings indicated considerable improvements under both EGb 761 and betahistine treatments (Table 2, Figures 2, 3, 4, and 5). There were no significant differences between the two treatment groups with respect to treatment-related changes. The size of treatment effects did not vary with age, gender, clinical neurootological findings, or severity of symptoms.

3.2. Safety. During the treatment period and a subsequent two-day washout period, 27 adverse events (AEs) were reported for 19 patients in the EGb 761 group and 39 AEs were

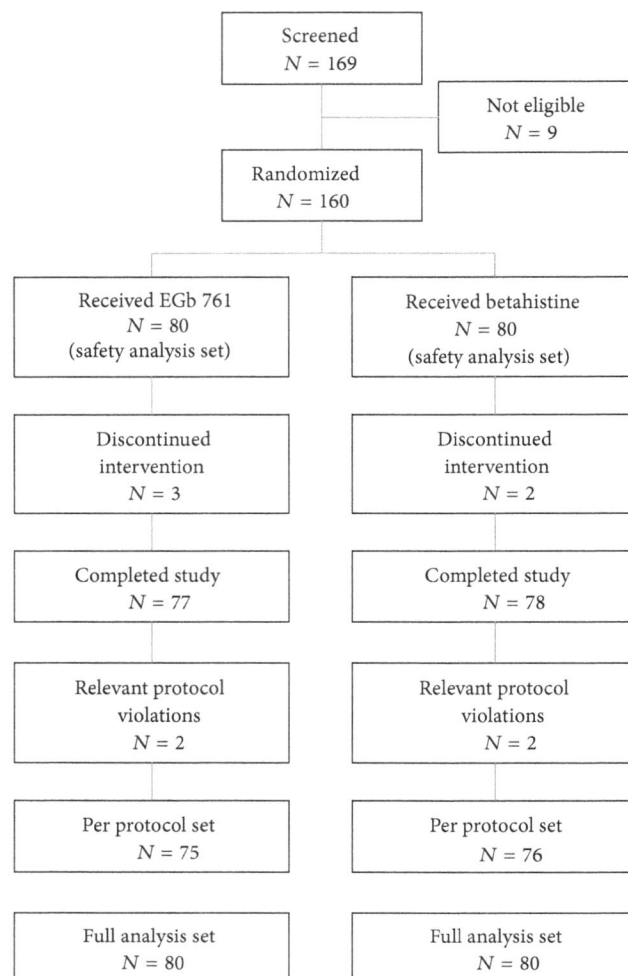

FIGURE 1: Patient disposition and analysis sets.

documented for 31 patients receiving betahistine. Blinded review could not rule out a causal relationship with the study medication for 6 AEs in 5 patients taking EGb 761 and for 18 AEs in 16 patients of the betahistine group. There was one serious AE in the betahistine group (spondylolisthesis) for which a causal relationship could be excluded. The most frequently observed types of AEs are listed in Table 3.

3.3. Discussion. In this randomized, double-blind, multicenter clinical trial, we found *Ginkgo biloba* extract EGb 761 and betahistine to be equally effective in the treatment of vertigo. We enrolled patients with unspecified vertigo, because, on one hand, specific vertiginous syndromes (e.g., Ménière's disease and benign paroxysmal positional vertigo) require specific treatments, and, on the other hand, both drugs are widely prescribed for vertigo not defined as part of a specific syndrome. In fact, betahistine is by far the most frequently prescribed drug for vertigo worldwide [6]. The results complement the findings from placebo-controlled trials of EGb 761 that demonstrated its clinical efficacy in vestibular and nonvestibular vertigo [15].

TABLE 1: Demographic data, rating scale scores, and clinical neurootological findings at enrollment; means ± standard deviations or numbers/percentages; P values (Wilcoxon test and Fisher's exact test*).

	EGb 761	Betahistine	P value
Gender			
Male	25/31%	22/27%	0.603*
Female	55/69%	58/73%	
Age [years]	57.5 ± 9.2	57.9 ± 8.4	0.561
Body mass index [kg/m^2]	27.0 ± 4.2	28.3 ± 4.2	0.082
Duration of symptoms [months]	25.1 ± 37.3	22.5 ± 31.2	0.633
NAS	5.4 ± 1.4	5.2 ± 1.2	0.644
VSS-SF total score	24.2 ± 8.9	22.6 ± 8.5	0.239
VSS-V subscore	10.6 ± 5.5	9.9 ± 5.4	0.433
VSS-A subscore	13.5 ± 5.6	12.6 ± 4.9	0.447
SDS total score	15.2 ± 5.4	14.2 ± 5.4	0.263
Spontaneous nystagmus	42/52.5%	44/55%	0.874
Romberg test			
No swaying	2/2.5%	5/6.3%	
Slight swaying	66/82.5%	68/85.0%	0.447
Swaying/foot movement	11/13.8%	6/7.5%	
Tendency to fall	1/1.3%	1/1.3%	
Unterberger's stepping test			
Rotation <30°	45/56.3%	46/57.5%	
Rotation 30°–60°	32/40.0%	32/40.0%	1.000
Rotation >60°	3/3.8%	2/2.5%	

TABLE 2: Changes during the 12-week treatment period; means ± standard deviations; P values (Wilcoxon test).

	EGb 761	Betahistine	P value
NAS	−3.5 ± 1.8	−3.3 ± 1.7	0.704
VSS-SF total score	−14.7 ± 7.8	−13.4 ± 8.5	0.319
VSS-V subscore	−7.6 ± 5.0	−7.0 ± 5.2	0.432
VSS-A subscore	−7.1 ± 4.1	−6.4 ± 4.6	0.446
SDS total score	−9.4 ± 5.7	−8.3 ± 5.7	0.260
CGI change score	1.9 ± 0.9	2.1 ± 0.9	0.237

More than 70% of the patients were rated "much improved" or "very much improved" by their physicians after the 12-week treatment period. Interestingly, the patients' ratings of overall improvement (NAS) closely match the degree of change assessed by the comprehensive symptom scale (VSS-SF), with about 60% improvement over the initial scores. The patients' subjective ratings and the physicians' global impressions of change were strongly supported by the objective findings from clinical neurootological examinations: swaying in the Romberg test and rotation in Unterberger's stepping test were decreased considerably and spontaneous nystagmus was no longer found in half of the patients who had nystagmus before treatment. Constraints in daily life due to vertigo, which were rated as moderate at enrollment, were reduced and perceived as not more than mild after treatment.

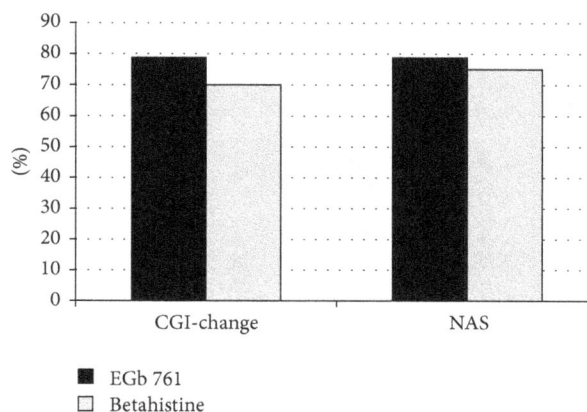

FIGURE 2: Response rates, defined as clinician's global impression (CGI) rated "much improved" or "very much improved" or patient's rating of NAS improvement at least 50%.

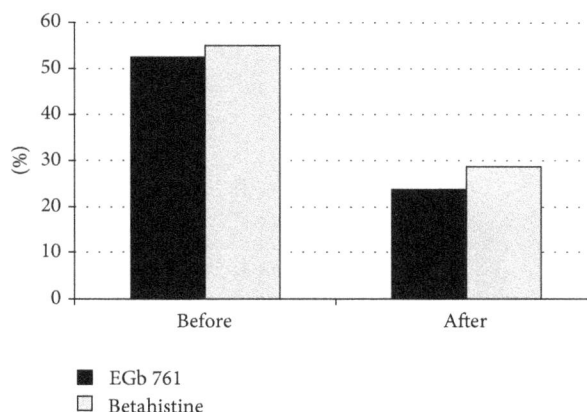

FIGURE 3: Proportion of patients with nystagmus before and after treatment.

With a sample size of 80 patients per treatment arm the study did not have statistical power to prove equivalence of the two treatments. The findings should therefore be interpreted as descriptive. Another limitation of our study is the lack of a placebo group as "negative" control. Taking into account that both treatments are evidence-based [7, 15] and high rates of marked spontaneous improvements are not very likely after an average duration of symptoms of approximately 2 years, there is reason to assume that the observed effects are mostly treatment-related and not mere placebo effects. There are numerically (not statistically significantly) more pronounced improvements in all outcome measures in the patients treated with EGb 761 compared to those receiving betahistine. As the likelihood of observing a difference between two treatment groups going in the same direction in 7 outcome measures just by chance when there is no real difference is less than 0.05, this could point to a slight superiority of EGb 761. However, subtle differences between the treatment groups in prognostic variables not documented at baseline and not completely balanced by randomization

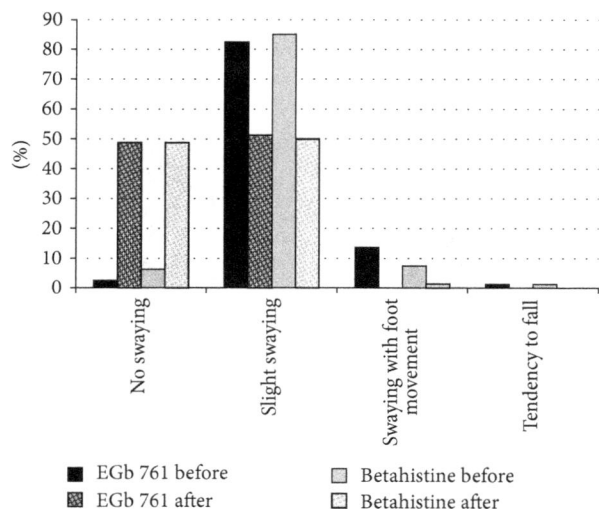

FIGURE 4: Proportion of patients with different grades of swaying in the Romberg test before and after treatment.

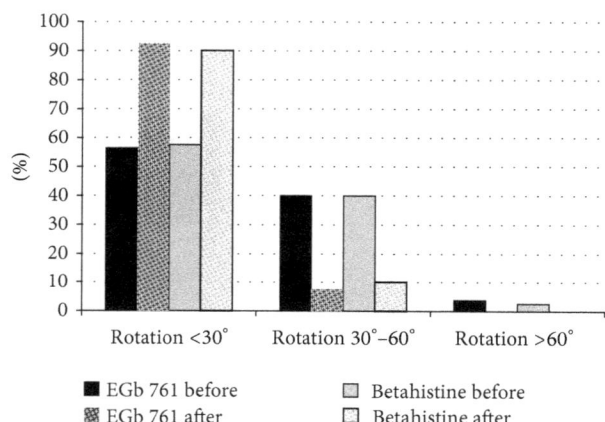

FIGURE 5: Proportion of patients with different grades of rotation in Unterberger's stepping test before and after treatment.

TABLE 3: The most frequently observed AEs in both treatment groups (at least three events in one treatment group).

System organ class—type of AE	EGb 761 (n)	Betahistine (n)
Gastrointestinal disorders:		
Dyspepsia and abdominal discomfort/pain	2	5
Nausea and vomiting	3	1
Diarrhea, frequent bowel movements infections, and infestations	1	3
Respiratory tract infections and nervous system disorders	5	9
Headache	3	5

[21]. We therefore believe that we used an appropriate dose for the symptomatic treatment of vertiginous syndromes.

In the light of recent research, one mechanism likely to be involved in the antivertiginous action of EGb 761 deserves attention. Vertigo and the sensation of dizziness may result from labyrinth dysfunction or disconnection or impaired processing of information within the central nervous networks (vestibular, ocular, oculomotor, cortical, and cerebellar) involved in equilibrium and posture control [22]. Aging-associated loss of cortical neurons and integrity of fiber tracts as well as a slowing of information processing [23] may contribute to or enhance such dysfunction. Impaired intrinsic and synaptic mechanisms of neuronal plasticity [22, 24] are likely to prevent full compensation of disturbances in the vestibular system and to play a role in long-lasting vertiginous syndromes. EGb 761 has been shown to enhance neuronal plasticity by stimulating neurogenesis, neurite outgrowth, synaptogenesis, and synaptic function [25]. Of note, Lacour and colleagues [26] observed an accelerated recovery of synaptic density in the medial vestibular nuclei of EGb 761-treated cats after unilateral vestibular neurectomy.

Regarding safety and tolerability, EGb 761 seems to have some advantage over betahistine. No patients withdrew from treatment due to adverse events, but the total number of adverse events as well as the number of patients who experienced an adverse event was lower in the EGb 761 group than in the betahistine group.

4. Conclusion

This study provides evidence that *Ginkgo biloba* extract EGb 761 is at least as effective as the world's most frequently prescribed antivertiginous agent, betahistine, in the treatment of unspecified vertiginous syndromes.

Disclosure

The clinical trial was sponsored by Dr. Willmar Schwabe GmbH & Co. KG, Karlsruhe, Germany. Larysa Sokolova and Tamara Mishchenko received investigator fees from the sponsor; Robert Hoerr is an employee of the sponsor receiving a fixed salary.

cannot be excluded, so this finding should be interpreted with caution.

The dosage of betahistine warrants some consideration, since, based on an open-label study, the use of higher daily doses has been suggested recently for the prevention of attacks of Ménière's disease [20]. This may be reasonable; a clear distinction must be made, however, between the prevention of attacks and the symptomatic treatment of existing vertigo. Systematic reviews found daily doses of 32 mg to 36 mg most effective in the symptomatic treatment of vertigo [7, 8]. While a review of trials in various vertiginous syndromes found similar effect sizes for 32 mg and 36 mg [7], the Cochrane review of betahistine in Ménière's disease found the strongest effects in high-quality placebo-controlled trials at 32 mg but no difference from placebo for 72 mg per day [8]. Similarly, another meta-analysis published recently found no advantage of 48 mg over 32 mg per day in parallel-group trials

Conflict of Interests

The authors declare that there is no conflict of interests regarding the publication of this paper.

References

[1] H. K. Neuhauser, A. Radtke, M. von Brevern, F. Lezius, M. Feldmann, and T. Lempert, "Burden of dizziness and vertigo in the community," *Archives of Internal Medicine*, vol. 168, no. 19, pp. 2118–2124, 2008.

[2] D. E. Newman-Toker, Y. Hsieh, C. A. Camargo Jr., A. J. Pelletier, G. T. Butchy, and J. A. Edlow, "Spectrum of dizziness visits to US emergency departments: Cross-sectional analysis from a nationally representative sample," *Mayo Clinic Proceedings*, vol. 83, no. 7, pp. 765–775, 2008.

[3] M. Strupp and T. Brandt, "Diagnosis and treatment of vertigo and dizziness," *Deutsches Ärzteblatt International*, vol. 105, no. 10, pp. 173–180, 2008.

[4] K. Hanley, T. O'Dowd, and N. Considine, "A systematic review of vertigo in primary care," *British Journal of General Practice*, vol. 51, no. 469, pp. 666–671, 2001.

[5] S. Okroglic, C. N. Widmann, H. Urbach, P. Scheltens, and M. T. Heneka, "Clinical symptoms and risk factors in cerebral microangiopathy patients," *PLoS ONE*, vol. 8, no. 2, Article ID e53455, 2013.

[6] S. Agus, H. Benecke, C. Thum, and M. Strupp, "Clinical and demographic features of vertigo: findings from the REVERT registry," *Frontiers in Neurology*, vol. 4, article 48, 2013.

[7] C. Della Pepa, G. Guidetti, and M. Eandi, "Betahistine in the treatment of vertiginous syndromes: a meta-analysis," *Acta Otorhinolaryngologica Italica*, vol. 26, no. 4, pp. 208–215, 2006.

[8] A. L. James and M. J. Burton, "Betahistine for Ménière's disease or syndrome," *Cochrane Database of Systematic Reviews*, no. 1, Article ID CD001873, 2001.

[9] W. D. Heiss and K. Zeiler, "Medikamentöse Beeinflussung der Hirndurchblutung [The influence on drugs on cerebral blood flow]," *Pharmakotherapie*, vol. 1, no. 3, pp. 137–144, 1978.

[10] B. Maass, J. Silberzahn, and R. Simon, "Zur Wirkung von Ginkgo-biloba—Extrakt (Tebonin) auf die Wasserstoff-Auswaschvorgänge an der Cochleabasis unter hypotensiver Ischämie," *Extracta Otorhinolaryngologica*, vol. 9, no. 5, pp. 169–172, 1987.

[11] S. Huang, C. Jeng, S. Kao, J. J. Yu, and D. Liu, "Improved haemorrheological properties by Ginkgo biloba extract (Egb 761) in type 2 diabetes mellitus complicated with retinopathy," *Deutsches Ärzteblatt International*, vol. 23, no. 4, pp. 615–621, 2004.

[12] F. Tchantchou, Y. Xu, Y. Wu, Y. Christen, and Y. Luo, "EGb 761 enhances adult hippocampal neurogenesis and phosphorylation of CREB in transgenic mouse model of Alzheimer's disease," *The FASEB Journal*, vol. 21, no. 10, pp. 2400–2408, 2007.

[13] R. Abdel-Kader, S. Hauptmann, U. Keil et al., "Stabilization of mitochondrial function by Ginkgo biloba extract (EGb 761)," *Pharmacological Research*, vol. 56, no. 6, pp. 493–502, 2007.

[14] B. A. Abdel-Wahab and S. M. Abd El-Aziz, "Ginkgo biloba protects against intermittent hypoxia-induced memory deficits and hippocampal DNA damage in rats," *Phytomedicine*, vol. 19, no. 5, pp. 444–450, 2012.

[15] K. F. Hamann, "Ginkgo special extract EGb 761 in vertigo: a systematic review of randomised , double-blind, placebo-controlled clinical trials," *The Internet Journal of Otorhinolaryngology*, vol. 6, no. 2, pp. 258–263, 2007.

[16] World Health Organization, *International Statistical Classification of Diseases and Related Health Problems*, World Health Organization, Geneva, Switzerland, 1992.

[17] L. Yardley, E. Masson, C. Verschuur, N. Haacke, and L. Luxon, "Symptoms, anxiety and handicap in dizzy patients: development of the Vertigo symptom scale," *Journal of Psychosomatic Research*, vol. 36, no. 8, pp. 731–741, 1992.

[18] D. V. Sheehan, *The Anxiety Disease*, Charles Scribner's Sons, New York, NY, USA, 1983.

[19] NIMH National Institute of Mental Health., "028 CGI. Clinical global impressions," in *ECDEU Assessment Manual for Psychopharmacology*, W. Guy, Ed., pp. 218–222, NIMH, Rockville, Md, USA, 1976.

[20] M. Strupp, D. Hupert, C. Frenzel et al., "Long-term prophylactic treatment of attacks of vertigo in Meniére's disease—comparison of a high with a low dosage of betahistine in an open trial," *Acta Oto-Laryngologica*, vol. 128, no. 5, pp. 520–524, 2008.

[21] J. J. P. Nauta, "Meta-analysis of clinical studies with betahistine in Ménière's disease and vestibular vertigo," *European Archives of Otorhinolaryngology*, vol. 271, no. 5, pp. 887–897, 2014.

[22] M. Beraneck and E. Idoux, "Reconsidering the role of neuronal intrinsic properties and neuromodulation in vestibular homeostasis," *Frontiers in Neurology*, vol. 3, article 25, 13 pages, 2012.

[23] S. Papegaaij, W. Taube, S. Baudry, E. Otten, and T. Hortobágyi, "Aging cuases a reorganization of cortical and spinal control of posture," *Frontiers in Aging Neuroscience*, vol. 6, article 28, 2014.

[24] M. Shao, J. C. Hirsch, and K. D. Peusner, "Plasticity of spontaneous excitatory and inhibitory synaptic activity in morphologically defined vestibular nuclei neurons during early vestibular compensation," *Journal of Neurophysiology*, vol. 107, no. 1, pp. 29–41, 2012.

[25] W. E. Müller, J. Heiser, and K. Leuner, "Effects of the standardized Ginkgo biloba extract EGb 761 on neuroplasticity," *International Psychogeriatrics*, vol. 24, supplement 1, pp. S21–S24, 2012.

[26] M. Lacour, L. Ez-Zaher, and J. Raymond, "Plasticity mechanisms in vestibular compensation in the cat are improved by an extract of Ginkgo biloba (EGb 761)," *Pharmacology Biochemistry and Behavior*, vol. 40, no. 2, pp. 367–379, 1991.

30

Sinonasal Cancer and Occupational Exposure in a Population-Based Registry

Carolina Mensi,[1] Dario Consonni,[1] Claudia Sieno,[1] Sara De Matteis,[2,3] Luciano Riboldi,[1] and Pier Alberto Bertazzi[1,3]

[1] *Department of Preventive Medicine, Fondazione IRCCS Ca' Granda—Ospedale Maggiore Policlinico, Via San Barnaba 8, 20122 Milan, Italy*
[2] *National Heart & Lung Institute, Department of Occupational & Environmental Medicine, Imperial College London, London SW3 6LR, UK*
[3] *Department of Clinical Science and Community Health, Università Degli Studi di Milano, Via San Barnaba 8, 20122 Milan, Italy*

Correspondence should be addressed to Carolina Mensi; carolina.mensi@unimi.it

Academic Editor: Peter S. Roland

We examined occupational exposures among subjects with sinonasal cancer (SNC) recorded in a population-based registry in the Lombardy Region, the most populated and industrialized Italian region. The registry collects complete clinical information and exposure to carcinogens regarding all SNC cases occurring in the population of the region. In the period 2008–2011, we recorded 210 SNC cases (137 men, 73 women). The most frequent occupational exposures were to wood (44 cases, 21.0%) and leather dust (29 cases, 13.8%), especially among men: 39 cases (28.5%) to wood and 23 cases (16.8%) to leather dust. Exposure to other agents was infrequent (<2%). Among 62 subjects with adenocarcinoma, 50% had been exposed to wood dust and 30.7% to leather dust. The proportions were around 10% in subjects with squamous cell carcinoma and about 20% for tumors with another histology. The age-standardized rates (×100,000 person-years) were 0.7 in men and 0.3 in women. Complete collection of cases and their occupational history through a specialized cancer registry is fundamental to accurately monitor SNC occurrence in a population and to uncover exposure to carcinogens in different industrial sectors, even those not considered as posing a high risk of SNC, and also in extraoccupational settings.

1. Introduction

Cancer of the nasal cavity and the paranasal sinuses, referred to as "sinonasal cancer" (SNC), is relatively uncommon in the general population, accounting for less than 1% of all neoplasms and less than 4% of those arising in the head and neck region [1–3]. SNC incidence is around $1 \times 100,000$ person-years in most developed countries [4]. In the period 1998–2002, the annual incidence rates in the United States were 0.8 and $0.6 \times 100,000$ in males and females, respectively [5]. In the same period, the RARECARE project, based on about 2200 cases of epithelial tumors of nasal cavities in Europe, showed an age-standardized rate of $0.36 \times 100,000$ [6]. The incidence rates in 1998–2002 estimated by the Italian network of cancer registries (Associazione Italiana

Registri Tumori, AIRTUM, http://www.registri-tumori.it/), which covers 40% of the whole population, were between 0.4 and 2.0 in males and 0.1 and $0.5 \times 100,000$ in females, with about 300 cases expected per year in the whole country; a high variability across Italian regions was reported.

Frequency, anatomical site, and histological type of SNCs vary across geographical areas due to several factors [3]. A history of chronic sinusitis, nasal polyps [7], use of nasal drug preparations, and smoking and occupational history of wood and leather working and nickel refining are reported as risk factors for the development of these tumors. A strong relationship between SNC and exposure to wood, leather dust, and nickel compounds has been established long time ago [8–11] and recently confirmed [12]. Other confirmed or suspected causative factors include hexavalent chromium compounds, welding fumes, arsenic, mineral oils, organic solvents, and textile dust [11, 13–16].

SNCs, particularly adenocarcinomas, are characterized by a high occupational etiologic fraction [17]. For this reason, in Italy, since 2008, their incidence and etiology are compulsorily surveyed in the whole Italian population (about 60 million people) through a nationwide cancer registry (ReNaTuNS), coordinated by the Italian Workers' Compensation Authority (Istituto Nazionale per l'Assicurazione contro gli Infortuni sul Lavoro, INAIL). ReNaTuNS collects information from a network of regional registries to monitor SNC incidence and to establish sources of occupational exposure (http://www.inail.it/). In the Lombardy region, northwest Italy, the most populated (almost 10 million residents at the 2011 census) and industrialized Italian region, the registry was established at the end of 2007. In this paper we present clinical characteristics and sources of occupational exposure for SNC cases recorded in the period 2008–2011. We also calculated Lombardy incidence rates of SNC for the period 2008-2009, in which registration of clinical and exposure information was complete.

2. Materials and Methods

2.1. Identification and Definition of SNC Cases. The Lombardy registry of sinonasal cancers (LRSNC) collects all SNC cases occurring among subjects with residence in the region (from about 9.6 million people in 2008 to about 9.9 million in 2011) at the time of first diagnosis.

The primary sources of information on SNC cases are the departments of diagnosis and treatment of SNC in regional hospitals (more than 100), particularly pathology, otolaryngology, maxillofacial surgery, and radiotherapy. Completeness of reporting is checked by periodic linkage made at LRSNC with databases of pathology departments (six-monthly), hospital discharge records (annual), mortality registries (annual), and occupational disease compensation records from INAIL (annual). This complex system virtually ensures complete ascertainment of SNC cases occurring in Lombardy residents and also allows the identification of the few patients admitted in hospitals outside the Lombardy region.

Diagnosis of SNC is established by a panel of experts at LRSNC based on complete clinical information (copy of clinical records, computed tomography and/or magnetic resonance imaging scans, pathology reports) according to the ReNaTuNS guidelines [18]. SNC cases include all newly diagnosed primary malignant epithelial cancers of the nasal cavity, code C30.0 of the International Classification of Diseases, Tenth Revision (ICD-10) and paranasal sinus, ICD-10 codes from C31.0 to C31.9. Histological types are defined according to the World Health Organization (WHO) classification [1].

2.2. Exposure Assessment. A standardized questionnaire is administered to patients or their next of kin by trained interviewers within the hospital in which diagnosis was made or at the occupational health services of the local health

units in Lombardy region. The questionnaire is designed to obtain a lifetime occupational history, including industrial sectors, plants, jobs, and specific task performed. Coding of the occupational history is performed according to the Italian Classification of Economic Activities. The questionnaire is then reviewed by occupational physicians and industrial hygienists who assess occupational exposure to agents with an established or suspected association with SNC: wood and leather dust, nickel and chromium compounds, polycyclic aromatic hydrocarbons (PAH), and cork dust. Also exposure to these agents in domestic setting or during hobby activities is evaluated. In case of exposure either in occupational or in other settings, the subjects is classified as occupationally exposed.

2.3. Statistical Analysis. For the period 2008–2011, to compare the distribution of demographics, clinical characteristics, and occupational exposures among SNC cases across gender and tumor morphology, we used the chi-square test. Age distribution across gender was evaluated using Mann-Whitney U test.

For the period 2008-2009, in which case registration was complete, we calculated age-standardized rates of SNC ($\times100,000$ person-years) separately for men and women using as standards either the Italian population in the year 2001 or the European population. Confidence intervals (CI) of standardized rates were calculated according to the formula proposed by Tiwari et al. [19, 20]. Analyses were performed with Stata 12 [21].

3. Results

In the period 2008–2011, we recorded 210 SNC cases, 137 (65.2%) among males and 73 (34.8%) among females (Table 1). Median age was around 68 years in either gender. About one-third of the tumors originated from the nasal cavity, one-fourth from the maxillary sinus, and one-fifth from multiple sites. The ethmoid sinus was affected in almost 25% of men and only about 7% of women. More than 40% of tumors were squamous cell carcinomas. Intestinal-type adenocarcinomas were especially frequent in men (26.3%). An interview was obtained for 200 cases (95.2%). The questionnaire was administered directly to the patient in 146 cases (69.5%) and to his/her relatives in 56 (26.6%). Ever smokers were almost 70% among males and about 40% among women. Smokers were more frequent in subjects with squamous cell carcinoma (63.9%) or adenocarcinoma (68.3%) than in subjects with other morphologies (56.1%). Current smokers were more frequent among subjects with squamous cell carcinomas (34.9%) than in subjects with adenocarcinoma (16.7%) or with other morphologies (15.8%). A history of nasal polyps was reported by 18 subjects (8.6%), 15 men and 3 women.

In the years 2008-2009, we recorded 82 SNC cases among men and 45 among women. In these years, registration was completed, while for the following two years (55 cases in men and 28 in women), completeness checks are still in progress. Using the Italian 2001 population as standard, in

TABLE 1: Characteristics of subjects with sinonasal cancer by gender; Lombardy region sinonasal cancer registry, 2008–2011.

	Men		Women		P value[a]
	No.	%	No.	%	
No. of subjects	137	100	73	100	
Age (median, min–max)	67.7	31.7–88.5	68.4	21.1–94.9	0.70
Cancer site of origin (ICD-10 code)					
Nasal cavity (C30.0)	44	32.1	27	37.0	0.01
Maxillary sinus (C31.0)	28	20.4	20	27.4	
Ethmoid sinus (C31.1)	32	23.4	5	6.8	
Frontal sinus (C31.2)	0	0.0	1	1.4	
Sphenoid sinus (C31.3)	3	2.2	6	8.2	
Multiple sites	30	21.9	14	19.2	
Cancer morphology					
Squamous cell carcinoma	54	39.4	34	46.6	0.002
Adenocarcinoma, unspecified	7	5.1	3	4.1	
Adenocarcinoma, intestinal type	36	26.3	8	11.0	
Adenocarcinoma, nonintestinal type	6	4.4	2	2.7	
Adenoid cystic carcinoma	8	5.8	12	16.4	
Neuroendocrine carcinoma	10	7.3	0	0.0	
Undifferentiated carcinoma	11	8.0	7	9.6	
Other	5	3.7	3	4.1	
Unknown	0	0.0	4	5.5	
Interview					
Patient	97	70.8	47	64.4	0.06
Relative	37	27.0	19	26.0	
Not performed	3	2.2	7	9.6	
Cigarette smoking					
Never	40	29.2	34	46.6	0.002
Former (>6 mo. before symptoms)	58	42.3	20	27.4	
Current	36	26.3	12	16.4	
Unknown	3	2.2	7	9.6	
Year of diagnosis					
2008 (complete)	32	23.4	23	31.5	0.10
2009 (complete)	50	36.5	22	30.1	
2010 (in progress)	37	27.0	12	16.4	
2011 (in progress)	18	13.1	16	21.9	

ICD-10: International Classification of Diseases, Tenth Edition
[a]From chi-square test, except for age (Mann-Whitney U test).

the years 2008-2009, the age-standardized rates ($\times$100,000 person-years) of SNC were 0.9 (95% CI: 0.7–1.1) in men and 0.4 (95% CI: 0.3–0.5) in women. Using the European population as standard, the SNC incidence rates were 0.7 (95% CI: 0.5–0.8) in men and 0.3 (95% CI: 0.2–0.4) in women. Age-specific rates had a peak over 60 years of age in both genders; however, rates began to increase at lower ages, especially in men (Figure 1).

Among men, occupational exposure to any of the six carcinogenic agents mentioned above was identified in 66 subjects (48.2%), while among women, the proportion was 15.1% (Table 2). Wood and leather dust particles were the most prevalent exposures, especially among males (28.5% and 16.8% of subjects, resp.). In women, the corresponding proportions were 6.9% and 8.2%. Exposure to other agents

was infrequent (<2%). Seven subjects (six men) had been ever exposed to wood dust and another agent: leather dust (four), nickel compounds (two), and chromium compounds (one subject). We also recorded extraoccupational exposure to a carcinogen for 8 subjects. In the first case, the subject had been exposed to leather dust in the domestic setting, where the mother produced leather buttons. The other seven cases had been exposed to wood dust during hobby activities (construction of furniture and wooden objects or hobby modeling), without using personal protective equipment.

Among subjects with adenocarcinoma, occupational exposure was recorded for the majority (77.4%) of subjects (Table 3). Half had been ever exposed to wood dust and almost one-third to leather dust. One case was exposed to cork dust. Among subjects with squamous cell carcinoma

TABLE 2: Occupational exposure to carcinogenic agents among subjects with sinonasal cancer, by gender; Lombardy region sinonasal cancer registry, 2008–2011 ($N = 200$ with interview).

Occupational exposure	Men		Women		P value[a]
	No.	%	No.	%	
Never exposed	68	50.7	55	83.3	Reference
Ever exposed (any agent)	66	49.3	11	16.7	<0.001
Wood dust	39	29.1	5	7.6	<0.001
Leather dust	23	17.2	6	9.1	0.02
Nickel compounds	4	3.0	0	0.0	0.08
Chromium compounds	4	3.0	0	0.0	0.08
PAH	2	1.5	0	0.0	0.21
Cork dust	0	0.0	1	1.5	0.27

PAH: polycyclic aromatic hydrocarbons.
[a]From chi-square test (reference: never exposed).
Note: a subject may have been exposed to more than one agent in his/her occupational history.

TABLE 3: Occupational exposure to carcinogenic agents among subjects with sinonasal cancer, by tumor morphology; Lombardy region sinonasal cancer registry, 2008–2011 ($N = 200$ with interview).

Occupational exposure	SCC		Adenocarcinoma		Other		P value[a]
	No.	%	No.	%	No.	%	
Never exposed	69	82.1	13	21.3	41	74.5	Reference
Ever exposed (any agent)	15	17.9	48	78.7	14	25.5	<0.001
Wood dust	6	7.1	31	50.8	7	12.7	<0.001
Leather dust	4	4.8	19	31.1	6	10.9	<0.001
Nickel compounds	1	1.2	1	1.6	1	1.8	0.44
Chromium compounds	2	2.4	1	1.6	1	1.8	0.65
PAH	2	2.4	0	0.0	0	0.0	0.46
Cork dust	0	0.0	1	1.6	0	0.0	0.02

PAH: polycyclic aromatic hydrocarbons, SCC: squamous cell carcinoma.
[a]From chi-square test (reference: never exposed).
Note: a subject may have been exposed to more than one agent in his/her occupational history.

and with tumors of other morphologies, the proportions of subjects ever exposed to any of the six carcinogens were 17.0% and 23.3%, respectively. Exposure to wood or leather dust was about 10% in the case of squamous cell carcinoma and about 20% for other morphologies.

Wood dust exposure occurred mainly (about 80%) in the wood and furniture industry, followed by building construction sectors (8%). The rest of the subjects were exposed in the metal-mechanic sector (construction of wood patterns, use of sawdust in metal polishing) or in a turkey farm (use of sawdust as bedding). Leather dust exposure occurred mainly in boot and shoe manufacture and repair (90%). A few workers were exposed in leather suit or sofa production. Subjects that worked in sofa production were also exposed to wood. Exposure to nickel compounds was recorded in the electroplating industry and in the paint manufacture. Exposure to hexavalent chromium was found for car painters using chromium paints and in the printing industry (use of chromic acid).

The mean length of occupational exposure was 26.6 years (range: 1 to 63) in the 66 men and 15.3 (1 to 38) in the 11 women. The mean latency was 53.3 years (min 18.2, max 74.4) in men and 42.1 years (min 13.6, max 74.6) in women.

Occupational exposure to any of the six carcinogens was relatively more frequent (51.3%) among former smokers (Table 4). Similar patterns were observed for each single agent. Occupational exposure was similarly distributed among the 18 subjects with a history of nasal polyps (8 cases, 44.4%) and among the 192 without (69 cases, 36.9%) (P value = 0.47).

4. Discussion

This study describes the findings of LRSNC, a dedicated SNC regional registry. For the first time, incidence of SNCs and the role of exposure to recognized carcinogens were examined in an Italian large population (nearly 10 million people), in a region where shoe/boot factories and repair shops, furniture production, and smelting and metal-mechanic industries are still widely present.

Incidence rates in men were more than twice as high as in women, probably reflecting differences in previous exposure to carcinogens. In this population-wide case series, we found that tumors originate more often (one-third) in the nasal cavities, while localization in maxillary (one-fourth) and

TABLE 4: Occupational exposure to carcinogenic agents among subjects with sinonasal cancer, by smoking status[a]; Lombardy region sinonasal cancer registry, 2008–2011 ($N = 200$ with interview).

Occupational exposure	Never smokers		Former smokers		Current smokers		P value[b]
	No.	%	No.	%	No.	%	
Never exposed	52	70.3	38	48.7	32	69.6	Reference
Ever exposed (any agent)	22	29.7	40	51.3	14	30.4	0.01
Wood dust	12	16.2	21	26.9	10	21.7	0.10
Leather dust	10	13.5	17	21.8	2	4.3	0.01
Nickel compounds	0	0.0	2	2.6	2	4.3	0.23
Chromium compounds	1	1.4	3	3.8	0	0.0	0.16
PAH	0	0.0	1	1.3	1	2.2	0.47
Cork dust	1	1.4	0	0.0	0	0.0	0.51

PAH: polycyclic aromatic hydrocarbons, SCC: squamous cell carcinoma.
[a]10 subjects with missing smoking history were excluded.
[b]From chi-square test (reference: never exposed).
Note: a subject may have been exposed to more than one agent in his/her occupational history.

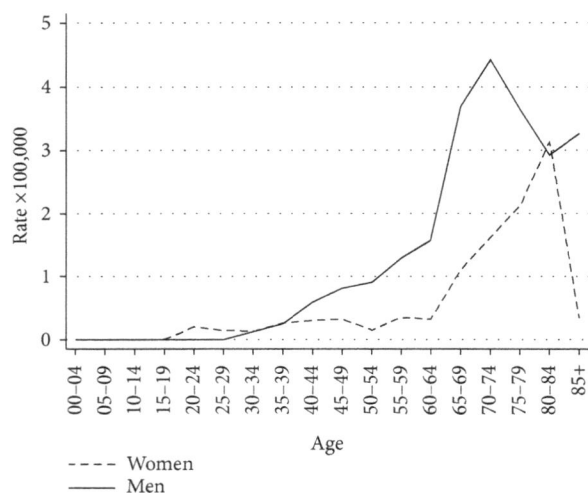

FIGURE 1: Age-specific sinonasal cancer rates (×100,000 person-years) by gender; Lombardy sinonasal cancer registry, 2008-2009.

ethmoid sinuses (almost one-fifth) was less frequent. This is in agreement with a recent review [2] which considered US and Italian cancer registries data (1998–2002), with a report from The Netherlands registry covering the period 1973–2009 [22], and with UK estimates for 2012 [23]. However, in about 20% of cases, we were not able to determine the site of tumor's origin because multiple sites were involved at first diagnosis. The most frequent morphology in our cases was squamous cell carcinoma. Again, this is in agreement with the mentioned US, Italian, Dutch, and British studies [2, 22, 23]. In our study, we found a closer association between smoking and squamous cell carcinomas and male gender. These were expected findings, in agreement with a European pooled study [24].

The literature estimates of the percentage of SNCs attributable to occupational exposures range from 25% to 41% [25]. In our study, the attributable fraction was 38.5%. In men the proportion of subjects ever exposed occupationally was

almost 50%, but also in women it was not negligible (15%). This finding underlines the need to investigate the exposure history, including occupation, of each case of SNC. We found a high frequency of exposure to wood and leather dust, especially among men and among subjects with adenocarcinoma. Although lower, the proportion of subjects with other histology (squamous cell carcinoma or other morphologies) exposed to wood or leather dust was not negligible (about 10–20%). This suggests that not only adenocarcinoma of ethmoid sinus can be induced by wood and leather dust exposure [17, 26].

This study had several merits. First, registration of cases in the LRSNC is quite complete, because the reporting of SNC cases by departments of diagnosis and treatment of SNC is supplemented by an active research which exploits all available information systems (databases of pathology departments, hospital discharge records, mortality registries, and occupational disease compensation records). For this reason, we are confident that the number of cases not identified through these sources is virtually zero. Second, diagnosis of SNC is established by experts based on complete clinical information. Third, diagnostic evaluation is made blind of exposure (the interview is performed after the diagnosis has been verified). Fourth, collection of exposure assessment was successful in 95% of subjects. The major limitation lies in the fact that the years 2010-2011 are still incomplete because some sources of data become available late after case occurrence. Therefore, the exposure profile of the current (in progress) case series might in theory be different from that calculated in the complete case series. However, when we restricted the analysis to the period 2008-2009, the exposure profile was quite similar to that observed in the whole 2008–2011 period (results not shown).

5. Conclusion

In conclusion, our study shows that complete collection of cases through a dedicated cancer registry can provide a clear picture of SNC occurrence in a population and of exposure to several relevant carcinogens, in different industrial sectors, including those not considered as posing a high risk of SNC, and also in extra-occupational settings. This allows the recognition of occupational diseases and ultimately compensation of the affected subjects.

Conflict of Interests

The authors declare that they have no conflict of interests.

Authors' Contribution

Carolina Mensi conceived the study and defined its design, participated in data collection and clinical and exposure evaluation, participated in the statistical analysis, and drafted the paper. Dario Consonni participated in the study design, performed the statistical analysis, and helped to draft the paper. Claudia Sieno participated in data collection and data management. Sara De Matteis performed the statistical analysis and revised the paper. Luciano Riboldi participated in data collection, helped in clinical and exposure evaluation, and revised the paper. Pier Alberto Bertazzi participated in study design and helped to draft the paper.

Acknowledgments

This work was partially funded by Grants from Lombardy Region, Direzione Generale Sanità, Environmental Epidemiology Program, Milan, Italy (14013-1/5/2010 and 8956-7/6/2006), and Ministero della Salute and INAIL, Rome, Italy (PMS/42/06). The authors wish to thank the personnel of the Departments of Pathology, Otorhinolaryngology, and Occupational Health of all the regional hospitals, the Occupational Health Services of the Local Health Units of the Lombardy Region, and Dr. Carlo Zocchetti, Direzione Generale Sanità, Lombardy Region, for providing hospital data.

References

[1] L. Barnes, *Pathology and Genetics of Head and Neck Tumours. World Health Organization Classification of Tumours*, vol. 9, IARC Press, Lyon, France, 2005.

[2] A. Franchi, L. Miligi, A. Palomba, L. Giovannetti, and M. Santucci, "Sinonasal carcinomas: recent advances in molecular and phenotypic characterization and their clinical implications," *Critical Reviews in Oncology Hematology*, vol. 79, no. 3, pp. 265–277, 2011.

[3] V. J. Lund, "Malignancy of the nose and sinuses. Epidemiological and aetiological considerations," *Rhinology*, vol. 29, no. 1, pp. 57–68, 1991.

[4] International Agency for Research on Cancer, *Cancer Incidence in Five Continents (Volume IX)*, vol. 160 of *IARC Scientific Publications*, IARC, World Health Organization, Geneva, Switzerland, 1993.

[5] National Cancer Institute (U.S.), "SEER program: National Cancer Institute (U.S.) Surveillance, epidemiology, and end results".

[6] B. A. C. Van Dijk, G. Gatta, R. Capocaccia, D. Pierannunzio, P. Strojan, and L. Licitra, "Rare cancers of the head and neck area in Europe," *European Journal of Cancer*, vol. 48, no. 6, pp. 783–796, 2012.

[7] K. Fukuda, A. Shibata, and K. Harada, "Squamous cell cancer of the maxillary sinus in Hokkaido, Japan: a case-control study," *British Journal of Industrial Medicine*, vol. 44, no. 4, pp. 263–266, 1987.

[8] *Wood, Leather, and Some Associated Industries*, vol. 25 of *IARC Monographs on the Evaluation of Carcinogenic Risk of Chemicals to Man*, International Agency for Research on Cancer, Lyon, France, 1981.

[9] *Wood Dust and Formaldehyde*, vol. 62 of *IARC Monographs on the Evaluation of Carcinogenic Risk of Chemicals to Man*, International Agency for Research on Cancer, Lyon, France, 1995.

[10] *Cadmium, Nickel, Some Epoxides, Miscellaneous Industrial Chemicals and General Considerations on Volatile Anaesthetics*, vol. 11 of *IARC Monographs on the Evaluation of Carcinogenic Risk of Chemicals to Man*, International Agency for Research on Cancer, Lyon, France, 1976.

[11] *Chromium, Nickel and Welding*, vol. 49 of *IARC Monographs on the Evaluation of Carcinogenic Risk of Chemicals to Man*, International Agency for Research on Cancer, Lyon, France, 1990.

[12] K. Straif, L. Benbrahim-Tallaa, R. Baan et al., "A review of human carcinogens C," *The Lancet Oncology*, vol. 10, no. 5, pp. 453–454, 2009.

[13] S. Samant and E. Kruger, "Cancer of the paranasal sinuses," *Current Oncology Reports*, vol. 9, no. 2, pp. 147–151, 2007.

[14] A. Leclerc, D. Luce, P. A. Demers et al., "Sinonasal cancer and occupation. Results from the reanalysis of twelve case-control studies," *American Journal of Industrial Medicine*, vol. 31, no. 2, pp. 153–165, 1997.

[15] A. d'Errico, S. Pasian, A. Baratti et al., "A case-control study on occupational risk factors for sino-nasal cancer," *Occupational and Environmental Medicine*, vol. 66, no. 7, pp. 448–455, 2009.

[16] D. Luce, A. Leclerc, D. Bégin et al., "Sinonasal cancer and occupational exposures: a pooled analysis of 12 case-control studies," *Cancer Causes and Control*, vol. 13, no. 2, pp. 147–157, 2002.

[17] G. Bimbi, M. S. Saraceno, S. Riccio, G. Gatta, L. Licitra, and G. Cantù, "Adenocarcinoma of ethmoid sinus: an occupational disease," *Acta Otorhinolaryngologica Italica*, vol. 24, no. 4, pp. 199–203, 2004.

[18] A. Marinaccio, A. Binazzi, G. Gorini, M. Pinelli, S. Iavicoli, and Gruppo di Lavoro ReNaTuNS, *Manuale Operativo per la Definizione di Procedure e Standard Diagnostici e Anamnestici per la Rilevazione, a Livello Regionale, dei Casi di Tumore dei Seni Nasali e Paranasali e Attivazione del Registro Nazionale ReNaTuNS*, Istituto Superiore per la Prevenzione e la Sicurezza del Lavoro, Rome, Italy, 2008.

[19] R. C. Tiwari, L. X. Clegg, and Z. Zou, "Efficient interval estimation for age-adjusted cancer rates," *Statistical Methods in Medical Research*, vol. 15, no. 6, pp. 547–569, 2006.

[20] D. Consonni, V. Coviello, C. Buzzoni, and C. Mensi, "A command to calculate age-standardized rates with efficient interval estimation," *Stata Journal*, vol. 12, no. 4, pp. 688–701, 2012.

[21] Stata Corp, *Stata: Release 12. Statistical Software*, Stata Corp LP, College Station, Tex, USA, 2011.

[22] J. H. Kuijpens, M. W. Louwman, R. Peters, G. O. Janssens, A. L. Burdorf, and J. W. Coebergh, "Trends in sinonasal cancer in The Netherlands: more squamous cell cancer, less adenocarcinoma.

A population-based study 1973–2009," *European Journal of Cancer*, vol. 48, pp. 2369–2374, 2012.

[23] R. Slack, C. Young, and L. Rushton, "Occupational cancer in Britain. Nasopharynx and sinonasal cancers," *British Journal of Cancer*, vol. 107, supplement 1, pp. S49–S55, 2012.

[24] A. t Mannetje, M. Kogevinas, D. Luce et al., "Sinonasal cancer, occupation, and tobacco smoking in European women and men," *American Journal of Industrial Medicine*, vol. 36, pp. 101–107, 1999.

[25] H. Rhif, "Cancers of the nasal cavity and paranasal sinuses: clinicopathological, etiological and therapeutic aspects," *Bulletin du Cancer*, vol. 99, no. 10, pp. 963–977, 2012.

[26] G. Cantu, C. L. Solero, L. Mariani et al., "Intestinal type adenocarcinoma of the ethmoid sinus in wood and leather workers: a retrospective study of 153 cases," *Head and Neck*, vol. 33, no. 4, pp. 535–542, 2011.

31

Communication Partners' Journey through Their Partner's Hearing Impairment

Vinaya K. C. Manchaiah,[1,2] **Dafydd Stephens,**[3] **and Thomas Lunner**[2,4]

[1] *Centre for Long Term and Chronic Conditions, College of Human and Health Sciences, Swansea University, Swansea SA2 8PP, UK*
[2] *Linnaeus Centre HEAD, Swedish Institute for Disability Research, Department of Behavioural Sciences and Learning, Linköping University, 58183 Linköping, Sweden*
[3] *Department of Psychological Medicine & Neurology, School of Medicine, Cardiff University, Cardiff CF14 4XN, UK*
[4] *Eriksholm Research Centre, Oticon A/S, 20 Rørtangvej, 3070 Snekkersten, Denmark*

Correspondence should be addressed to Vinaya K. C. Manchaiah; v.k.c.manchaiah@swansea.ac.uk

Academic Editor: B. J. Yates

The objective of this study was to further develop the Ida Institute model on communication partners' (CPs) journey through experiences of person with hearing impairment (PHI), based on the perspectives of CPs. Nine CPs of hearing aid users participated in this study, recruited through the Swansea hearing impaired support group. Semi-structured interviews were conducted, the data were analysed using qualitative thematic analysis and presented with the use of process mapping approach. Seven main phases were identified in the CP journey which includes: (1) contemplation, (2) awareness, (3) persuasion, (4) validation, (5) rehabilitation, (6) adaptation, and (7) resolution. The Ida Institute model (based on professionals' perspective) was compared with the new template developed (based on CPs' perspectives). The results suggest some commonalities and differences between the views of professionals and CPs. A new phase, adaptation, was identified from CPs reported experiences, which was not identified by professionals in the Ida Institute model. The CP's journey model could be a useful tool during audiological enablement/rehabilitation sessions to promote discussion between the PHI and the CP. In addition, it can be used in the training of hearing healthcare professionals.

1. Introduction

Communication partners (CPs) are those with whom the person with hearing impairment (PHI) communicates on a regular basis. The term communication partner has been used to refer to the significant others which may include their spouse, siblings, children, friends, relatives, colleagues, and carers.

Hearing impairment is a communication problem which affects everyone in the communication situation, not only the PHI [1]. It can result in various physical, mental, and psychosocial effects on PHI and their CPs. According to the World Health Organisation-International Classification of Functioning, Disability, and Health (WHO-ICF), spouses of PHI, although they do not have a health condition themselves, may experience activity limitations and participation restrictions due to their spouses' health condition which is referred to as a "third-party disability" [2]. Studies have

shown that CPs may undergo various experiences through their partners' hearing loss, and this may often influence the help-seeking behaviour of the PHI [3–6]. Our recent review identified various impacts that CPs can have due to their partners' hearing loss, and suggesting the need to involve CPs in the audiological enablement/rehabilitation which will result in mutual advantages for both the PHI and their CPs [7]. Moreover, exploring the journey of CPs through the PHI's hearing loss was identified as one of the key research questions.

Ida Institute at Denmark is a non-profit organisation with a mission to foster better understanding of human dynamics of hearing loss. The institute conducts various activities to create and share innovative, actionable knowledge to help hearing care professionals address the psychological and social challenges of hearing loss and implement patient-centered care practices. The institute with collaborative effort from hearing healthcare professionals around the world

TABLE 1: Demographic details of communication partners of PHI.

No.	Age	Sex	Relationship with PHI	Duration of contact with PHI	Duration of PHI's hearing loss	Accompanied PHI to audiological session at least on one occasion
1	52	Male	Colleague/friend	15 years	>20 years	No
2	58	Female	Daughter	58 years	>30 years	Yes
3	74	Female	Spouse	48 years	30 years	Yes
4	31	Female	Spouse	4 years	15 years	No
5	75	Female	Spouse	46 years	12 years	No
6	19	Female	Carer	1 year	>10 years	No
7	19	Female	Friend	7 years	>10 years	No
8	53	Male	Spouse	33 years	6 years	No
9	19	Female	Daughter	19 years	>20 years	Yes

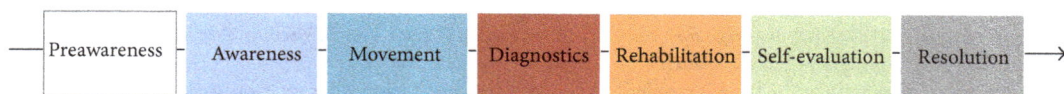

FIGURE 1: Patient's journey model of adults with gradual-onset acquired hearing impairment [10].

developed the possible CP journey model [8]. However, this model was based only on professionals perspectives and includes six main phases: (1) what is going on?, (2) awareness, (3) persuasion, (4) validation, (5) rehabilitation, and (6) maintenance. Further details of this model are presented in Section 3. It was suggested that this model/template recognises the emotional reactions and practical activities the CPs experience during the onset of their partner's hearing loss, successful management and learning to live with the condition. However, studies from medical anthropologists and also from our previous studies on patient journey of PHI have shown differences in professionals' and patients' perspectives [9–11]. This may indicate that the professionals' and the CPs' perception of the CP journey could be different.

In a recent international study that focused on exploring the perspectives of the PHI, it was highlighted that PHI use their life experiences rather than clinical encounters to describe the hearing help-seeking and hearing rehabilitation process [12]. In addition, it was suggested that the patients did not report their experiences on clinical encounters towards hearing help-seeking and rehabilitation as a connected process. This may be because they may have not made an attempt to think about the help-seeking and hearing rehabilitation in the temporal order, and to some extent, they may have even forgotten some of the experiences. Whilst there are studies focusing on the impact of the person's hearing impairment on CPs [7, 13, 14], we were unable to identify any studies that focused on the perspectives and experiences of CPs through their partner's hearing help-seeking and rehabilitation process. In addition, we believe that such an effort to map the process over time and understand the journey of CPs may give some insights into how CPs are affected by PHIs' hearing loss, how they might cope with these effects, and how they may influence the journey and the help-seeking behaviour of the PHI. Such journey models of PHIs and CPs could

be helpful during the audiological enablement/rehabilitation process to prompt the discussion between PHIs and CPs and potentially in developing the relationship-centered care (RCC).

In our previous studies, we have explored the journey of PHI [10, 11]. Figure 1 shows the typical patient's journey model of adults with gradual-onset acquired hearing impairment which has seven main phases: (1) preawareness, (2) awareness, (3) movement, (4) diagnostics, (5) rehabilitation, (6) self-evaluation, and (7) resolution. These phases correspond quite well with stages of the transtheoretical model of change which demonstrates individual's readiness to act on a new health behaviour [15, 16].

The aim of the current study was to further develop the Ida Institute model on the CP journey through their partner's hearing impairment, based on the perspectives of CPs and to examine the relationship between the perspectives of hearing healthcare professionals and of CPs.

2. Method

2.1. Participants. Ethical clearance was obtained from Departmental Research Ethics Committee, College of Human and Health Sciences, Swansea University. A purposeful sampling strategy [17] (usually used in theory-driven or theory-developing qualitative research) was used in order to recruit CPs of the hearing aid users through the Swansea Hard of Hearing Support Group. Most members of this group are healthcare users of National Health Services, experienced hearing aid users (i.e., over 2 years), and they meet once a month for few hours in a designated place. The participants included 9 CPs which involved spouses, children, friends, colleague and a carer. Whilst the participants include a wide range of people, all were reported to spend a significant amount of time communicating with the PHI (i.e., during most days of the week). However, CPs typically do not attend the support group meetings. Table 1 presents the demographic details of participants. There were 7 females and 2 males with a mean age of 44.4 years (ranging from 19 to 74 years). The duration of contact of the CP with the PHI varied from 1 year to 58 years with an average of 25.6 years and the duration of PHI's hearing loss varied from 6 years to >30 years. Only 3 of the 9 CPs in the study had accompanied the PHI to an audiological appointment on at least one occasion. All PHI were reported to have bilateral hearing loss with mild to severe degree. However, we were unable to obtain the exact degree of hearing loss in each case.

2.2. Data Collection. All the participants were supplied with an information sheet usually a week before the interview and scheduled an appointment. In addition, on the day of interview, they were given a short introduction to the study, an opportunity was given to ask questions, they were informed about confidentiality, and a written consent was obtained. The data were collected through semistructured interviews. A questionnaire was developed based on the literature review and from our previous experience of studies on the journey of PHI, which was used as a guide during the interview (see the appendix for details). Initially, CPs were asked to narrate their journey (tell their story) through their partner's/friend's/father's hearing loss. This was followed by some general questions (i.e., all the questions in the questionnaire were asked to each participant) to explore the CPs' experiences broadly. In addition, more directed questions based on their reports during the interview were asked to obtain an in-depth understanding of their experiences. Interviews typically lasted for about 60–90 minutes. The interviews were recorded using portable digital recorders to recheck the notes taken by the researcher. It was noticed that many CPs had prepared notes about their experiences before the interview, even though it was not requested in the information sheet.

2.3. Data Analysis. The data collection and the data analysis were conducted by the first author. Thematic analysis which involves identifying, analyzing, and reporting patterns within the data was employed to analyse the data [18]. The main task in thematic analysis is to identify a limited number of themes which adequately reflect the data. A hybrid of inductive and deductive approaches was used for the coding and the development of themes [19]. The Ida Institute CP's journey model was used as a theoretical base [8]. Such an approach allowed the researcher to focus on important aspects of the data based on theory and also to look for new themes which emerged from the data.

The main steps in data analysis included: familiarization with the data by repeated reading of notes and by listening to the voice recordings repeatedly, generating the initial codes (i.e., the participants' reports were shortened to simple and meaningful units), categorising the data and searching for subthemes and themes, ongoing review, defining and naming of themes and subthemes (the Ida model acted as

an inspiration for naming the themes), and identifying some extracts which could be used in reporting the data. The subthemes were categorised into most (i.e., approximately two thirds), many (i.e., approximately half), several, and/or few (i.e., less than half) based on how frequently they were reported by the participants. Moreover, the rule of most of participants reporting was considered for a theme (i.e., phase) and many participants reporting for a subtheme (i.e., stage). The working model with seven main phases was developed with the interview data of seven participants. Two new participants were interviewed to check for data saturation, and the data collection was stopped as there were no new themes (i.e., phases) being identified (i.e., data saturation— no significant new data emerging from the data in relation to research question) [20, 21].

A total of 58 unique subthemes that were related to the study were identified through 9 interviews. However, only 31 of them that were reported by most and many participants were considered for the development of CP's journey model. An ongoing matching of subthemes was done with Ida Institute model to see if the same code names can be assigned. However, where new subthemes (i.e., stages) were identified, new names were assigned to reflect the meaning and essence of the reported experiences. The subthemes were grouped together to identify themes, and the themes were further confirmed by repeatedly listening to participants' interviews to check if the identified themes capture the reported experiences. The process mapping (i.e., a way of representing a sequence of actions involved in a process) was used to define these themes in appropriate phases to represent the CP's journey model [22]. Process maps can be an effective way to demonstrate either individual or organisational process about virtually any aspect. The visual approach used in presenting the information makes it easier for readers to understand the process and may also help in identifying any constraints and/or bottle necks. Whilst the use of process mapping in healthcare seems to be relatively new, it has increased mainly in clinical audits to identify how we manage the patient's journey, using patient's perspectives to identify issues and suggested improvements to healthcare [23, 24]. Such an approach to presenting qualitative data about the patient's journey has also been used in our previous studies and also by others [10, 11, 25].

3. Results

Seven main phases and various stages were identified. Figure 2 shows the CPs' perspective on their journey through their partners' hearing loss. In this section, we present the phases and stages of the CP's journey in a logical order. Whilst there was some temporal order to participants' narratives, not all the CPs reported them in this order. For example, many participants went back and forth while talking about a particular theme. However, those who consistently maintained the temporal order are the ones who usually had prepared notes for this interview after reading the participant's information sheet. This may suggest that there is generally a temporal order to participants' reported stories; however, their ability

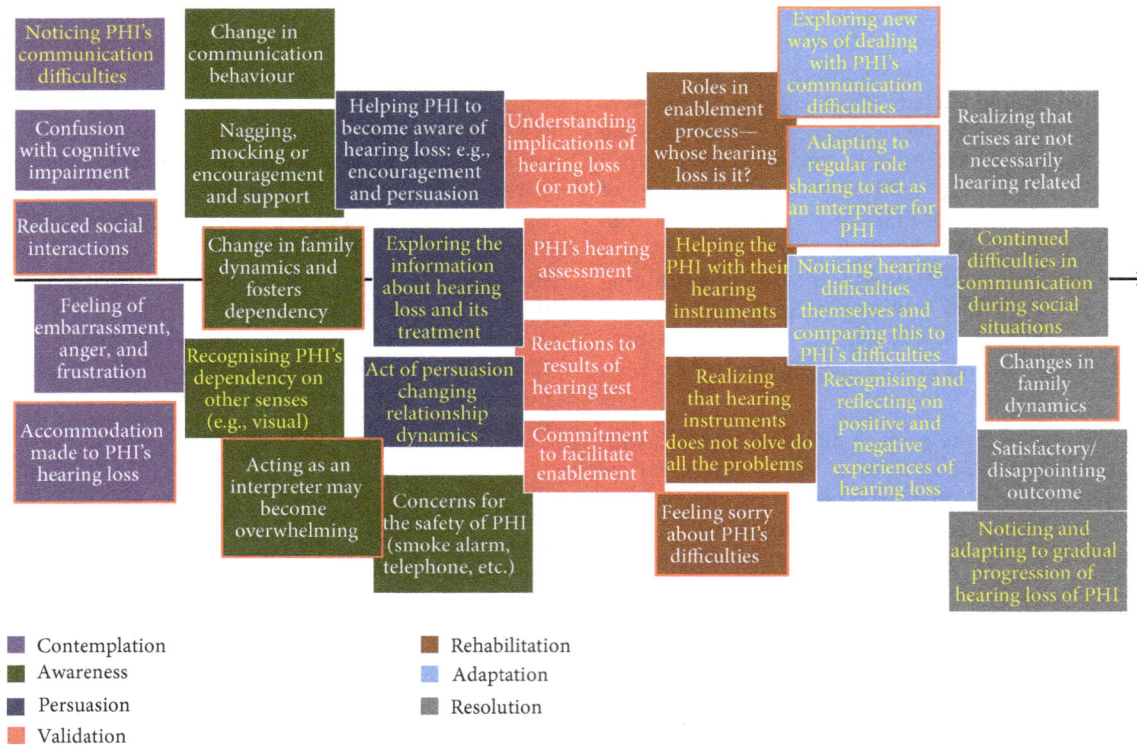

FIGURE 2: Communication partner's perspectives of their journey through their partners' hearing impairment (stages identified only by CPs are highlighted in yellow text, and stages which are reported in multiple phases are highlighted with red outline).

to remember the fine details and articulate the experiences may have influenced this. Based on data from this study and also our previous studies on patient's journey, we suggest that there is a journey through this process. For this reason, we decided to present them in a linear fashion using process mapping, even though not all reported them in such a systematic manner. In addition, some stages were reported in more than one phase. For example, role sharing and relationship dynamics that were reported both in initial and later phases of the journey. CPs talked more about contemplation, awareness, adaptation, and resolution phases compared to other phases (i.e., persuasion, validation, and rehabilitation). Moreover, the reported experience of one of the CPs (participant 9) was quite unique compared to the others. In this case, the CP had grown up through her father's hearing loss rather than starting to notice the hearing loss when the PHI initially started developing it. In that case, whilst she did not report a contemplation stage, she reported how she started becoming aware of her father's hearing loss as she got older and also the reported experiences in all the other phases.

3.1. Contemplation (or What Is Going On?). In this phase, CPs may start noticing the PHI's communication difficulties and reduced social interactions. This may sometimes result in feeling embarrassed, angry, and frustrated. Initially, the CPs might attribute some of the problems noticed to possible cognitive impairments, attentions and concentration. Moreover,

the CPs may also start making some accommodation, to the PHI's hearing loss.

The following statement made by the CP of a PHI shows how, in the initial phase of the PHI's hearing loss, the CP may think that the communication difficulties noticed were due to attention and concentration rather than to poor hearing. This highlights the fact that the identification of hearing loss is not straightforward.

> *Initially I thought a lot of it was due to his attention...! I could say something to him and if it was not of his interest, I could see that he has not heard it, or he will repeat what I said five minutes later, and I would say.....I just told you that..! ....* *Even though I had experience with deafness due to others in the family, I could not realise he had problem straightaway.*

3.2. Awareness. In this phase, CPs become aware that the PHI has genuine difficulties with their hearing. This may be by noticing clear changes in the PHI's communication behaviour, PHI's dependency on other senses, noticing that PHI was not hearing the smoke alarm, telephone, and so forth, and more importantly, by noticing changes in the family dynamics. They may start nagging the PHI (or indirectly persuading the PHI to seek help) or provide support and encouragement, and they may start acting as an interpreter for the PHI. However, this new role of acting as an interpreter may become overwhelming.

This description below shows how a CP confirmed their speculation about the PHI's hearing loss (elements of contemplation and awareness phases). It also highlights how this awareness may change the family dynamics.

> I can remember a few things which can put the picture together...The first thing I noticed was that he was shouting on the telephone. I could be in there with the doors shut and could hear him. I say to him, do you realise that you were shouting on the telephone?, I do not think I was.. You cannot say anything to that one...... and the other thing is shouting at public places, for example, shouting in the restaurant.

> ....after it was confirmed to me with these observations, I told my children what I noticed and they agreed, especially the elder daughter, and she started making some adjustments...

The following statement made by a CP highlights the change in their communication roles, a change in family dynamics and the dependency of the PHI on the CP for everyday activities in relation to communication.

> After I started noticing his difficulties...I almost started acting like his secretary...it could be very tiring sometimes...especially later in the day...!!

3.3. *Persuasion.* After CPs become aware of the PHIs hearing loss, they often start making attempts to make the PHI aware of their communication problems. In addition, they may also start searching for information related to hearing loss and start persuading them to seek help. In the initial stages, this could be indirect. However, there could be some triggering factors for the CPs which make them start directly persuading the PHI to seek help.

The following quote confirms that the CPs could act as drivers (or facilitators) to the PHI seeking help. The CP's expression in this makes it clear that this task is not always straightforward. They may start with indirect persuasion and move to more direct persuasion as time progresses.

> I have to be very diplomatic you know. ..... [Chuckle].... I got a bit of adverse reaction on one occasion. He said to me speak up you are mumbling, and I said to him you are not hearing me properly and asked him to get his hearing checked. ...... [Chuckle].... He said to me 'you get your hearing checked', you don't hear something that I say to you... Once he said that I have to back off for a while obviously....work with it for a while and then change my approach...

> ....I think I nagged him to such an extent that he went to get a hearing test... he was not hearing the telephone, once he did not hear the alarm and ......once it got to that stage I have to tell him..!!

3.4. *Validation.* This phase was not widely discussed by the CPs. However, in this phase, CPs mainly confirm whether or not the PHI had hearing loss. The results of hearing assessment of the PHIs may or may not surprise the CPs. Even though most CPs were not very keen about the hearing assessment, some accompanied the PHI for hearing assessment and made an attempt to understand the hearing test results and what they may indicate. However, almost all of them made commitments to support the PHIs.

In this statement, the CP talks about the PHI's reaction to the hearing test and acceptance of hearing loss. However, this also indirectly implies that the CP confirmed that their assessment was correct. There are also elements of later stages being mentioned, for example, the rehabilitation phase (i.e., starting to wear hearing aids).

> After the hearing test, the realisation made him do something about it. ...after he consulted he started wearing hearing aids, getting them fixed regularly, adjusts them, and it has made a great difference to us.

3.5. *Rehabilitation.* In this phase, most CPs were relieved that the PHIs were seeking help. However, they started realising that they also have an important role to play in the rehabilitation process, mainly in supporting the PHI (e.g., in using hearing aids). They soon realised that hearing instrument may not solve all the problems, which made them feel sympathy for the PHI's difficulties.

The following description highlights that soon after the PHI is fitted with hearing aids, they will start realising that they may not solve all the problems. In addition, the coping strategies used and the way in which the CP would support the PHI are evident.

> He wears hearing aids, but I still have to shout and I say things six times....oh....I have to say six times very often..! You hear what I said then?....He will say no.. oh....right....I will start again then. So, it's again my temperament....I don't get cross over him... I would say...oh... for goodness sake...you listening now?....[chuckle]...watch my lips... .[chuckle]...

The following statement made by a CP is an example of what may happen at a dinner table when they have big family dinner. This may suggest that they feel sorry for the PHI as they feel helpless in some occasions.

> I feel a bit guilty sometime....Everyone having a conversation...having a laugh and everything....I feel guilty sometime if he can't join in sometime, and if he is sitting in the corner...and everyone don't realise that.

3.6. *Adaptation.* This was a new phase identified from CP's reports when compared to the Ida Institute professionals' perspectives of the communication partners' journey [8]. This phase was noticed soon after the hearing assessment and rehabilitation session, when CPs started exploring new ways to communicate with the PHI, adapting to regular role of sharing, and reflecting on positive and negative consequences of the hearing impairment and the audiological management. Many elderly CPs also reported having started noticing hearing problems themselves and started comparing their own problems to those of the PHI.

The spouse of a PHI made the following statement in relation to how they started exploring new ways of communication after he was confirmed as having hearing loss.

> *I do repeat things for him, yes, he said such and such...sometime he will ask to me what did he say, when he misses a bit...the other day I repeated three times and eventually I say, I spell it out...because if they don't get it after three times....then we just spell it out.*

The following quote was made while the CP was talking about how he adapted to dealing with the PHI which demonstrates that the CP is able to identify some positive aspects of hearing loss.

> *It's not like he is missing a lot, because we talk after the meeting, what is been said, and it's not like he is missing anything. In fact, there is another person in the office who just can't be bothered, who goes to meeting and ....dreams. Whereas he [name of PHI] is different, he concentrates on what is being said and pays attention. Maybe it's been a benefit to him in that respect, because, he is hard of hearing he got to concentrate on hearing it.*

3.7. Resolution. This was a more stable phase which most of the CPs reported during the course of the interview. In this phase, CPs started noticing continued difficulties experienced by the PHI in social situations and started realising that crisis may not necessarily hearing related. They also gradually started noticing the increasing difficulties of the PHI, possibly due to the worsening of their hearing loss. Some CPs had positive temperaments and reported satisfactory outcomes. However, others reported frustrating and disappointing outcomes. Changes in family dynamics (more of relationship dynamics) seemed like a dynamic process which was noticed even in this phase. Moreover, in this phase, most CPs were more stable, and hearing loss had just become a way of life compared to the earlier phase (i.e., adaptation) in which they were exploring new ways of communication to improve the situation.

The following statement shows that the CP has started using a certain way of communicating rather than exploring new ways of communication.

> *We have a way of talking to him now. We have a certain way. We sometime do it with normal hearing people when I talk to them, and they say why are you speaking to me like this? I am so used to being around dad. It does change our lives.*

A daughter of a PHI made this statement indicating how her life had changed, and the crisis was not only hearing related.

> *It's our responsibility now...because, we can't expect him to do everyday things now. He will pick up the phone and ring me. Nine out of ten times he does not understand what we say. Few times now, since my mother has died and he lives on his own, if we don't get a response from him on the telephone we have to go there to check if he's alright.*

3.8. Other Interesting Observations. A few interesting observations were made while analysing the data. The progression of CPs from one phase to other phase varied in terms of time scale (i.e., a few weeks to a few years). For example, in the case of a carer, there was very limited time between the contemplation and adaptation phase. Moreover, each CP had different expectations of their PHI and most CPs reported that they had taken additional responsibilities after their partner developed hearing impairment (e.g., answering the telephone and interpreting conversations in difficult listening situations). Whilst CPs may need to continually adapt to life situations (as the hearing loss of PHI progressed, changes in the use of technology, etc.), in the initial phases of the journey, CPs reported having explored ways to improve their communication behaviour (i.e., exploring coping strategies). However, as time progressed, they became used to dealing with the PHI rather than finding new ways to improve their communication. Such observations also acted as the key difference between adaptation and resolution phase.

CPs, who reported less psychosocial consequences and who were coping well, appeared to have had a positive temperament (or attitude) towards life and also had some experience of dealing with other chronic conditions. However, this was not measured using any standard scale but only a subjective interpretation of the researcher. More research is needed to understand the relationship between such factors as CP temperament and personality and their influence on the success of audiological rehabilitation of the PHI.

3.9. Comparison to Professionals' Perspectives of the CP's Journey. Figure 3 shows the professionals' perspectives of the CPs' journey [8]. This was developed by collaborative efforts of 75 hearing healthcare professionals from around the world who attended the seminars of Enabling Communication Partnerships conducted by the Ida Institute in Denmark during 2009-2010.

Table 2 shows the differences and similarities in the key phases and/or stages identified by CPs and professionals. This suggests that the unique stages identified only by professionals were relatively few. Moreover, there were some stages which were identified by the professionals but were coded differently when we analysed the experiences reported by CPs. For example, in the contemplation phase, professionals identified that less social interaction leads to frustration or anger. However, CPs reported "reduced social interactions" and "feeling of embarrassment, anger, and frustration." This is because there were other reasons (e.g., communication breakdown) which also resulted in the feeling of frustration and anger. Moreover, the CPs have highlighted the fact that

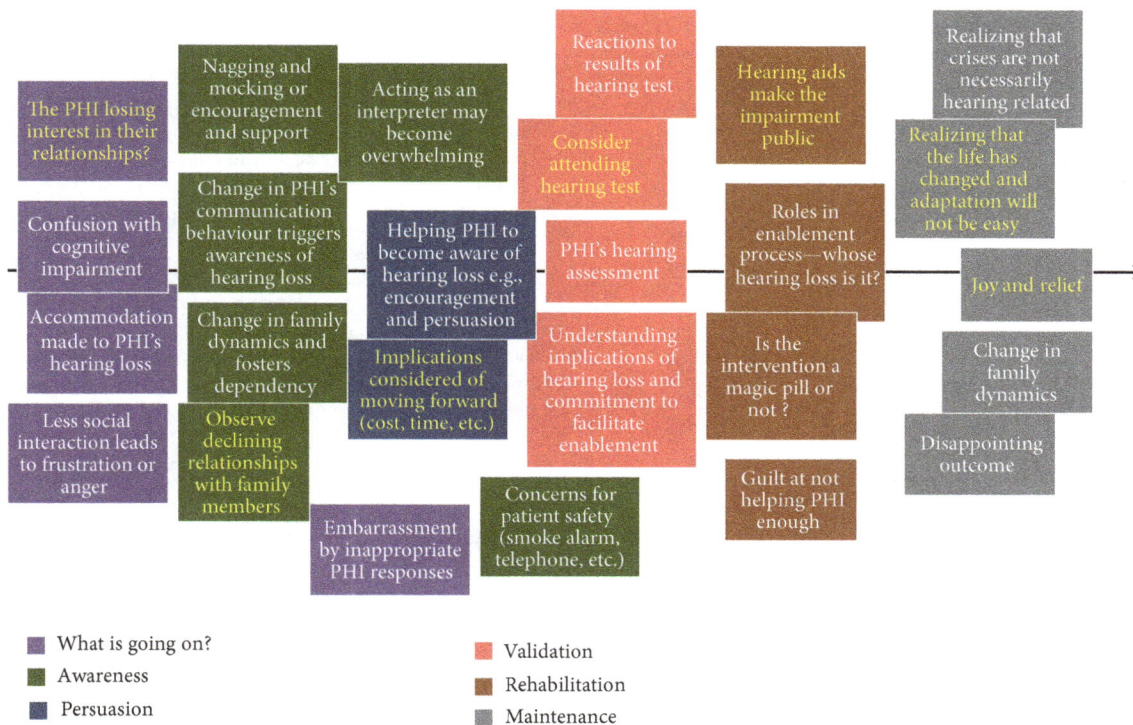

FIGURE 3: Professionals' perspective of the communication partners' journey (stages identified only by professionals are highlighted in yellow text) [8].

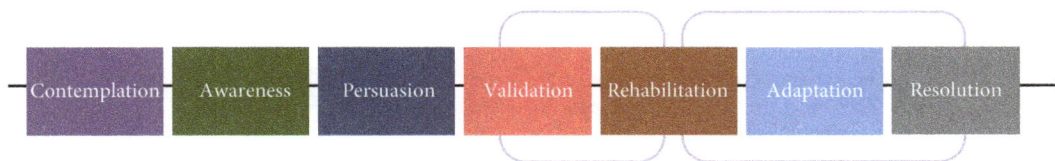

FIGURE 4: Main phases of communication partners' journey through their partner's hearing impairment (various stages are not drawn to any scale in regard to duration, and time spent in each phase may vary between individuals).

some stages may occur in more than one phase (e.g., reduced social interactions, changes in family dynamics, and acting as interpreter may become overwhelming).

4. Discussion

Figure 4 shows the main phases of the CPs' journey through their partners' hearing loss. Seven main phases were identified which include (1) contemplation, (2) awareness, (3) persuasion, (4) validation, (5) rehabilitation, (6) adaptation, and (7) resolution.

CPs referred more to the initial and later phases in their journey through their partner's hearing loss. Similar results have also been found in studies focusing on experiences of PHI [10, 12]. These findings strengthen the argument that patients and their CPs use their life experiences to relate to the chronic condition rather than the experiences during clinical encounters. This has important clinical implications in that clinicians may have to employ the strategy of talking more about life experiences to find common ground between the

PHI and CPs rather than about the disease, clinical tests, and other technical details. The observations, such as CPs having different expectations from the PHI, need more exploration in terms of new ways to improve their communication with the PHI at the beginning of the condition. Moreover, the fine differences between adaptation and resolution phases may highlight the fact that it is important to involve CPs in audiological enablement/rehabilitation at the earliest stage to give them support (i.e., social and emotional) and to teach them communication strategies. Moreover, studies suggest that there is considerable variation in how caregivers adapt to their care-giving demands [26]. For this reason, it is important to better understand CPs' experiences through PHI's hearing loss.

The study highlights the fact that the professionals failed to identify an important phase adaptation of the CPs' journey. Possible reasons for this may be that the professionals paid less attention to the subjective experiences of the PHI and CP during the rehabilitation process and/or professionals not being able to differentiate between adaptation and resolution

TABLE 2: Differences and similarities between phases/stages identified by CPs and professionals.

Phases	Stages identified only by CPs	Stages identified only by professionals	Stages identified by both CPs and professionals
Contemplation (or what is going on?)	Noticing the PHI's communication difficulties	Is the PHI losing interest in their relationship?	Confusion with cognitive impairment; accommodation made to the PHI's hearing loss; less social interaction leads to frustration and anger; embarrassment by inappropriate PHI responses; feeling of embarrassment, anger, and frustration
Awareness	Recognising the PHI's dependency on other senses (e.g., visual)	Observe declining relationships with family members	Nagging and mocking or encouragement and support; changes in the PHI's communication behaviour; changes in family dynamics and fosters dependency; acting as an interpreter may become overwhelming; concerns for the safety of PHI (smoke alarm, telephone, etc.)
Persuasion	Exploring the information about hearing loss and its treatment; act of persuasion changing relationship dynamics	Implications considered of moving forward (cost, time, etc.)	Helping PHI to become aware of hearing loss, for example, encouragement and persuasion
Validation		Consider attending a hearing test	Understanding the implications of hearing loss (or not); commitment to facilitate enablement; PHI's hearing assessment; reactions to results of hearing test
Rehabilitation	Helping the PHI with their hearing instruments; Realising that hearing instruments do not solve all the problems	Hearing aids make the impairment public	Roles in enablement process—whose hearing loss is it? feeling sorry about the PHI's difficulties
Adaptation	Exploring new ways of dealing with the PHI's communication difficulties; adapting to regular role sharing to act as an interpreter for the PHI; noticing hearing difficulties themselves and comparing this to the PHI's difficulties; recognising and reflecting on positive and negative experiences of hearing loss		
Resolution (or maintenance)	Continued difficulties in communication during social situations; noticing and adapting to gradual progression of hearing loss of PHI	Realizing that life has changed and adaptation is not easy; joy and relief	Realizing that crises are not necessarily hearing related; changes in family dynamics; satisfactory/disappointing outcome

phases. Similar results were seen in our previous study on the patient's journey of adults with gradual-onset acquired hearing impairment where professionals did not identify the self-evaluation phase [10]. In addition, some indications of what is described as adaptation and self-evaluation were also seen in studies by Engelund in her thesis which was focused on defining the process of help-seeking in PHI [27].

4.1. Applications of the Study. The current study has number of clinical and research implications. This is because the model helps to see the bigger picture about experiences of CPs and how they change over time, which is the most important in managing chronic conditions such as hearing impairment. Considering most of the research focuses on specific question (which may only provide fragments of information about CPs

experiences), this innovative approach may help organising such information using the proposed model. Whilst the way in which the data presented in this study is quite unique to qualitative research, it appears to be a format which is relatively easy for both professionals and nonprofessionals to understand and remember (i.e., organisation of information chronologically which is the format generally used in story-telling). Furthermore, the study highlights that it is important to understand the perspectives of both professionals and CPs as there are differences and commonalities.

More specifically, in this study, the data reflected personal stories of CPs through PHI's hearing loss which was used to develop typical journey model of CPs. This may suggest that the narrative (i.e., storytelling/listening) approach appeared to be a simple and useful way to gather data from CPs (similar to our previous study findings on PHIs) [28]. We suggest that this model could be helpful for clinicians to identify which phase (e.g., contemplation, awareness, and persuasion) the CPs might be during clinical encounters by taking in-depth history. This model can be presented to PHIs and CPs to make them think about their journey, and as a starting point in history taking, clinicians could ask CPs to describe their stories. Understanding how the experiences of CPs change over time and what phases CPs are at could be important for clinicians during counselling in order to tailor the information provided to meet the individual CP's needs. Moreover, it is important for hearing healthcare professionals to understand the journey of both the PHI and their CPs in order to facilitate their partnership during audiological enablement/rehabilitation. For this reason, CP's journey model could be used in training hearing healthcare professionals.

Aspects such as the frequency of communication and emotional closeness played an important role in the extent to which the CP was affected by the person's hearing impairment. For example, three of the participants (a carer, a friend, and a colleague) reported very few psychological consequences on them. In addition, three of the CPs (two daughters and a friend) talked about the impact of the PHI on their spouse and expressed the fact that the spouses of PHI were most affected in communication, social, and emotional aspects. This identifies the need for understanding more about the social networks of the PHI and their communication behaviour with CPs. For this purpose, tools such as "communication world" and/or "communication rings" could be helpful [1, 29].

In addition, the identification of a new phase (i.e., adaptation phase in the CP's journey, and self-evaluation phase in the PHI's journey from our previous study) [10] is significant in terms of clinical practice which may highlight the need of having review appointments soon after the initial assessment and rehabilitation' session. These sessions should be focused on assessing and modifying expectations, providing psychosocial support, and teaching communication tactics to CPs. Moreover, the literature suggests positive outcomes of involving CPs in the audiological rehabilitation sessions [30, 31].

4.2. Limitations of the Model.
In general, the intensity of psychological, emotional, and social consequences reported by each CP varied. For example, to what degree the CPs experienced communication difficulties during social situations. Whilst the CP's journey model represents the main experience of CPs through their partner's hearing loss (i.e., phases and stages) over a period of time, it may not clearly differentiate to what extent individual CPs were affected. This may suggest that this model provides us with an understanding of CPs experiences over time. For this reason, informal questioning, use of open-ended questionnaires, and use of structured questionnaires such as Significant Other Assessment of Communication (SOAC), Hearing Handicap Inventory for Elderly for Spouses (HHIE-SP), and the Significant Other Scale for Hearing Disability (SOS-HEAR) can

be useful during clinical encounters to gather information about the effect of the PHI's hearing loss on CPs in different dimensions [32–35]. It is important to note that informal questioning during clinical encounters generally focuses on some elements of CP's and PHI's experiences which may be of clinical interest due to the limited time. Structured questionnaires (e.g., SOAC, HHIE-SP, etc.) focus on the problems experienced at a particular point in time and the intensity to which they are experienced. The use of structured questionnaires before and after treatment and/or management may provide information about the effectiveness of treatment and/or management (i.e., outcome measure). However, the main focus in our approach was to understand how the experiences change over time (i.e., process of change or process evaluation) [36]. For this reason, the combination of such approaches may be necessary in practice, and they may act as complementary to each other. Moreover, this model is one of a variety of ways in which the CP's experiences can be illustrated [8]. Nevertheless, even though this model may not exactly represent each individual CPs' journey, it can be used as a tool to promote discussion with the PHI and CPs to explore their journeys further.

4.3. Advantages and Shortcomings of the Study.
The study's methodology has some advantages and drawbacks which may have influenced the results and the development of the model. For example, whilst thematic analysis offers theoretically flexible approach to the analysis of the data, other approaches such as narrative or other biographical approaches may have tapped into different aspects of the data (i.e., being able to retain a sense of continuity and contradiction through any individual account) [18]. However, thematic analysis helped in focusing on specific themes derived from the data and highlighting overlaps in themes in the journey model (i.e., stages appearing in multiple phases).

Considering the nature of the study, the data collection and analysis were conducted by the first author, and the analyses was discussed with other two authors. This allowed consistency in the method but may have failed to provide multiple perspectives and rechecking the coding. In addition, using notes and voice recordings for data analysis when compared to transcribing the recordings may have some advantages and disadvantages. For example, having the transcription of the interviews may have made the process of coding the data into themes and subthemes easier. However, considering that the data were collected and analysed by the same researcher, we would argue that the researcher was sufficiently familiarised to establish themes and subthemes. Moreover, listening to voice recordings repeatedly rather than looking at the transcriptions allowed the researchers to rethink and reperform parts of the analysis and helped in identifying the differences in intensity of reported psychological, emotional, and social consequences at different points which are not clearly reflected in the proposed model.

4.4. Further Research.
The reported experience of CPs may vary, based on differences in cultural aspects, social structures, healthcare structures, educational background, and so

on. For this reason, it would be interesting to study the CP's journey from other social and cultural backgrounds. Furthermore, an important question would be to explore how PHI's and their CPs' interactions may influence each other's journey. In the current study, most of the CPs were in the resolution stage and the journey reported was retrospectively based on what they could remember. However, it would be important to investigate the CP's journey longitudinally, by interviewing the CPs at different points of time. More importantly, whilst this exploratory study provides a model of CPs' journey, it should be validated using appropriate quantitative methods on a large sample size.

5. Conclusions

The study highlighted commonalities and differences in perspectives of CPs and professionals. The CP's journey model could be a useful tool during audiological enablement/rehabilitation sessions to promote the discussion between PHI and CPs. In addition, it can be used in training the hearing healthcare professionals. The CP's model was developed from a relatively small sample and may not represent the diverse group of CPs' experiences. Moreover, even though the CP's journey model illustrates CPs' experience through their partner's hearing loss, it may not cover all the complex dimensions. For this reason, the model should be used as a starting point to explore the CP's journey further in clinical situations.

Appendix

Interview Questionnaire

(1) Tell me about yourself and also tell me the story of your journey through your partner's/friend's/father's hearing loss.

(2) How did you confirm that your partner/friend/father had hearing loss?

(3) What were your immediate reactions to your partner's/friend's/father's hearing loss?

(4) What were the reactions of your partner/friend/father towards their hearing loss?

(5) What did you and your partner/friend/father think about hearing assessment, management, and rehabilitation sessions? Did you do anything in particular during and/or after these sessions?

(6) What life adjustments did you have to make because of your partner's/friend's/father's hearing loss?

(7) What effects does the hearing loss of your partner/friend/father have on your quality of life?

(8) Have you had any positive experiences due to your partner's/friend's/father's hearing loss?

(9) What are your strategies to cope with your partner's/friend's/father's hearing loss?

(10) What are the main stages (or important milestones) you went through with your partner's/friend's/father's hearing loss?

Conflict of Interests

The authors declare that they have no conflict of interests.

Acknowledgments

The authors wish to acknowledge the participants for their time and the Ida Institute for letting them use the professionals' perspective of communication partners' journey template. This study was partially funded by the Oticon Foundation.

References

[1] M. Gregory, "Tools for enabling communication partners," *Hearing Journal*, vol. 64, no. 5, pp. 44–49, 2011.

[2] WHO, *International Classification of Functioning, Disability and Health, ICF*, World Health Organisation, Geneva, Switzerland, 2001.

[3] N. Donaldson, L. Worrall, and L. Hickson, "Older people with hearing impairment: a literature review of the spouse's perspective," *Australian and New Zealand Journal of Audiology*, vol. 26, no. 1, pp. 30–39, 2004.

[4] J. A. Duijvestijn, L. J. C. Anteunis, C. J. Hoek, R. H. S. Van Den Brink, M. N. Chenault, and J. J. Manni, "Help-seeking behaviour of hearing-impaired persons aged ≥ 55 years; effect of complaints, significant others and hearing aid image," *Acta Oto-Laryngologica*, vol. 123, no. 7, pp. 846–850, 2003.

[5] C. F. O Mahoney, S. D. G. Stephens, and B. A. Cadge, "Who prompts patients to consult about hearing loss?" *British Journal of Audiology*, vol. 30, no. 3, pp. 153–158, 1996.

[6] R. H. S. Van den Brink, H. P. Wit, G. I. J. M. Kempen, and M. J. G. Van Heuvelen, "Attitude and help-seeking for hearing impairment," *British Journal of Audiology*, vol. 30, no. 5, pp. 313–324, 1996.

[7] V. K. C. Manchaiah, D. Stephens, F. Zhao et al., "The role of communication partners in the audiological enablement/rehabilitation of a person with hearing impairment: a discussion paper," *Audiological Medicine*, vol. 10, pp. 21–30, 2012.

[8] Ida Institute, "Communication partner journey," 2012, http://idainstitute.com/fileadmin/user_upload/Tools%20for%20Website%202011/Partner%20Journey%20-%20Ida%20Institute%20Tool.pdf.

[9] L. M. Hunt and N. H. Arar, "An analytical framework for contrasting patient and provider views of the process of chronic disease management," *Medical Anthropology Quarterly*, vol. 15, no. 3, pp. 347–367, 2001.

[10] V. K. C. Manchaiah, D. Stephens, and R. Meredith, "The patient journey of adults with hearing impairment: the patients' view," *Clinical Otolaryngology*, vol. 36, pp. 227–234, 2011.

[11] V. K. C. Manchaiah and D. Stephens, "The patient journey of adults with sudden-onset acquired hearing impairment: a pilot study," *The Journal of Laryngology & Otology*, vol. 126, pp. 471–485, 2012.

[12] A. Laplante-Lévesque, L. V. Knudsen, J. E. Preminger et al., "Hearing help-seeking and rehabilitation: perspectives of adults

with hearing impairment," *International Journal of Audiology*, vol. 51, pp. 93–102, 2012.

[13] N. Scarinci, L. Worrall, and L. Hickson, "The ICF and third-party disability: its application to spouses of older people with hearing impairment," *Disability and Rehabilitation*, vol. 31, no. 25, pp. 2088–2100, 2009.

[14] N. Scarinci, L. Worrall, and L. Hickson, "The effect of hearing impairment in older people on the spouse," *International Journal of Audiology*, vol. 47, no. 3, pp. 141–151, 2008.

[15] J. O. Prochaska and W. F. Velicer, "The transtheoretical model of health behavior change," *American Journal of Health Promotion*, vol. 12, no. 1, pp. 38–48, 1997.

[16] J. O. Prochaska and C. C. DiClemente, "Stages and processes of self-change of smoking: toward an integrative model of change," *Journal of Consulting and Clinical Psychology*, vol. 51, no. 3, pp. 390–395, 1983.

[17] M. Q. Patton, *Qualitative Evaluation and Research Methods*, Sage, Newbury Park, Calif, USA, 2nd edition, 1990.

[18] V. Braun and V. Clarke, "Using thematic analysis in psychology," *Qualitative Research in Psychology*, vol. 3, no. 2, pp. 77–101, 2006.

[19] J. Fereday and E. Muir-Cochrane, "Demonstrating rigor using thematic analysis: a hybrid approach of inductive and deductive coding and theme development," *International Journal of Qualitative Methods*, vol. 5, no. 1, pp. 80–92, 2006.

[20] J. M. Morse, "The significance of saturation," *Qualitative Health Research*, vol. 5, pp. 147–149, 1995.

[21] L. V. Knudsen, A. Laplante-Lévesque, L. Jones et al., "Conducting qualitative research in audiology: a tutorial," *International Journal of Audiology*, vol. 51, pp. 93–92, 2012.

[22] R. Damelio, *The Basics of Process Mapping*, Productivity Press, Cambridge, Mass, USA, 1996.

[23] B. Kollberg, J. J. Dahlgaard, and P. O. Brehmer, "Measuring lean initiatives in health care services: issues and findings," *International Journal of Productivity and Performance Management*, vol. 56, no. 1, pp. 7–24, 2007.

[24] T. M. Trebble, N. Hansi, T. Hydes, M. A. Smith, and M. Baker, "Practice pointer: process mapping the patient journey: an introduction," *British Medical Journal*, vol. 341, no. 7769, pp. 394–397, 2010.

[25] N. Macdonald, A. Shapiro, C. Bender et al., "Experiences and perspectives on the GIST patient journey," *Journal of Patient Preference and Adherence*, vol. 5, pp. 653–662, 2012.

[26] P. Raina, M. O'Donnell, H. Schwellnus et al., "Caregiving process and caregiver burden: conceptual models to guide research and practice," *BMC Pediatrics*, vol. 4, article 1, 2004.

[27] G. Engelund, *Time for hearing—recognising process for the individual [Ph.D. thesis]*, University of Copenhagen, Eriksholm, Denmark, 2006.

[28] V. K. C. Manchaiah and D. Stephens, "The Patient journey: living with hearing impairment," *Journal of the Academy of Rehabilitative Audiology*, vol. 44, pp. 29–40, 2011.

[29] V. K. C. Manchaiah and D. Stephens, "Models to represent communication partners within the social networks of people with hearing impairment," *Journal of Audiological Medicine*, vol. 9, pp. 103–109, 2011.

[30] J. E. Preminger, "Should significant others be encouraged to join adult group audiologic rehabilitation classes?" *Journal of the American Academy of Audiology*, vol. 14, no. 10, pp. 545–555, 2003.

[31] J. E. Preminger and S. Meeks, "Evaluation of an audiological rehabilitation program for spouses of people with hearing loss," *Journal of the American Academy of Audiology*, vol. 21, no. 5, pp. 315–328, 2010.

[32] R. L. Schow and M. A. Nerbonne, "Communication screening profile: use with elderly clients," *Ear and Hearing*, vol. 3, no. 3, pp. 135–147, 1982.

[33] C. W. Newman and B. E. Weinstein, "The hearing handicap inventory for the elderly as a measure of hearing aid benefit," *Ear and Hearing*, vol. 9, no. 2, pp. 81–85, 1988.

[34] D. Stephens, L. France, and K. Lormore, "Effects of hearing impairment on the patient's family and friends," *Acta Oto-Laryngologica*, vol. 115, no. 2, pp. 165–167, 1995.

[35] N. Scarinci, L. Worrall, and L. Hickson, "The effect of hearing impairment in older people on the spouse: development and psychometric testing of the Significant Other Scale for Hearing Disability (SOS-HEAR)," *International Journal of Audiology*, vol. 48, no. 10, pp. 671–683, 2009.

[36] V. K. C. Manchaiah, B. Danermark, J. Rönnberg, and T. Lunner, "Importance of "process evaluation": examples from studies on hearing impairment," unpublished.

32

Long-Term Effect of Enzyme Replacement Therapy with Fabry Disease

Manabu Komori,[1] **Yuika Sakurai,**[1] **Hiromi Kojima,**[1]
Toya Ohashi,[2,3] **and Hiroshi Moriyama**[1]

[1] Department of Otorhinolarygology, The Jikei University School of Medicine, 3-25-8 Nishishinbashi Minato-ku, Tokyo 105-8461, Japan
[2] Department of Gene Therapy, Institute of DNA Medicine, The Jikei University School of Medicine, Tokyo 105-8461, Japan
[3] Department of Pediatrics, The Jikei University School of Medicine, Tokyo 105-8461, Japan

Correspondence should be addressed to Manabu Komori; m_komori@jikei.ac.jp

Academic Editor: Bill Yates

Objective. To determine the effects of enzyme replacement therapy (ERT) on the hearing acuity in patients with Fabry disease. *Materials.* The study sample comprised 34 ears of 17 affected patients who underwent pure-tone audiometry before and after ERT. *Methods.* The patients were studied in relation to factors such as changes in hearing, presence of accompanying symptoms, status of renal and cardiac function, age, and gender. Data of pure-tone audiometry obtained before ERT and at the final examination were compared. *Results.* At the end of the follow-up period, no significant worsening of hearing acuity was noted at the end of the follow-up period. SSNHL was detected in 10 ears of 6 patients. Steroid therapy successfully cured the disease in 9 of the 10 ears. *Conclusions.* No significant worsening of hearing acuity was noted from the beginning to the end of ERT. The rate of improvement in SSNHL of Fabry disease was excellent in the treated patients. Hearing loss is a factor that causes marked deterioration of the patients' quality of life, and it is desirable that the hearing acuity of patients be periodically evaluated and prompt treatment of SSNHL be administered, if available.

1. Introduction

Fabry disease is a genetic inborn error of metabolism in which the enzymatic activity of α-galactosidase (α-Gal), a hydrolytic enzyme present in lysosomes, is decreased due to a gene mutation; this results in the accumulation of glycolipids, mainly in the vascular endothelium. This disorder was first reported in 1898 by 2 independent investigators, namely, Anderson from the UK and Fabry from Germany [1, 2]. The disease is acquired by X chromosome-linked inheritance, and male and female patients with Fabry disease are hemizygous and heterozygous, respectively. Further, male patients with Fabry disease can either present with the classic type of the disease or the late-onset subtype.

The disease mainly involves the kidney, heart, and brain, and accordingly, affected patients often die in their 40 s or 50 s because of renal failure, heart failure, or cerebral infarction.

In addition, angiokeratoma and hypohidrosis are present, with a variety of neurologic symptoms, including severe pain in the extremities, burning sensation, headache, dizziness, hearing loss, lack of motivation, and neurosis. According to the published literature, 54.5% [3] to 80% [4] of patients with Fabry disease experience hearing loss. In a previous study, we examined the relationship between hearing acuity and complications occurring in Fabry disease patients treated at our institution and found that 44.4% of the patients had hearing loss [5]. We reported that flat-type hearing loss was predominant in both male and female patients, that all patients with renal dysfunction had hearing impairment, and that the incidence of hearing impairment was higher in men than in women [5].

As agents for enzyme replacement therapy (ERT), α-Galβ (Fabrazyme) and α-Galα (Replagal) were approved in Europe in 2001 and in the USA in 2003. In Japan, Fabrazyme was

TABLE 1: Grades of severity of hearing loss. In Japan, the severity of SSNHL has been classified as follows.

Grade 1	Less than 40 dB
Grade 2	More than 40 dB, less than 60 dB
Grade 3	More than 60 dB, less than 90 dB
Grade 4	90 dB or more

TABLE 2: Criteria for improvement. In Japan, outcome of therapy has been classified as follows.

(1) Healing	(1) When hearing level at 0.25, 0.5, 1, 2, 4 kHz returned to less than 20 dB. (2) When hearing level returned to the same as that in the other side.
(2) Marked recovery	When the value of the arithmetic means of the hearing levels at the five above-mentioned frequencies was greater than 30 dB.
(3) Recovery	When the value of the arithmetic means of the hearing levels at the five above-mentioned frequencies was less than 30 dB and greater than 10 dB.
(4) Unchangeable	When the value of the arithmetic means of the hearing levels at the five above-mentioned frequencies was less than 10 dB. (Including exacerbation)

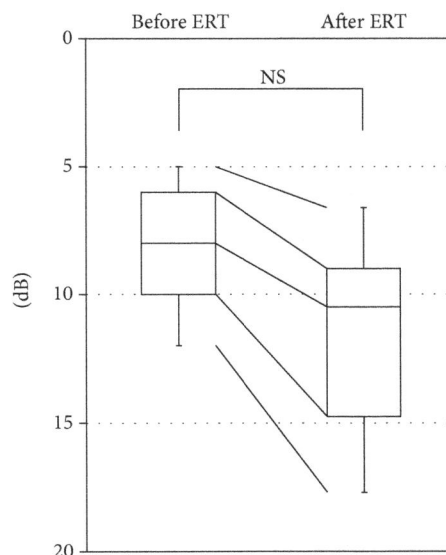

FIGURE 1: Changes in the hearing level after ERT. None of the patients showed significant worsening of hearing from the beginning of ERT until the end of followup.

approved in 2004 and Replagal in 2007. Early initiation of ERT has been reported to prevent or improve renal failure and heart failure [6, 7]. Studies from Europe and North America have reported the beneficial effect of ERT on hearing impairment, as long as it was not very severe [4, 8]. However, the course of changes in hearing remains unclear. With this in view, we sought to determine the changes in hearing affected by ERT in patients who had normal hearing acuity before the initiation of the therapy.

2. Materials

In this study, we examined 34 ears of 17 patients (8 men and 9 women) with Fabry disease, who underwent pure-tone audiometry before and after ERT. All these patients had a normal mean hearing level of less than 20 dB before the initiation of ERT. The mean age of the patients at the first visit was 35.0 years (31.0 years in men, 38.6 years in women), and the mean follow-up period was 46.6 months (8–90 months).

3. Methods

The patients were investigated for the course of changes in hearing and the severity of accompanying symptoms (sudden sensorineural hearing loss (SSNHL), tinnitus, and vertigo); different groups of patients were compared in terms of factors such as renal and cardiac functions, age, and gender. Hearing impairment was evaluated by pure-tone audiometry by using the five-division method, (250 Hz + 500 Hz + 1000 Hz + 2000 Hz + 4000 Hz)/5, according to the diagnostic criteria for sudden hearing loss in Japanese patients. The results

of pure-tone audiometry performed before starting ERT and at the final follow-up examination were compared. The severity of SSNHL and the outcome of therapy were classified according to the classification criteria set for assessing sudden hearing loss in Japanese patients (Tables 1 and 2). When the difference between the mean hearing levels recorded before and after ERT exceeded 5 dB, hearing impairment was deemed present. Renal failure was defined by increased levels of serum urea nitrogen (>20 mg/dL), increased levels of serum creatinine level (>1.2 mg/dL), or if the patient received renal dialysis. To evaluate cardiac function, patients were examined for myocardial hypertrophy in terms of the thickness of the myocardium in the interatrial septum and posterior wall, as determined by echocardiography or cardiac MRI. Cardiac damage was diagnosed when the patient had a history of myocardial hypertrophy, cardiac ischemic events, or pacemaker implantation. This study was approved by the Jikei University School of Medicine Ethics Committee.

4. Results

4.1. Overview. Data collected over the study period are presented in Table 3. Hearing impairment was noted in 7 ears of 5 patients (>5 dB) at the end of the follow-up period. The impairment had progressed slowly in the case of 4 (all in men) of the 7 ears, whereas SSNHL occurred in the remaining 3 ears (1 man and 2 women). However, the mean hearing level was less than 30 dB in all these 5 patients, thereby eliminating the need for hearing aids. None of the patients showed significant worsening of hearing (>5 dB) from the beginning of ERT until the end of followup (Figure 1; χ^2 test). Thirteen of the 17 patients had tinnitus, while 9 (4 men, 5 women) had vertigo. SSNHL was found in 10 ears of 6 patients (3 men, 3 women).

TABLE 3: Results along a time series. Thirteen of the 17 patients had tinnitus, while 9 had vertigo. SSNHL was found in 10 ears of 6 patients. Repetitive SSNHL was found in 3 of the 6 patients with SSNHL. The incidence of SSNHL tended to increase over the follow-up period, and all patients with renal dysfunction had SSNHL.

ID	Sex	Age	Fabry type	Tinnitus	Vertigo	SSNHL	Time to onset	SSNHL outcome	Hearing outcome	Hearing change	Renal function	Heart function	Period	Before ERT (dB)	After ERT (dB)
1	F	40	Hetero	–	–	–	–	–	–	–	–	–	8 M	8.0 / 6.0	6.0 / 5.0
2	F	52	Hetero	+	–	–	–	–	–	–	–	–	12 M	8.0 / 10.0	10.0 / 12.0
3	F	31	Hetero	+	–	–	–	–	–	–	–	–	12 M	14.0 / 14.0	17.0 / 15.0
4	M	55	Heart	+	+	–	–	–	Worth	Slow	–	–	17 M	8.0 / 6.0	11.0 / 13.0
5	M	14	Classical	–	–	–	–	–	–	–	–	–	26 M	6.0 / 6.0	9.0 / 9.0
6	M	38	Classical	+	–	–	–	–	Worth / Worth	Slow / Slow	–	–	27 M	6.0 / 9.0	24.0 / 15.0
7	F	23	Hetero	+	+	–	–	–	–	–	–	–	28 M	8.0 / 11.0	11.0 / 10.0
8	F	30	Hetero	+	+	–	–	–	–	–	–	–	36 M	5.0 / 5.0	10.0 / 9.0
9	M	25	Classical	–	+	–	–	–	–	–	–	Worth	43 M	9.0 / 11.0	8.0 / 8.0
10	F	47	Hetero	+	+	Grade 1 / Grade 1	54 M / 41 M	Healing / Healing	–	Sudden / Sudden	–	Worth	58 M	10.0 / 10.0	11.0 / 9.0
11	F	41	Hetero	+	+	–	–	–	Worth	Sudden	–	–	67 M	12.0 / 12.0	18.0 / 15.0
12	F	34	Hetero	+	–	Grade 1	64 M	Healing	–	Sudden	–	–	67 M	4.0 / 4.0	9.0 / 8.0
13	F	49	Hetero	+	+	Grade 1 / Grade 3	20 / 67 M	Healing / Healing	Worth	Sudden	Worth	Worth	68 M	10.0 / 14.0	21.0 / 14.0
14	M	35	Classical	+	–	Grade 1	48 M	Healing	–	Sudden	–	–	68 M	6.0 / 6.0	9.0 / 11.0
15	M	30	Classical	+	+	Grade 1	66 M	Healing	–	Sudden	Worth	Worth	77 M	8.0 / 9.0	9.0 / 11.0
16	M	39	Classical	+	+	Grade 1	84 M	No change	Worth / Worth	Slow / Sudden	Worth	–	88 M	8.0 / 7.0	15.0 / 21.0
17	M	12	Classical	–	–	Grade 1	90 M	Healing	Stable	Sudden	–	–	90 M	2.0 / 5.0	3.0 / 5.0

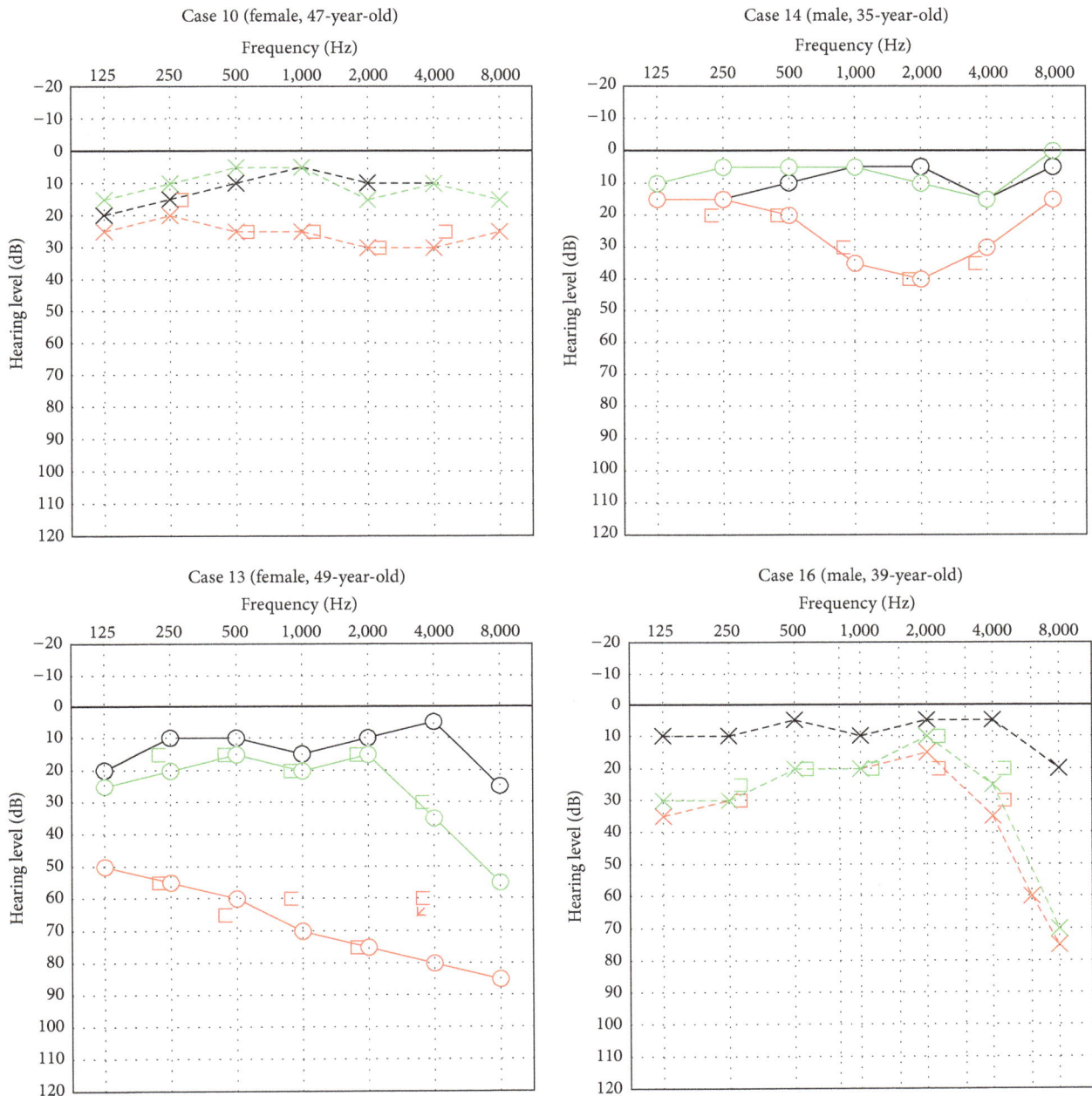

FIGURE 2: Four cases of sudden sensorineural hearing loss. Black line: at the first visit (before ERT). Red line: at the onset of SSNHL. Green line: after steroid treatment.

The severity of SSNHL was grade 1 in 9 ears and grade 3 in 1 ear. The condition was judged as cured in 9 of the 10 ears after steroid therapy, on the basis of our criteria for improvement. Repetitive SSNHL was found in 3 (1 man and 2 women) of the 6 patients with SSNHL. The incidence of SSNHL tended to increase over the follow-up period, and all patients with renal dysfunction had SSNHL.

4.2. *Patients with SSNHL.* The findings of typical cases of SSNHL are presented in Figure 2. Various patterns of hearing loss were noted among the patients, such as whole-area involvement, valley-type hearing loss, and sudden drop in high-frequency hearing.

4.2.1. *Case 10 (A 47-Year-Old Woman).* The patient developed SSNHL (grade 1) on 1 side at 41 months of age and on the opposite side at 54 months of age; at both instances, the patient was cured by steroid therapy.

4.2.2. *Case 14 (A 35-Year-Old Man).* SSNHL (grade 1) first occurred when the patient was 48 months of age and then again reoccurred at the opposite side at 60 months of age;

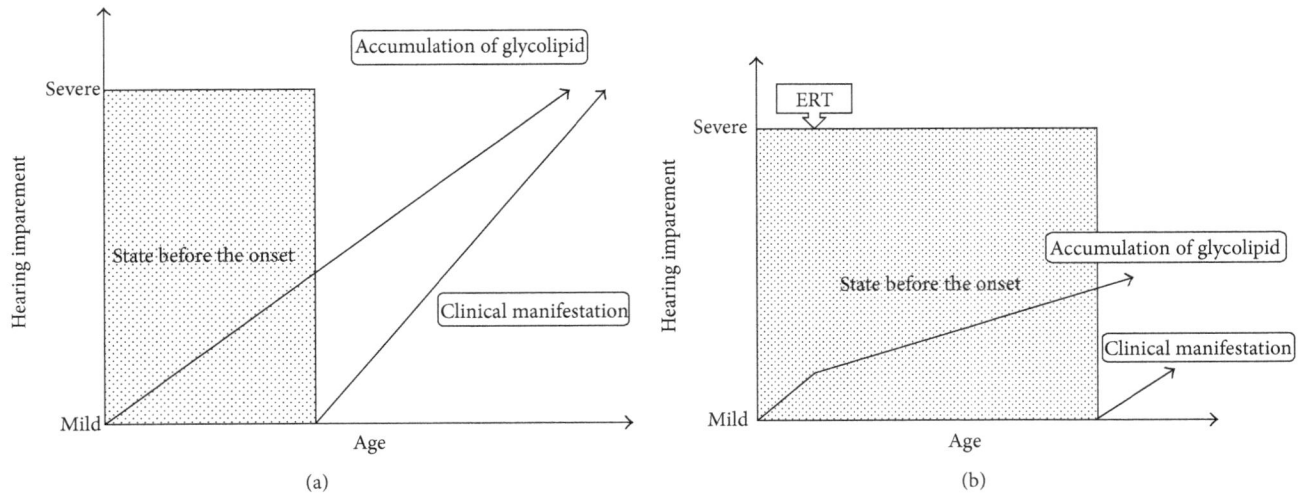

FIGURE 3: Hypothesis of the effect of ERT. (a) Natural history of Fabry disease. (b) Effect of ERT with Fabry disease.

both ears responded to steroid therapy. This patient showed no symptoms of the Fabry disease other than hearing loss.

4.2.3. Case 13 (A 49-Year-Old Woman). In this case, the patient developed SSNHL first at 20 months of age with grade 1 severity and then at 67 months with grade 3 severity. The condition was successfully treated with steroid therapy at both instances.

4.2.4. Case 16 (A 39-Year-Old Man). SSNHL (grade 1) occurred at 84 months of age and did not respond to steroid therapy.

5. Discussion

Since the Fabry disease is rare and shows diverse symptoms in the initial stages of manifestation, the definitive diagnosis of this disease was often delayed in the past. However, in recent years, Fabry disease has become more widely recognized, and therefore the disease is now increasingly detected at an early stage and ERT is soon initiated. In this study, all the enrolled patients had normal hearing of less than 20 dB before ERT, and the mean follow-up period was approximately 4 years.

Because the model of Fabry disease showed a densely-stained material accumulation in the inner ear stria vascularis cell [9] and organ damage is reported to be improved by ERT [6, 7], it is reasonable for otorhinolaryngologists to expect that ERT may prevent hearing loss. Hearing loss is a symptom that markedly impairs patients' quality of life (QOL), and therefore the prevention of hearing loss is expected to contribute to the maintenance of QOL in patients with Fabry disease. On the basis of the pathologic features of Fabry disease, we hypothesized that the decrease in the accumulation of glycolipids brought about by ERT would inhibit, or delay, the manifestation of symptoms (Figure 3). Further, the progression of Fabry disease is known to vary among different individuals; these differences have been

attributed to factors such as the type of Fabry disease, discrepancy in enzymatic activity, and antibodies to ERT.

Some important findings of this study were that no eventual worsening of hearing occurred while the patients received ERT and that the incidence of SSNHL was obviously higher in this population than the incidence of sudden hearing loss in the general population. None of the patients required hearing aids, with the mean hearing level of the patients being less than 30 dB even for those who showed more than 5 dB decrease in hearing acuity. The pathologic status of SSNHL in Fabry disease remains unclear; however, some type of vascular disorder is believed to occur, similar to that observed in cerebral infarction. Although the incidence of SSNHL was higher among patients who were followedup for more than 3 years, mild cases of grade 1 severity were predominant, and the cure rate was as high as 90%. These results suggest that ERT inhibits the onset of hearing loss and SSNHL and decreases the severity of the latter. However, since this study did not include a placebo control group, the results cannot be compared against patients not receiving the therapy. Therefore, the results of the therapy over a longer period of observation should be studied before reaching a conclusion as to whether ERT is truly effective.

In our previous study, several patients had severe hearing loss [5]. These were patients who already had severe hearing loss at the beginning of ERT and had other progressive symptoms of Fabry disease [5]. In contrast, all patients in the present study had normal hearing acuity at the beginning of ERT. Taking these features into account, the following 2 points need to be considered. First, it is possible that ERT decreases the severity of hearing loss. Second, gradually progressing hearing loss and SSNHL may have different mechanisms of onset. This speculation is supported by the finding that gradually progressing hearing loss is irreversible, whereas the cure rate of SSNHL is very high, as observed in this study. In other words, SSNHL in Fabry disease is a reversible disorder.

The results of this study indicate that patients with Fabry disease should be periodically evaluated for hearing acuity and administered prompt treatment of SSNHL, if available, in order to maintain their QOL. A new finding of this study is that repeated hearing loss was observed as the only symptom of Fabry disease, albeit in 1 case (Case 14). This is suggestive of the diversity of the clinical presentation of Fabry disease and possibly points towards the existence of the auditory subtype of this disease, in addition to the renal subtype and the cardiac subtype. Further investigations of the pathologic condition of this disease in the light of these findings are desirable.

6. Conclusions

No significant worsening of hearing acuity was noted until the end of ERT.

The incidence of SSNHL tended to be higher in patients who were followed up for a longer duration and who had renal dysfunction. SSNHL that occurred in patients on ERT for Fabry disease was relatively mild, and the cure rate for steroid therapy was 90%. The results suggest that ERT delays the onset of hearing loss and reduces the severity of SSNHL. Periodic evaluation of hearing acuity and prompt treatment of SSNHL, if any, are desirable to maintain patients' QOL.

Conflict of Interests

Toya Ohashi has active research support from Genzyme Japan K.K. Dainippon Sumitomo Pharma K.K. and Shire Japan K.K. These activities have been fully disclosed and are managed under a Memorandum of Understanding with the Conflict of Interest Resolution Board of The Jikei University School of Medicine.

References

[1] W. Anderson, "A case of angio-keratoma," *British Journal of Dermatology*, vol. 10, no. 4, pp. 113–117, 1898.

[2] J. Fabry, "Beitrag zur Kennthis der Purpura heamorrhagica nodularis," *Archives of Dermatology and Syphilology*, vol. 43, pp. 187–200, 1898.

[3] D. P. Germain, P. Avan, A. Chassaing, and P. Bonfils, "Patients affected with Fabry disease have an increased incidence of progressive hearing loss and sudden deafness: an investigation of twenty-two hemizygous male patients," *BMC Medical Genetics*, vol. 3, p. 10, 2002.

[4] D. Hajioff, S. Hegemannn, G. Conti et al., "Agalsidase alpha and hearing in Fabry disease: data from the fabry outcome survey," *European Journal of Clinical Investigation*, vol. 36, no. 9, pp. 663–667, 2006.

[5] Y. Sakurai, H. Kojima, M. Shiwa, T. Ohashi, Y. Eto, and H. Moriyama, "The hearing status in 12 female and 15 male Japanese Fabry patients," *Auris Nasus Larynx*, vol. 36, no. 6, pp. 627–632, 2009.

[6] C. M. Eng, N. Guffon, W. R. Wilcox et al., "International collaborative Fabry disease study group. Safety and efficacy of recombinant human alpha-galactosidase A—replacement therapy in Fabry's disease," *New England Journal of Medicine*, vol. 5, no. 1, pp. 9–16, 2001.

[7] B. L. Thurberg, H. Rennke, R. B. Colvin et al., "Globotriaosylceramide accumulation in the fabry kidney is cleared from multiple cell types after enzyme replacement therapy," *Kidney International*, vol. 62, no. 6, pp. 1933–1946, 2002.

[8] G. Conti and B. Sergi, "Auditory and vestibular findings in Fabry disease: a study of hemizygous males and heterozygous females," *Acta Paediatrica*, vol. 92, supplement 443, pp. 33–37, 2003.

[9] Y. Sakurai, R. Suzuki, R. Yoshida et al., "Inner ear pathology of alpha-galactosidase A deficient mice, a model of Fabry disease," *Auris Nasus Larynx*, vol. 37, no. 3, pp. 274–280, 2010.

33

Diagnosis and Management of Extracranial Head and Neck Schwannomas: A Review of 27 Cases

Ryuji Yasumatsu, Torahiko Nakashima, Rina Miyazaki, Yuichi Segawa, and Shizuo Komune

Department of Otorhinolaryngology, Graduate School of Medical Sciences, Kyushu University, 3-1-1 Maidashi, Higashi-ku, Fukuoka 812-8582, Japan

Correspondence should be addressed to Ryuji Yasumatsu; yasuryuj@qent.med.kyushu-u.ac.jp

Academic Editor: Peter S. Roland

Objectives. Clinical records of 27 patients with extracranial head and neck schwannoma were retrospectively reviewed. *Methods.* Ultrasonography (US) was performed in all cases. Seven patients underwent CT. Twenty-five patients underwent MRI. Fine needle aspiration cytology (FNAC) was performed for 12 of the 27 patients. Clinical history, surgical data, and postoperative morbidity were analyzed. *Results.* The images of US showed a well-defined, hypoechoic, primarily homogeneous solid mass. At CT, only one of 7 cases (14%) was able to suggest the diagnosis of schwannoma. At MRI, twenty of 25 cases (80%) suggested the diagnosis of schwannoma. Only three of 12 cases (25%) displayed a specific diagnosis of schwannoma rendered on FNAC. The distribution of 27 nerves of origin was 10 (37%) vagus nerves, 6 (22%) sympathetic trunks, 5 (19%) cervical plexuses, 3 (11%) brachial plexuses, 2 (7%) hypoglossal nerves, and 1 (4%) accessory nerve. Complete tumor resection was performed in 11 patients, and intracapsular enucleation of the tumor was performed in 16 patients. The rate of nerve palsy was 100 (11/11) and 31% (5/16). *Conclusions.* MRI is sensitive and specific in the diagnosis of schwannoma. Intracapsular enucleation was an effective and feasible method for preserving the neurological functions.

1. Introduction

Schwannoma is a benign neural sheath tumor, and it occurs in overall body areas including the head and neck region. As a slowly growing benign tumor, it has been reported that 25 to 45% of schwannomas were located in the extracranial head and neck region [1]. It involves the cranial nerves such as V, VII, X, XI, and XII or sympathetic and peripheral nerves [2].

Preoperative diagnostic investigations included ultrasonography (US), computed tomography (CT), magnetic resonance imaging (MRI), and fine needle aspiration cytology (FNAC) [3–5]. However, the preoperative diagnosis of schwannoma is difficult and should be suggested by clinical features and supported by investigations.

As for the management of schwannomas, multiple treatment options exist including observation, complete tumor excision, and intracapsular enucleation [6, 7]. For tumors arising from the major cranial nerves, complete tumor resection renders lifelong morbidity to the patients. On the other hand, the nerve-preserving excision method, such as intracapsular enucleation, does not guarantee intact nerve function after surgery. Because of the substantial chance of nerve palsy after operation, obtaining an accurate preoperative diagnosis, and preferably, with the identification of the nerve of origin is crucial to the management of the disease.

In the present study, clinical records of 27 cases with extracranial head and neck schwannoma treated at our department were retrospectively reviewed.

2. Methods

Between 2003 and 2010, 27 patients with extracranial head and neck schwannoma were operated on in the Department of Otorhinolaryngology at Kyushu University Hospital.

TABLE 1: Demographic data, radiological findings, and fine needle aspiration cytology.

Case	Gender	Age	Nerve origin	Tumor size	CT	MRI	FNAC
1	M	54	Vagus nerve	50 × 42 × 40 mm	ND	Schwannoma	Schwannoma
2	M	40	Vagus nerve	100 × 45 × 40 mm	ND	Glomus tumor or schwannoma	ND
3	M	58	Vagus nerve	45 × 35 × 33 mm	ND	Glomus tumor or schwannoma	ND
4	F	37	Vagus nerve	50 × 40 × 42 mm	ND	Schwannoma	Nondiagnostic
5	F	68	Vagus nerve	80 × 35 × 35 mm	Schwannoma	Schwannoma	ND
6	F	32	Vagus nerve	20 × 18 × 15 mm	Cervical tumor	Schwannoma	Nondiagnostic
7	F	80	Vagus nerve	30 × 25 × 25 mm	Cervical tumor	Schwannoma	ND
8	F	61	Vagus nerve	30 × 28 × 20 mm	Cervical tumor	Schwannoma	Nondiagnostic
9	M	54	Vagus nerve	27 × 25 × 25 mm	Cervical tumor	ND	ND
10	F	49	Vagus nerve	30 × 25 × 25 mm	ND	Glomus tumor or schwannoma	Nondiagnostic
11	M	52	Sympathetic trunk	70 × 35 × 35 mm	ND	Schwannoma	ND
12	M	47	Sympathetic trunk	30 × 28 × 22 mm	ND	Schwannoma	ND
13	M	79	Sympathetic trunk	45 × 25 × 20 mm	ND	Schwannoma	ND
14	F	35	Sympathetic trunk	40 × 30 × 25 mm	ND	Glomus tumor or schwannoma	ND
15	F	54	Sympathetic trunk	30 × 28 × 25 mm	ND	Schwannoma	ND
16	M	62	Sympathetic trunk	35 × 25 × 20 mm	ND	Glomus tumor	ND
17	F	42	Cervical plexus	60 × 35 × 33 mm	ND	Schwannoma	Schwannoma
18	M	50	Cervical plexus	35 × 30 × 30 mm	Cervical tumor	Schwannoma	ND
19	M	21	Cervical plexus	40 × 35 × 33 mm	ND	Schwannoma	Nondiagnostic
20	F	55	Cervical plexus	68 × 45 × 40 mm	ND	Schwannoma	Schwannoma
21	F	54	Cervical plexus	20 × 18 × 15 mm	ND	Schwannoma	Nondiagnostic
22	F	31	Brachial plexus	20 × 15 × 15 mm	ND	Schwannoma	Nondiagnostic
23	M	34	Brachial plexus	30 × 30 × 25 mm	ND	Schwannoma	ND
24	M	60	Brachial plexus	45 × 40 × 25 mm	ND	Schwannoma	Schwannoma
25	M	32	Hypoglossal nerve	50 × 35 × 35 mm	ND	Schwannoma	ND
26	F	57	Hypoglossal nerve	30 × 30 × 25 mm	Submandibullar gland tumor	ND	Nondiagnostic
27	F	69	Accessory nerve	40 × 30 × 30 mm	ND	Schwannoma	ND

ND: not done.

The data for the 27 patients, consisting of 14 males and 13 females, were analyzed. The subjects' ages ranged from 21 to 80 years, with a median age of 51 years. All cranial nerves were normal, and no Horner's syndrome was noted. Clinical history, surgical data, and postoperative morbidity were obtained. US were performed in all cases. Seven patients underwent CT with or without MRI. Twenty-five patients underwent MRI. Fine needle aspiration cytology (FNAC) was performed for 12 of the 27 patients after imaging. Tumor location, size, and demographic data are described in Table 1. The medical records of these patients were reviewed.

3. Results

3.1. Imaging Findings. The images of US typically showed a well-defined, ovoid or round, hypoechoic, and primarily homogeneous solid mass with or without a moderate posterior acoustic enhancement. None of them showed a direct connection to the nerve.

Seven of 27 patients underwent CT. Five patients (71%) had tumors that were hypoattenuated, with poor enhancement compared with adjoining skeletal muscles. Two tumors (29%) were isoattenuated to skeletal muscle. Only one of seven cases (14%) was able to suggest the diagnosis of schwannoma.

At MRI, all 25 schwannomas revealed relatively low signal intensity on T1-weighted imaging and signal hyperintensity on T2-weighted imaging, with 11 tumors (44%) showing homogeneously high intensity, and 14 tumors (56%) showing heterogeneously high intensity. There were no flow voids seen in any of the tumors. Twenty (80%) suggested the diagnosis of schwannoma. Figure 1 demonstrates the characteristic features of schwannomas on T1- and T2-weighting MRI. Depending on the site, a number of differential diagnoses were suggested including carotid body tumor, branchial cervical cyst, submandibular tumor, and metastases.

3.2. Fine Needle Aspiration Cytology (FNAC). From these 27 patients, 12 received fine needle aspiration cytology. Only

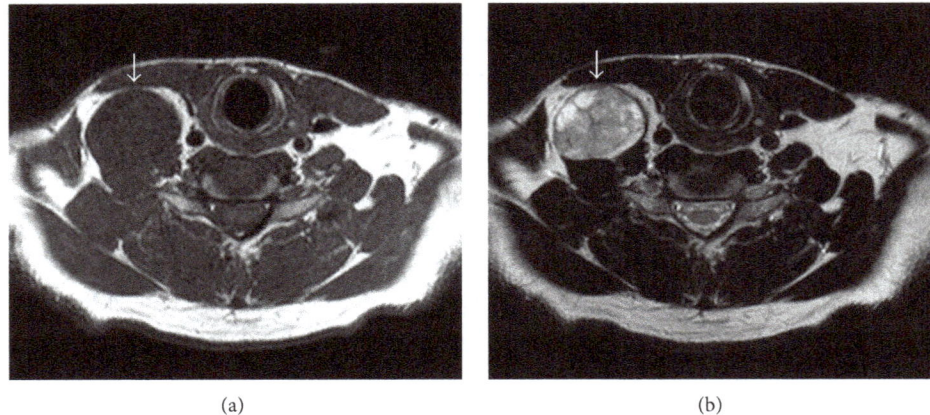

(a)   (b)

FIGURE 1: MRI findings for case 24. (a) Axial T1-weighted imaging showed a mass with signal hypointensity (arrow). (b) Axial T2-weighted imaging showed a mass with heterogeneous signal hyperintensity (arrow).

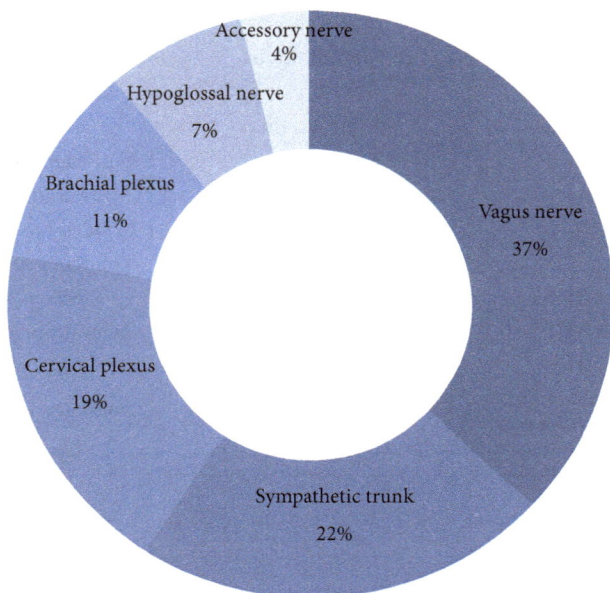

FIGURE 2: The nerve of origin of 27 extracranial head and neck schwannomas.

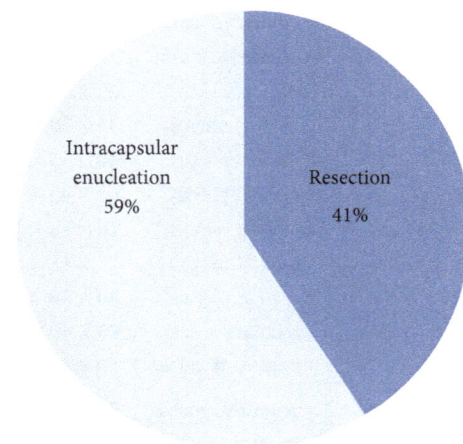

FIGURE 3: Operation method.

three cases (25%) displayed a specific diagnosis of schwannoma rendered on preoperative FNAC.

3.3. Treatment and Neural Function Outcome. All of the tumors were resected through a transcervical approach. The nerve of origin was mainly determined by the postoperative neurological findings. The distribution of 27 nerve of origins was 10 (37%) vagus nerves, 6 (22%) sympathetic trunks, 5 (19%) cervical plexuses, 3 (11%) brachial plexuses, 2 (7%) hypoglossal nerves, and 1 (4%) accessory nerve (Figure 2).

Complete tumor resection was performed on 11 patients, and intracapsular enucleation of the tumor was performed on 16 patients (Figure 3). The preoperative and postoperative neurological functions were evaluated. The rate of nerve palsy at 6 months after complete tumor resection and intracapsular

enucleation was 100 (11/11) and 31% (5/16), respectively. In the cases treated with intracapsular enucleation, only one case (20%) maintained normal postoperative neurological function of the five vagal schwannomas. Of the two sympathetic schwannomas, one case (50%) maintained normal postoperative neurological function. In the case of cervical plexus, brachial plexus, and accessory nerve schwannomas, there were no aggravated neurological deficits. In the cases with postoperative nerve palsy treated by intracapsular enucleation, 6 of 11 cases recovered from the palsy within 6 months after operation (Table 2).

4. Discussion

Schwannomas are benign tumors that originate from the Schwann cells of the nerve sheath. Schwann cells are neural crest-derived glial cells that are responsible for providing myelin insulation to peripheral nervous system axons [8]. There are several important issues relating to the diagnosis and management of these tumors.

TABLE 2: Neural function outcome after tumor intracapsular enucleation.

Case	Nerve origin	Preoperative status	Postoperrative status	6 months after operation
6	Vagus nerve	Normal	Vocal cord paralysis	Vocal cord paralysis
7	Vagus nerve	Normal	Vocal cord paralysis	Vocal cord paralysis
8	Vagus nerve	Normal	Vocal cord paralysis	Vocal cord paralysis
9	Vagus nerve	Normal	Vocal cord paralysis	Vocal cord paralysis
10	Vagus nerve	Normal	Normal	Normal
14	Sympathetic trunk	Normal	Ptosis	Ptosis
15	Sympathetic trunk	Normal	Ptosis	Normal (improved)
17	Cervical plexus	Normal	Paralysis	Normal (improved)
18	Cervical plexus	Normal	Paralysis	Normal (improved)
19	Cervical plexus	Normal	Normal	Normal
20	Cervical plexus	Normal	Normal	Normal
21	Cervical plexus	Normal	Normal	Normal
22	Brachial plexus	Normal	Paralysis	Normal (improved)
23	Brachial plexus	Normal	Paralysis	Normal (improved)
24	Brachial plexus	Normal	Paralysis	Normal (improved)
27	Accessory nerve	Normal	Normal	Normal

The first of these is difficulty with obtaining a preoperative diagnosis, since symptoms are usually nonspecific [9]. Symptoms, such as severe pain or cranial nerve palsy, would be unusual for these tumors. On examination, these benign masses are typically palpable. In treating schwannoma patients, it is critical to determine the origin of the tumor to preserve nerve function. Some authors suggest that preoperative evaluation with imaging modalities like CT and MRI in determining the nerve of origin may reduce the postoperative neural deficits [5, 10].

In terms of preoperative investigations, FNAC, US, and radiographic imaging with CT or MRI are usually performed. However, schwannomas are frequently difficult to characterize on FNAC. Liu et al. reported that the accuracy of FNAC was only 20% [11]. Our results also showed that only three cases (25%) displayed a specific diagnosis of schwannoma. It was not found to be of help in diagnosis.

In the current study, US, was performed in all cases. King et al. showed that schwannomas are highly vascular tumors with an abundance of vessels and blood flow, and the direct connection to the nerve is specific to neurogenic tumors [12]. Although two of five cases showed a direct connection to the nerve in other literature [5], these findings were not detected on US in our cases and were not sensitive enough to use this method.

On noncontrast CT, it was reported that schwannomas were typically hypodense versus muscle; with contrast, these lesions tended to show some peripheral enhancement [10]. Only one case (14%) in our study was able to suggest the diagnosis of schwannoma by CT and clinical features. On the other hand, MRI consistently identifies these lesions on both T1- and T2-weighted imaging. T1-weighted images display low signal intensity, and T2-weighted images show high intensity [5, 10, 13]. Hirano et al., also reported that MRI was especially useful for the diagnosis and peripheral hyperintense rim with central low intensity on enhanced T1 images of MRI [14]. The relationship between the schwannoma and its nerve of origin can be better appreciated with MRI than CT. In addition, MRI appears to be the investigation of choice for diagnosis and identification of nerve of origin. In our cases, twenty cases (80%) suggested the diagnosis of schwannoma. These results indicate that MRI is most sensitive and specific in the diagnosis of schwannoma [5]. The authors propose an algorithm for the management of extracranial head and neck schwannoma (Figure 4).

The decision of operation should be based on the balance between the risk and benefit of the surgery, that is, the severity of preoperative symptomatology and the anticipated postoperative neurological deficit. Surgical excision is the treatment of choice, but slow growth and the noninvasive nature of schwannomas of the neck also allow an observational approach. The preferred method of removing a schwannoma is intracapsular enucleation. Complications are usually transient and in most cases do not require treatment. According to the study by Valentino et al., intracapsular enucleation while preserving the nerve fibers preserved its function by more than 30% when compared to complete tumor resection [7]. In our cases, the rate of nerve palsy at 6 months after complete tumor resection and intracapsular enucleation was 100% and 31%, and none of them recurred more than two years from the operation. These results suggested that intracapsular enucleation was an effective and feasible method for preserving the neurological functions.

In conclusion, cervical schwannomas are rare neck tumors that are not widely discussed in the core surgical literature. Physicians who evaluate neck masses need to be aware of the diagnostic work-up, surgical treatment, and likely complications of this pathology. In addition, treatments assuring the preservation of neurological functions are needed, since surgical resection may cause fatal nerve damage unlike other tumors. An accurate preoperative diagnosis with identification of the nerve of origin, therefore, allows

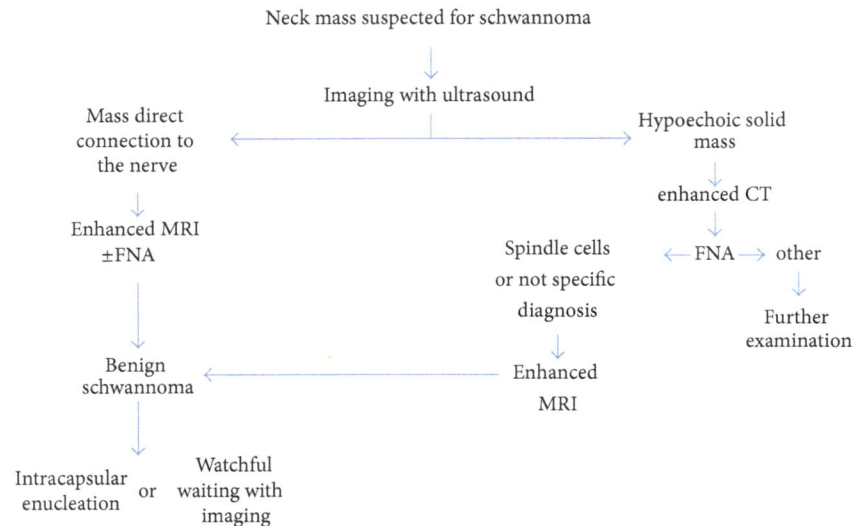

FIGURE 4: Diagnostic and treatment algorithm for the extracranial head and neck schwannoma.

patients to make an informed decision on whether to undergo operation or observation. In addition, before the surgical procedure, we could explain the possible nerve damages to patients.

References

[1] B. S. Ducatman, B. W. Scheithauer, D. G. Piepgras, H. M. Reiman, and D. M. Ilstrup, "Malignant peripheral nerve sheath tumors: a clinicopathologic study of 120 cases," *Cancer*, vol. 57, no. 10, pp. 2006–2021, 1986.

[2] M. P. Colreavy, P. D. Lacy, J. Hughes et al., "Head and neck schwannomas—a 10 year review," *Journal of Laryngology and Otology*, vol. 114, no. 2, pp. 119–124, 2000.

[3] Y. S. Leu and K. C. Chang, "Extracranial head and neck schwannomas: a review of 8 years experience," *Acta Oto-Laryngologica*, vol. 122, no. 4, pp. 435–437, 2002.

[4] R. N. Satarkar, S. S. Kolte, and S. K. Vujhini, "Cystic schwannoma in neck: fallacious diagnosis arrived on fine needle aspiration cytology," *Diagnostic Cytopathology*, vol. 39, pp. 866–867, 2011.

[5] Y. N. Kami, T. Chikui, K. Okamura et al., "Imaging findings of neurogenic tumours in the head and neck region," *Dentomaxillofacial Radiology*, vol. 41, pp. 18–23, 2012.

[6] M. J. Gibber, J. P. Zevallos, and M. L. Urken, "Enucleation of vagal nerve schwannoma using intraoperative nerve monitoring," *Laryngoscope*, vol. 122, pp. 790–792, 2012.

[7] J. Valentino, M. A. Boggess, J. L. Ellis, T. O. Hester, and R. O. Jones, "Expected neurologic outcomes for surgical treatment of cervical neurilemomas," *Laryngoscope*, vol. 108, no. 7, pp. 1009–1013, 1998.

[8] M. A. Shugar, W. W. Montgomery, and E. J. Reardon, "Management of paranasal sinus schwannomas," *Annals of Otology, Rhinology and Laryngology*, vol. 91, no. 1, pp. 65–69, 1982.

[9] J. D. Suh, V. R. Ramakrishnan, P. J. Zhang et al., "Diagnosis and endoscopic management of sinonasal schwannomas," *ORL—Journal for Otorhinolaryngology and Its Related Specialties*, vol. 73, pp. 308–312, 2011.

[10] G. Anil and T. Y. Tan, "Imaging characteristics of schwannoma of the cervical sympathetic chain: a review of 12 cases," *American Journal of Neuroradiology*, vol. 31, no. 8, pp. 1408–1412, 2010.

[11] H. L. Liu, S. Y. Yu, G. K. Li, and W. I. Wei, "Extracranial head and neck schwannomas: A Study of the Nerve of Origin," *European Archives of Oto-Rhino-Laryngology*, vol. 268, pp. 1343–1347, 2011.

[12] A. D. King, A. T. Ahuja, W. King, and C. Metreweli, "Sonography of peripheral nerve tumors of the neck," *American Journal of Roentgenology*, vol. 169, no. 6, pp. 1695–1698, 1997.

[13] T. Tomita, H. Ozawa, K. Sakamoto, K. Ogawa, K. Kameyama, and M. Fujii, "Diagnosis and management of cervical sympathetic chain schwannoma: a review of 9 cases," *Acta Oto-Laryngologica*, vol. 129, no. 3, pp. 324–329, 2009.

[14] S. Hirano, H. Kitamura, K. Miyata et al., "Extracranial neurinomas of head and neck," *Jibiinkouka Rinsyo*, vol. 87, pp. 253–257, 1994 (Japanese).

34

The Effect of Topical Application of Royal Jelly on Chemoradiotherapy-Induced Mucositis in Head and Neck Cancer: A Preliminary Study

Kohichi Yamauchi, Yasunao Kogashiwa, Yorihisa Moro, and Naoyuki Kohno

Department of Otolaryngology, Head and Neck Surgery, Kyorin University School of Medicine, 6-20-2 Shinkawa, Mitaka, Tokyo 181-8611, Japan

Correspondence should be addressed to Naoyuki Kohno; sukohno@kyorin-u.ac.jp

Academic Editor: David W. Eisele

Purpose. One of the common side effects experienced by head and neck cancer patients on chemoradiotherapy is mucositis. Severe mucositis may be controllable by limiting cancer therapy, but it has resulted in decreasing the completion rate of chemoradiotherapy. The efficacy of royal jelly (RJ) as prophylaxis against chemoradiotherapy-induced mucositis was evaluated through clinical scoring of oral and pharyngeal mucositis. *Methods.* In this randomized, single-blind (physician-blind), clinical trial, 13 patients with head and neck cancer requiring chemoradiation were randomly assigned to two groups. Seven patients assigned to the study group received RJ, and 6 patients were assigned to the control group. RJ group patients took RJ three times per day during treatment. The patients in both groups were evaluated twice a week for the development of mucositis using Common Terminology Criteria for Adverse Events version 3.0. *Results.* A significant reduction in mucositis was seen among RJ-treated patients compared with controls ($P < 0.001$). *Conclusion.* This study demonstrated that prophylactic use of RJ was effective in reducing mucositis induced by chemoradiotherapy in head and neck cancer patients. However, further studies are needed because of the small sample size and the absence of double blinding.

1. Introduction

Chemoradiotherapy for head and neck cancer induces mucositis, and it can also cause ulcers. Patients may experience pain, dysphagia, and dysphonia. As patients lose their oral feeding ability, they require external nutrition support. Strong early side effects of chemoradiotherapy may be controllable by limiting cancer therapy, but this has resulted in decreasing the chemoradiotherapy completion rate.

Many authors have reported the prophylactic use of bee products such as honey, royal jelly (RJ), and propolis for oral mucositis [1–7]. Kohno et al. reported the prophylactic use of honey extract as concurrent chemoradiotherapy for head and neck cancer patients [8]. Suemaru et al. also evaluated their effects on 5-fluorouracil-induced experimental oral mucositis in hamsters [9]. Erdem and Gungormus evaluated the effect of RJ on oral mucositis in patients undergoing radiotherapy and chemotherapy, and they reported that the mean time to resolution of oral mucositis was significantly shorter in the RJ group than in the control group [10].

The results suggested that the topical application of royal jelly may have a healing effect on severe oral mucositis induced by chemotherapy. Therefore, the efficacy of RJ as prophylaxis against chemoradiotherapy-induced mucositis was evaluated.

2. Materials and Methods

2.1. Design. The objective of this study was to evaluate the efficacy of RJ as prophylaxis against chemoradiotherapy-induced mucositis through clinical scoring of oral and pharyngeal mucositis in head and neck cancer patients.

This study was approved by the Ethics Committee of Kyorin University. All patients provided their written, informed consent. Head and neck squamous cell carcinoma patients were enrolled. Eligible patients were aged >18 years with a performance status of 0 to 1. Patients were randomly assigned to the control and RJ groups in this single-blind (physician-blind), clinical trial.

2.2. Induction Chemotherapy. The regimen was as follows. Nedaplatin ($80 \, \text{mg/m}^2$) was administered on day 1, and S-1 was simultaneously administered to patients orally twice daily at an initial dose of $65 \, \text{mg/m}^2/\text{day}$ (patients with body surface area (BSA) $> 1.5 \, \text{m}^2$ received $100 \, \text{mg/day}$; patients with $1.25 \, \text{m}^2 < \text{BSA} < 1.5 \, \text{m}^2$ received $80 \, \text{mg/day}$) for 2 weeks (days 1–14).

2.3. Concomitant Chemotherapy and Radiotherapy. Three chemotherapy regimens were used.

Weekly Nedaplatin and Docetaxel Regimen. During radiotherapy, weekly nedaplatin ($15 \, \text{mg/m}^2$) and docetaxel ($10 \, \text{mg/m}^2$) were administered for 6 courses intravenously.

S-1 Regimen. S-1 was administered at a dose of $80 \, \text{mg/day}$ on alternate days for 6 weeks.

Cisplatin Regimen. This was a form of selective arterial chemotherapy. Cisplatin ($5 \, \text{mg/m}^2$) was administered with the catheter in the vessel feeding the tumor on Monday to Friday (5 days/week) for 6 weeks.

Radiotherapy was administered to both groups: $2.0 \, \text{Gy/day}$ fractions on Monday to Friday for 33 to 35 fractions, for a total dose of 66 to 70 Gy by Linac.

2.4. RJ Group. RJ was prepared by Yamada Apiculture Center, Inc. (Okayama, Japan). RJ was collected from *Apis mellifera* L. that fed primarily on nectar and pollen from several flowers in Zhejiang, China. This product complies with the organic standards of the European Union. The product name is "organic royal jelly-gen nyu." It has the consistency of an ointment and contains a 1 gram measuring spoon that patients used to apply the RJ. The RJ group took 1 gram of RJ three times a day (3 g/day) during radiation treatment.

2.5. Control Group. The control group did not take any RJ.

2.6. Evaluation. Evaluation was done during the radiation period and 1 month after radiation. Patients were evaluated twice a week from the mouth to the pharynx by inspection and fiberscope examination. The reaction of the mucosa was graded using the Common Terminology Criteria for Adverse Events version 3.0 (CTCAE). The mucositis was graded as follows: Grade 1, erythema of the mucosa; Grade 2, patchy ulcerations or pseudomembranes; Grade 3, confluent ulcerations or pseudomembranes, bleeding with minor trauma; Grade 4, tissue necrosis, significant spontaneous bleeding, life-threatening consequences; and Grade 5, death.

2.7. Statistical Analysis. Data are shown as means ± standard deviation. Statistical significance was analyzed using the nonparametric Mann-Whitney U test for 2 groups. $P < 0.05$ was considered significant.

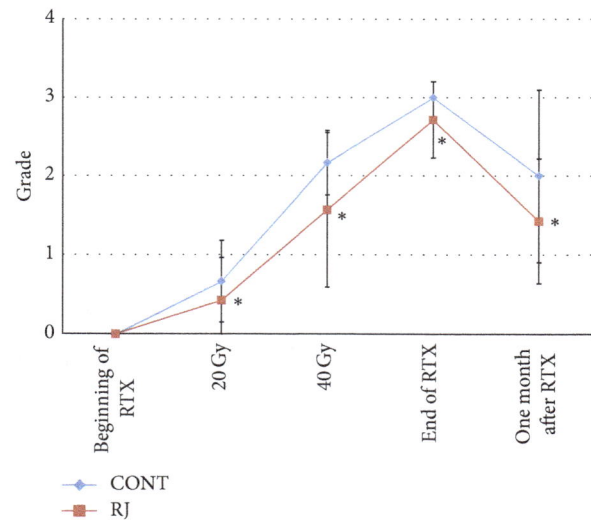

FIGURE 1: Grades of mucositis. Each data point represents the mean ± SD. Mann-Whitney U test: $^*P < 0.001$ versus control. RTX: radiotherapy.

3. Results

3.1. Patients' Characteristics. This study was done at Kyorin University Hospital, Japan, between 2009 and 2010. Thirteen patients (12 males, 1 female; median age 65.0 years; age range, 51–84 years) diagnosed with head and neck cancer were enrolled in the trial. The primary cancer site was hypopharyngeal in 5 patients, oropharyngeal in 4, laryngeal in 2, oral cavity in 1, and maxillary sinus in 1. The patients' characteristics are shown in Table 1. Seven patients were assigned to the RJ group and 6 to the control group.

There were no side effects such as allergy, irritation, or toxicity during treatment. All patients of both groups completed planned chemoradiotherapy.

3.2. Mucositis. Four patients received induction chemotherapy. All had no sign of mucositis at the beginning of concomitant chemoradiotherapy.

At the end of radiation, in the RJ group, Grade 3 mucositis was observed in 71.4% (5/7), and Grade 2 was seen in 28.6% (2/7). In the control group, Grade 3 mucositis was seen in 100% (6/6). In the control group, one case progressed to Grade 4 one month after treatment.

Figure 1 shows the grades of mucositis at the beginning of radiation, after 20 Gy, after 40 Gy, at the end of radiation, and 1 month after radiation. A significant difference was observed between the groups in the grade of mucositis at each point.

Figure 2 shows the average time to progress to Grade 2 mucositis from the beginning of radiation in both groups. The average time was 25.9 ± 9.6 days in the RJ group and 19.0 ± 4.1 days in the control group. The average time was significantly longer in the RJ group ($P < 0.001$).

Figure 3 shows the average time to progress to grade 3 mucositis from the beginning of radiation in both groups. The average time was 37.4 ± 11.8 days in the RJ group and

TABLE 1: Patients' profile.

Case	Group	Tumor site	Sex	Age (year)	TNM stage	IC	CRT
1	RJ	Larynx	M	59	T2N0M0	—	S-1
2	RJ	Oropharynx	M	84	T3N2cM0	—	S-1
3	RJ	Hypopharynx	M	62	TXN3M0	S1 + N	N + T
4	RJ	Hypopharynx	M	58	T1N3M0	S1 + N	N + T
5	RJ	Larynx	F	75	T2N0M0	—	S-1
6	RJ	Oropharynx	M	65	T4aN2bM0	—	CDDP
7	RJ	Hypopharynx	M	51	T2N2bM0	—	N + T
8	CONT	Hypopharynx	M	84	T2N0M0	—	S-1
9	CONT	Oropharynx	M	63	T1N2bM0	—	N + T
10	CONT	Oropharynx	M	62	T1N2aM0	—	CDDP
11	CONT	Oropharynx	M	65	T4aN0M0	S1 + N	N + T
12	CONT	Hypopharynx	M	66	T2N1M0	S1 + N	S-1
13	CONT	Maxillary sinus	M	78	T4aN0M0	—	CDDP

RJ: royal jelly, CONT: control, M: male, and F: female.
IC: induction chemotherapy.
CRT: chemoradiotherapy.
S1 + N: S1 + nedaplatin.
S1: S-1 regimen.
N + T: Weekly nedaplatin and docetaxel regimen.
CDDP: Cisplatin regimen.

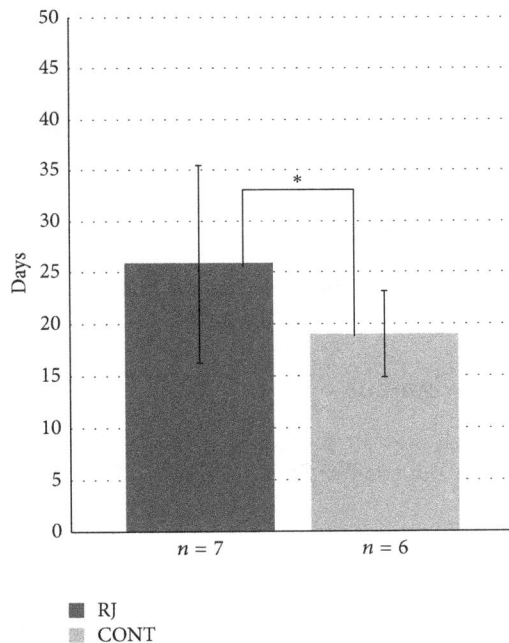

FIGURE 2: Time to progress to G2 mucositis. Each data point represents the mean ± SD. Mann-Whitney U test: $^{*}P < 0.001$ versus control.

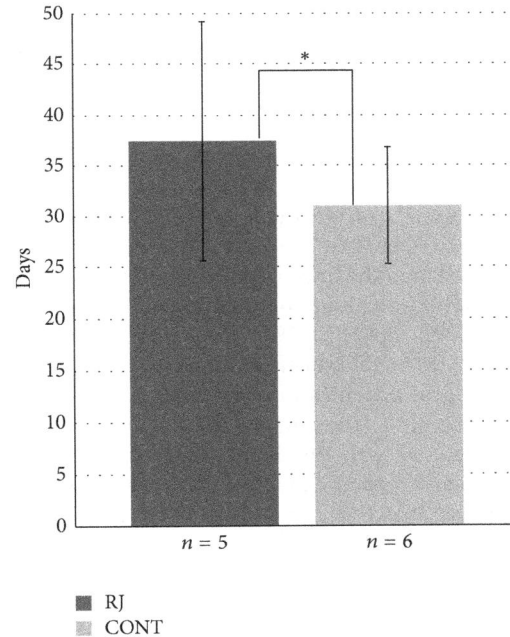

FIGURE 3: Time to progress to G3 mucositis. Each data point represents the mean ± SD. Mann-Whitney U test: $^{*}P < 0.001$ versus control.

31.0 ± 5.8 days in the control group. The average time was significantly longer in the RJ group ($P < 0.001$).

The results shown in Figures 1 and 2 suggest that applying RJ may prevent or reduce the severity of chemoradiotherapy-induced mucositis.

4. Discussion

Oral mucositis occurs in 15–40% of patients receiving standard chemotherapy, and 100% of patients receiving radiation therapy for head and neck cancer develop oral mucositis of varying degrees [11, 12]. The mechanism by which mucositis occurs is based on the fact that the oral mucosa has a high level of mitotic activity and high cell turnover. Due to the high degree of cell desquamation, there is a continuous need for cell multiplication to recover the oral mucosa. Tissues with high levels of mitotic activity respond rapidly to radiation, since the most sensitive phases of the cell cycle are G2 and mitosis. Thus, the mucosa is rapidly affected [13]. The same is true for chemotherapeutic drugs such as cisplatin, S-1, nedaplatin, and docetaxel. Chemoradiotherapy causes various changes in normal tissues, depending on the closely interrelated factors of total dose, fractionation schedule, and volume treated. Until now, there has been no way to prevent chemoradiotherapy-induced mucositis using only gargling and analgesics.

Bee products are commonly used traditionally to treat not only mucositis, but also skin disorders like cuts and burns as traditional wound healing agents [14–17]. Bee products are not artificial, but natural resources. This point results in easy acceptance among many cancer patients because they must always take so many artificial medicines. Therefore, this study evaluated the efficacy of bee products for mucositis induced by chemoradiotherapy.

The first issue that needed to be resolved was which kind of bee product would be best for mucositis. Suemaru et al. already evaluated three bee products (honey, RJ, and propolis) for 5-fluorouracil-induced experimental oral mucositis in hamsters [9]. They reported that only the RJ ointments significantly improved recovery from chemotherapy-induced mucositis in a dose-dependent manner. These results suggested that topical application of RJ has a healing effect on severe oral mucositis induced by chemotherapy. This is the reason why RJ was selected for this study.

RJ is mainly secreted by the hypopharyngeal and mandibular glands of worker honeybees between the sixth and twelfth days of their life, and it is an essential food for the development of the queen honeybee. RJ is a complex substance containing a unique combination of proteins (12–15%), sugars (10–12%), lipids (3–7%), amino acids, vitamins, and minerals [18]. RJ has also been demonstrated to possess many pharmacological activities in experimental animals, including antitumor [19], antioxidant [20, 21], anti-inflammatory [22], antibacterial [23], antiallergic [24], antiaging [25], and antihypertensive properties [26]. Recently, many authors have reported that the antioxidant effect is important for wound healing [27–29]. In this respect, RJ is an ideal agent. Inoue et al. reported the effect of dietary RJ on tissue DNA oxidative damage in mice [20]. In mice that were fed a dietary supplement of RJ, the levels of a marker of oxidative stress, 8-hydroxy-2-deoxyguanosine, were significantly reduced in kidney DNA and serum.

Furthermore, Kohno et al. suggested that RJ has anti-inflammatory actions through inhibiting proinflammatory cytokine production by activated macrophages [22]. They named the factor honeybee RJ-derived anti-inflammatory factor.

Watanabe et al. reported that RJ showed scavenging activity for 1,1-diphenyl-2-picrylhydrazyl (DPPH) radicals, superoxide radicals, and hydroxylradicals. Therefore, in the healing effect of RJ on mucositis, radical scavenging activity

is more important than keratinocyte growth factor generation [30].

RJ also has antibacterial actions. Royalisin found in the RJ of *Apis mellifera* is an antimicrobial peptide. It plays an important role in protecting wounds from being infected [23].

The present study showed that RJ prevented progression of mucositis from the early phase, and the average time to progress to Grade 2 mucositis was 25.9 ± 9.6 days versus 19.0 ± 4.1 days (RJ versus control). The average time to progress to Grade 3 was 37.4 ± 11.8 days versus 31.0 ± 5.8 days (RJ versus control). A significant reduction in mucositis occurred among RJ-treated patients compared with controls ($P < 0.001$).

At the end of radiation, Grade 3 mucositis was observed in 71.4% (5/7) in the RJ group and 100% (6/6) in the control group. These results suggest that topical application of RJ is effective in preventing accelerated mucositis induced by chemoradiotherapy.

In this study, only RJ was evaluated for mucositis, but Nakajima et al. reported that, of all bee products, propolis is the most powerful antioxidant [21]. An antioxidant effect is important in the mucositis healing process. Although we would have liked to evaluate propolis, propolis extracted with water was not available. Propolis extracted with ethanol is not good for mucositis due to stimulation by alcohol. In the future, we would like to evaluate propolis extracted with water.

Thus, further studies are needed to evaluate the effect of RJ on mucositis and elucidate the precise mechanisms of action. Nevertheless, it is possible to say that RJ tends to prevent progression of mucositis.

Conflict of Interests

The authors declare that there is no conflict of interests regarding the publication of this paper.

Acknowledgment

This research was supported by Yamada Research Grant (2009) from Yamada Bee Farm in Japan.

References

[1] M. Abdulrhman, N. Samir El Barbary, D. Ahmed Amin, and R. Saeid Ebrahim, "Honey and a mixture of honey, beeswax, and olive oilpropolis extract in treatment of chemotherapy-induced oral mucositis: a randomized controlled pilot study," *Pediatric Hematology and Oncology*, vol. 29, no. 3, pp. 285–292, 2012.

[2] J. Bardy, A. Molassiotis, W. D. Ryder et al., "A double-blind, placebo-controlled, randomised trial of active manuka honey and standard oral care for radiation-induced oral mucositis," *British Journal of Oral and Maxillofacial Surgery*, vol. 50, no. 3, pp. 221–226, 2012.

[3] B. M. Biswal, A. Zakaria, and N. M. Ahmad, "Topical application of honey in the management of radiation mucositis: a preliminary study," *Supportive Care in Cancer*, vol. 11, no. 4, pp. 242–248, 2003.

[4] B. Khanal, M. Baliga, and N. Uppal, "Effect of topical honey on limitation of radiation-induced oral mucositis: an intervention study," *International Journal of Oral and Maxillofacial Surgery*, vol. 39, no. 12, pp. 1181–1185, 2010.

[5] M. Motallebnejad, S. Akram, A. Moghadamnia, Z. Moulana, and S. Omidi, "The effect of topical application of pure honey on radiation-induced mucositis: a randomized clinical trial," *Journal of Contemporary Dental Practice*, vol. 9, no. 3, pp. 40–47, 2008.

[6] U. M. Rashad, S. M. Al-Gezawy, E. El-Gezawy, and A. N. Azzaz, "Honey as topical prophylaxis against radiochemotherapy-induced mucositis in head and neck cancer," *Journal of Laryngology and Otology*, vol. 123, no. 2, pp. 223–228, 2009.

[7] J. J. Song, P. Twumasi-Ankrah, and R. Salcido, "Systematic review and meta-analysis on the use of honey to protect from the effects of radiation-induced oral mucositis," *Advances in Skin and Wound Care*, vol. 25, no. 1, pp. 23–28, 2012.

[8] N. Kohno, S. Kitahara, E. Tamura, and T. Tanabe, "Concurrent chemoradiotherapy with low-dose cisplatin plus 5-fluorouracil for the treatment of patients with unresectable head and neck cancer," *Oncology*, vol. 63, no. 3, pp. 226–231, 2002.

[9] K. Suemaru, R. Cui, B. Li et al., "Topical application of royal jelly has a healing effect on 5-fluorouracil-induced experimental oral mucositis in hamsters," *Methods and Findings in Experimental and Clinical Pharmacology*, vol. 30, no. 2, pp. 103–106, 2008.

[10] O. Erdem and Z. Gungormus, "The effect of royal jelly on oral mucositis in patients undergoing radiotherapy and chemotherapy," *Holistic Nursing Practice*, vol. 28, pp. 242–246, 2014.

[11] D. Das, S. K. Agarwal, and H. M. Chandola, "Protective effect of Yashtimadhu (*Glycyrrhiza glabra*) against side effects of radiation/chemotherapy in head and neck malignancies," *Ayu*, vol. 32, pp. 196–199, 2012.

[12] A. V. S. Suresh, P. P. Varma, S. Sinha et al., "Risk-scoring system for predicting mucositis in patients of head and neck cancer receiving concurrent chemoradiotherapy [rssm-hn]," *Journal of Cancer Research and Therapeutics*, vol. 6, no. 4, pp. 448–451, 2010.

[13] R. C. S. Santos, R. S. Dias, A. J. Giordani, R. A. Segreto, and H. R. C. Segreto, "Mucositis in head and neck cancer patients undergoing radiochemotherapy," *Revista da Escola de Enfermagem*, vol. 45, no. 6, pp. 1338–1344, 2011.

[14] B. K. Boekema, L. Pool, and M. M. Ulrich, "The effect of a honey based gel and silver sulphadiazine on bacterial infections of in vitro burn wounds," *Burns*, vol. 39, no. 4, pp. 754–759, 2013.

[15] S. Farsaei, H. Khalili, and E. S. Farboud, "Potential role of statins on wound healing: review of the literature," *International Wound Journal*, vol. 9, no. 3, pp. 238–247, 2012.

[16] S. S. Gupta, O. Singh, P. S. Bhagel, S. Moses, S. Shukla, and R. K. Mathur, "Honey dressing versus silver sulfadiazene dressing for wound healing in burn patients: a retrospective study," *Journal of Cutaneous and Aesthetic Surgery*, vol. 4, no. 3, pp. 183–187, 2011.

[17] M. K. Tan, D. S. Hasan Adli, M. A. Tumiran, M. A. Abdulla, and K. M. Yusoff, "The efficacy of Gelam honey dressing towards excisional wound healing," *Evidence-Based Complementary and Alternative Medicine*, vol. 2012, Article ID 805932, 6 pages, 2012.

[18] H. Morita, T. Ikeda, K. Kajita et al., "Effect of royal jelly ingestion for six months on healthy volunteers," *Nutrition Journal*, vol. 11, no. 1, article 77, 2012.

[19] G. F. Townsend, J. F. Morgan, S. Tolnai, B. Hazlett, H. J. Morton, and R. W. Shuel, "Studies on the in vitro antitumor activity of fatty acids. I. 10-Hydroxy-2-decenoic acid from royal jelly," *Cancer research*, vol. 20, pp. 503–510, 1960.

[20] S.-I. Inoue, S. Koya-Miyata, S. Ushio, K. Iwaki, M. Ikeda, and M. Kurimoto, "Royal Jelly prolongs the life span of C3H/HeJ mice: correlation with reduced DNA damage," *Experimental Gerontology*, vol. 38, no. 9, pp. 965–969, 2003.

[21] Y. Nakajima, K. Tsuruma, M. Shimazawa, S. Mishima, and H. Hara, "Comparison of bee products based on assays of antioxidant capacities," *BMC Complementary and Alternative Medicine*, vol. 9, article 4, 2009.

[22] K. Kohno, I. Okamoto, O. Sano et al., "Royal jelly inhibits the production of proinflammatory cytokines by activated macrophages," *Bioscience, Biotechnology and Biochemistry*, vol. 68, no. 1, pp. 138–145, 2004.

[23] J.-M. Tseng, J.-R. Huang, H.-C. Huang, J. T. C. Tzen, W.-M. Chou, and C.-C. Peng, "Facilitative production of an antimicrobial peptide royalisin and its antibody via an artificial oil-body system," *Biotechnology Progress*, vol. 27, no. 1, pp. 153–161, 2011.

[24] I. Okamoto, Y. Taniguchi, T. Kunikata et al., "Major royal jelly protein 3 modulates immune responses in vitro and in vivo," *Life Sciences*, vol. 73, no. 16, pp. 2029–2045, 2003.

[25] H. M. Park, M. H. Cho, Y. Cho, and S. Y. Kim, "Royal jelly increases collagen production in rat skin after ovariectomy," *Journal of Medicinal Food*, vol. 15, no. 6, pp. 568–575, 2012.

[26] K.-H. Tokunaga, C. Yoshida, K.-M. Suzuki et al., "Antihypertensive effect of peptides from Royal Jelly in spontaneously hypertensive rats," *Biological and Pharmaceutical Bulletin*, vol. 27, no. 2, pp. 189–192, 2004.

[27] M. Deniz, H. Borman, T. Seyhan, and M. Haberal, "An effective antioxidant drug on prevention of the necrosis of zone of stasis: N-acetylcysteine," *Burns*, vol. 39, no. 2, pp. 320–325, 2013.

[28] C.-Y. Hsiao, C.-Y. Hung, T.-H. Tsai, and K.-F. Chak, "A study of the wound healing mechanism of a traditional chinese medicine, *Angelica sinensis*, using a proteomic approach," *Evidence-Based Complementary and Alternative Medicine*, vol. 2012, Article ID 467531, 14 pages, 2012.

[29] Y.-H. Lee, J.-J. Chang, C.-T. Chien, M.-C. Yang, and H.-F. Chien, "Antioxidant sol-gel improves cutaneous wound healing in streptozotocin-induced diabetic rats," *Experimental Diabetes Research*, vol. 2012, Article ID 504693, 11 pages, 2012.

[30] S. Watanabe, K. Suemaru, K. Takechi, H. Kaji, K. Imai, and H. Araki, "Oral mucosal adhesive films containing royal jelly accelerate recovery from 5-fluorouracil-induced oral mucositis," *Journal of Pharmacological Sciences*, vol. 121, no. 2, pp. 110–118, 2013.

Permissions

All chapters in this book were first published in IJOTO, by Hindawi Publishing Corporation; hereby published with permission under the Creative Commons Attribution License or equivalent. Every chapter published in this book has been scrutinized by our experts. Their significance has been extensively debated. The topics covered herein carry significant findings which will fuel the growth of the discipline. They may even be implemented as practical applications or may be referred to as a beginning point for another development.

The contributors of this book come from diverse backgrounds, making this book a truly international effort. This book will bring forth new frontiers with its revolutionizing research information and detailed analysis of the nascent developments around the world.

We would like to thank all the contributing authors for lending their expertise to make the book truly unique. They have played a crucial role in the development of this book. Without their invaluable contributions this book wouldn't have been possible. They have made vital efforts to compile up to date information on the varied aspects of this subject to make this book a valuable addition to the collection of many professionals and students.

This book was conceptualized with the vision of imparting up-to-date information and advanced data in this field. To ensure the same, a matchless editorial board was set up. Every individual on the board went through rigorous rounds of assessment to prove their worth. After which they invested a large part of their time researching and compiling the most relevant data for our readers.

The editorial board has been involved in producing this book since its inception. They have spent rigorous hours researching and exploring the diverse topics which have resulted in the successful publishing of this book. They have passed on their knowledge of decades through this book. To expedite this challenging task, the publisher supported the team at every step. A small team of assistant editors was also appointed to further simplify the editing procedure and attain best results for the readers.

Apart from the editorial board, the designing team has also invested a significant amount of their time in understanding the subject and creating the most relevant covers. They scrutinized every image to scout for the most suitable representation of the subject and create an appropriate cover for the book.

The publishing team has been an ardent support to the editorial, designing and production team. Their endless efforts to recruit the best for this project, has resulted in the accomplishment of this book. They are a veteran in the field of academics and their pool of knowledge is as vast as their experience in printing. Their expertise and guidance has proved useful at every step. Their uncompromising quality standards have made this book an exceptional effort. Their encouragement from time to time has been an inspiration for everyone.

The publisher and the editorial board hope that this book will prove to be a valuable piece of knowledge for researchers, students, practitioners and scholars across the globe.

List of Contributors

Guilherme Machado de Carvalho, Alexandre C. Guimaraes, Alexandre S.M. Duarte, Eder B. Muranaka, Marcelo N. Soki, Renata S. Zanotello Martins, Walter A. Bianchini, Jorge R. Paschoal and Arthur M. Castilho
Otology, Audiology and Implantable Ear Prostheses, Ear, Nose, Throat and Head & Neck Surgery Department, P.O. Box 6111, Campinas University, UNICAMP, 13081-970 S~ao Paulo, SP, Brazil

Pietro Canzi, Anna Berardi, Fabio Pagella and Marco Benazzo
Department of Otorhinolaryngology, University of Pavia and IRCCS Policlinico San Matteo Foundation, Viale Camillo Golgi 19, 27100 Pavia, Italy

Carmine Tinelli
Biometrics Unit, University of Pavia and IRCCS Policlinico San Matteo Foundation, Viale Camillo Golgi 19, 27100 Pavia, Italy

Filippo Montevecchi and Claudio Vicini
ENT Unit, Department of Special Surgery, Morgagni-Pierantoni Hospital, Via Forlanini 34, 47121 Forlí, Italy

Ahmad Nasrat Al-juboori
Ibn Sina College ofMedicine, Al-IraqiaUniversity, Baghdad, Iraq

Emily Papsin and Adrienne L. Harrison
Auditory Science Laboratory, Neuroscience and Mental Health Program, The Hospital for Sick Children, 555 University Avenue, Toronto, ON, Canada M5G 1X8

Mattia Carraro
Auditory Science Laboratory, Neuroscience and Mental Health Program, The Hospital for Sick Children, 555 University Avenue, Toronto, ON, Canada M5G 1X8
Institute of Biomaterials and Biomedical Engineering, University of Toronto, Toronto, ON, Canada M5S 1A1

Robert V. Harrison
Auditory Science Laboratory, Neuroscience and Mental Health Program, The Hospital for Sick Children, 555 University Avenue, Toronto, ON, Canada M5G 1X8
Institute of Biomaterials and Biomedical Engineering, University of Toronto, Toronto, ON, Canada M5S 1A1
Department of Otolaryngology-Head and Neck Surgery, University of Toronto, 190 Elizabeth Street, Toronto, ON, Canada M5G 2N2

Kazuhiro Nomura
Department of Otorhinolaryngology, Jikei University School of Medicine, 3-25-8 Nishishinbashi, Minato-ku, Tokyo 105-8461, Japan
Department of Otolaryngology-Head and Neck Surgery, Tohoku University Graduate School of Medicine, 1-1 Seiryo-cho, Aoba-ku, Sendai, Miyagi 980-8574, Japan

Daiya Asaka, Tsuguhisa Nakayama, Tetsushi Okushi, Yoshinori Matsuwaki, Tsuyoshi Yoshimura, Mamoru Yoshikawa Nobuyoshi Otori and Hiroshi Moriyama
Department of Otorhinolaryngology, Jikei University School of Medicine, 3-25-8 Nishishinbashi, Minato-ku, Tokyo 105-8461, Japan

Toshimitsu Kobayashi
Department of Otolaryngology-Head and Neck Surgery, Tohoku University Graduate School of Medicine, 1-1 Seiryo-cho, Aoba-ku, Sendai, Miyagi 980-8574, Japan

J. C. Bewick, M. A. Buchanan and A. C. Frosh
Department of ENT, East and North Hertfordshire NHS Trust, Lister Hospital, Corey's Mill Lane, Stevenage SG1 4AB, UK

E. Thibaudeau, O. Abboud, L. Guertin, A. Christopoulos and J. Tabet
Department of Head and Neck Surgery, Centre Hospitalier de l'Université de Montréal, HôpitalNotre-Dame, 1560 Sherbrooke Est, Montreal (Quebec), Canada H2L 4M1

B. Fortin
Department of Radiation Oncology, Hôpital Maisonneuve-Rosemont, 5415 Boulevard de l'Assomption, Montréal (Quebec), Canada H1T 2M4

F. Coutlée
Department of Microbiology, Centre Hospitalier de l'Université de Montréal, Hôpital Notre-Dame, 1560 Sherbrooke Est, Montreal (Quebec), Canada H2L 4M1

P. Nguyen-Tan
Department of Radiation Oncology, Centre Hospitalier de l'Université de Montréal, Hôpital Notre-Dame, 1560 Sherbrooke Est, Montreal (Quebec), Canada H2L 4M1

X. Weng and M.-L. Audet
Department of Haematology and Medical Oncology, Centre Hospitalier de l'Université de Montréal, Hôpital Notre-Dame, 1560 Sherbrooke Est, Montreal (Quebec), Canada H2L 4M1

D. Soulières
Department of Haematology and Medical Oncology, Centre Hospitalier de l'Université de Montréal, Hôpital Notre-Dame, 1560 Sherbrooke Est, Montreal (Quebec), Canada H2L 4M1
Laboratoire de Biologie Moléculaire et Hématologie Spéciale, Département d'Hématologie, Hématologue et Oncologue Médical, Centre Hospitalier de l'Université de Montréal, HôpitalNotre-Dame, 1560 Sherbrooke Est, Montreal (Quebec), CanadaH2L 4M1

Saad Musbah Alasil
Department of Microbiology, Faculty of Medicine, MAHSA University, 59100 Kuala Lumpur, Malaysia

Rahmat Omar
Pantai Hospital Cheras, 56100 Kuala Lumpur, Malaysia

Salmah Ismail
Institute of Biological Science, Faculty of Science, University of Malaya, 50603 Kuala Lumpur, Malaysia

Mohd Yasim Yusof and Ghulam N. Dhabaan
Department of Medical Microbiology, Faculty of Medicine, University of Malaya, 50603 Kuala Lumpur, Malaysia

Mahmood Ameen Abdulla
Department of Biomedical Science, Faculty of Medicine, University of Malaya, 50603 Kuala Lumpur, Malaysia

Abdul Latif Hamdan and Jad Jabour
Department of Otolaryngology-Head & Neck Surgery, American University of Beirut Medical Center, P.O. Box 110-236, Beirut, Lebanon

Sami T. Azar
Department of Otolaryngology-Head & Neck Surgery, American University of Beirut Medical Center, P.O. Box 110-236, Beirut, Lebanon
Department of Internal Medicine, Division of Endocrinology and Metabolism, American University of Beirut Medical Center, P.O. Box 110-236, Beirut, Lebanon

Sangeet Kumar Agarwal, Satinder Singh, Shalabh Sharma and Asish Kr. Lahiri
Department of Otorhinolaryngology and Head, Neck Surgery, Sir Ganga Ram Hospital, New Delhi 110049, India

Samarjit Singh Ghuman
Department of Radiology, Sir Ganga Ram Hospital, New Delhi 110049, India

Benson Wahome Karanja
University of Nairobi, P.O. Box 2209-00202, KNH, Nairobi, Kenya

Herbert Ouma Oburra
Department of Surgery, University of Nairobi, P.O. Box 30197-00100, G.P.O. Nairobi, Kenya

Peter Masinde
ENT Department, Kenyatta National Hospital (KNH), University of Nairobi, P.O. Box 20723-00202, Nairobi, Kenya

Dalton Wamalwa
Department of Pediatrics and Child Health, University of Nairobi, P.O. Box 19676-00202, Nairobi, Kenya

K. L. Tremblay and C. W. Miller
Department of Speech and Hearing Sciences, University of Washington, Seattle, WA 98105, USA

Tamer S. Sobhy
Faculty of Medicine, Ain Shams University, 15 Khalifa Maamoon, Heliopolis, Cairo, Egypt

Nobuo Ohta, TomooWatanabe, Tsukasa Ito, Toshinori Kubota, Yusuke Suzuki, Akihiro Ishida, Masaru Aoyagi and Seiji Kakehata
Department of Otolaryngology, Head and Neck Surgery, Faculty of Medicine, Yamagata University, 2-2-2 Iida-nishi, Yamagata 990-9585, Japan

AtsushiMatsubara
Department of Otorhinolaryngology, Hirosaki University Graduate School of Medicine, Hirosaki 036-8562, Japan

Kenji Izuhara
Division of Medical Biochemistry, Department of Biomolecular Sciences, Faculty of Medicine, Saga University, Saga 840-8502, Japan

Samira Anderson
Auditory Neuroscience Laboratory, Northwestern University, Evanston, IL 60208, USA
Department of Communication Sciences, Northwestern University, Evanston, IL 60208, USA
Department of Hearing and Speech Sciences, University of Maryland, 0100 Lefrak Hall, College Park, MD 20742, USA

Nina Kraus
Auditory Neuroscience Laboratory, Northwestern University, Evanston, IL 60208, USA
Department of Communication Sciences, Northwestern University, Evanston, IL 60208, USA
Department of Neurobiology and Physiology, Northwestern University, Evanston, IL 60208, USA
Department of Otolaryngology, Northwestern University, Evanston, IL 60208, USA

Aqeel Absalan and Ibrahim Pirasteh
Audiology Department, Faculty of Rehabilitation, Zahedan University of Medical Sciences & Health Services, Zahedan, Iran

Gholam Ali Dashti Khavidaki
Otolaryngology (ENT) Department, Zahedan University of Medical Sciences & Health Services, Zahedan, Iran

Azam Asemi rad
Department of Anatomical Sciences, Shahid Beheshti University of Medical Sciences, Tehran, Iran

Ali Akbar Nasr Esfahani
Audiology Department, Faculty of Rehabilitation, Tehran University of Medical Sciences & Health Services, Tehran, Iran

Mohammad Hussein Nilforoush
Audiology Department, Faculty of Rehabilitation, Isfahan University of Medical Sciences, Isfahan, Iran

Tolga Ersözlü
Department of Otorhinolaryngology Head and Neck Surgery, Elbistan State Hospital, 46300 Kahramanmaras, Turkey

Yavuz Selim YJldJrJm
Department of Otorhinolaryngology and Head and Neck Surgery, Faculty of Medicine, Bezmialem Vakif University, Adnan Menderes Bulvarı, Vatan Caddesi Fatih, 34093 Istanbul, Turkey

Selman Sarica
Department of Otorhinolaryngology Head and Neck Surgery, Afs¸in State Hospital, 46300 Kahramanmaras, Turkey

CatherineM. McMahon
Centre for Language Sciences, Australian Hearing Hub, 16 University Dve, Macquarie University, North Ryde, NSW2109, Australia
HEARing Cooperative Research Centre, 550 Swanston St, Audiology, Hearing and Speech Sciences University of Melbourne, VIC 3010, Australia

Paul Mitchell and Bamini Gopinath
Centre for Vision Research, Department of Ophthalmology andWestmead Millennium Institute, The University of Sydney, Westmead Hospital,Westmead, NSW2145, Australia

Julie Schneider and Stephen R. Leeder
Menzies Centre for Health Policy, Victor Coppleson Building,The University of Sydney, NSW2006, Australia

Jennifer Reath
School of Medicine, University ofWestern Sydney, Penrith, NSW2751, Australia

Louise Hickson
HEARing Cooperative Research Centre, 550 Swanston St, Audiology, Hearing and Speech Sciences University of Melbourne, VIC 3010, Australia
School of Health and Rehabilitation Sciences, St Lucia Campus, University of Queensland, Brisbane, QLD 4072, Australia

Robert Cowan
HEARing Cooperative Research Centre, 550 Swanston St, Audiology, Hearing and Speech Sciences University of Melbourne, VIC 3010, Australia
School of Audiology, 550 Swanston St, Audiology, Hearing and Speech Sciences, University of Melbourne, VIC 3010, Australia

Masafumi Ohki
Department of Otolaryngology, Saitama Medical Center, 1981 Kamoda, Kawagoe-shi, Saitama 350-8550, Japan

Masanobu Shinogami
Department of Otolaryngology, Tokyo Metropolitan Police Hospital, 4-22-1 Nakano, Nakano-ku, Tokyo 164-8541, Japan

Aamir Yousuf, Zafarullah Beigh, Raja Salman Khursheed, Aleena Shafi Jallu and Rafiq Ahmad Pampoori
Department of ENT and HNS, Government Medical College, Srinagar, Jammu and Kashmir 190001, India

Russel Kahmke, Richard L. Scher and Ramon M. Esclamado
Division of Otolaryngology-Head and Neck Surgery, Department of Surgery, Duke University Medical Center, Duke University, Durham, NC 27710, USA

Walter T. Lee and Liana Puscas
Division of Otolaryngology-Head and Neck Surgery, Department of Surgery, Duke University Medical Center, Duke University, Durham, NC 27710, USA
Section of Otolaryngology-Head and Neck Surgery, Department of Surgery, Durham VA Medical Center, Durham, NC 27705, USA

Michael J. Shealy
Division of Pathology Clinical Services, Department of Pathology, Duke University Medical Center, Duke University, Durham, NC 27710, USA

Warner M. Burch
Division of Endocrinology, Metabolism, and Nutrition, Department of Medicine, Duke University Medical Center, Duke University, Durham, NC 27710, USA

Mustafa Sahin
Department of Otorhinolaryngology, Diskapi Yildirim Beyazit Research and Training Hospital, Irfan Bastug Street, Dıskapi, 06110 Ankara, Turkey

Cem Bilgen and RasitMidilli
Department of Otorhinolaryngology, Ege University School of Medicine, İzmir, Turkey

M. Sezai Tasbakan and Ozen K. Basoglu
Department of Chest Diseases, Ege University School of Medicine, İzmir, Turkey

Eric Bissada, Olivier Abboud, Zahi Abou Chacra, Louis Guertin, Jean-Claude Tabet and Ève Thibaudeau
Department of Head and Neck Surgery, Centre Hospitalier de l'Université de Montréal (CHUM), Montreal, QC, Canada

Phuc Félix Nguyen-Tan, Louise Lambert and Bernard Fortin
Department of Radiation Oncology, CHUM, Montreal, QC, Canada

Xiaoduan Weng, Marie-Lise Audet and Denis Soulières
Department of Hematology and Medical Oncology, CHUM, Montreal, QC, Canada

Anja Lieder and Wolfgang Issing
Department of Otorhinolaryngology, Freeman Hospital, Freeman Road, High Heaton, Newcastle upon Tyne NE7 7DN, UK

Owen PyekoMenach and Herbert Ouma Oburra
Department of Surgery, ENT Division, University of
Nairobi, P.O. Box 330-00202, Nairobi, Kenya
ENT Head & Neck Department, Kenyatta National
Hospital, P.O. Box 20723-00202, Nairobi, Kenya

Asmeeta Patel
ENT Head & Neck Department, Kenyatta National
Hospital, P.O. Box 20723-00202, Nairobi, Kenya

**Tsutomu Nomura, YoshimiMakizumi, Tsuyoshi
Yoshida and Tatsuya Yamasoba**
Department of Otolaryngology and Head and Neck
Surgery, Faculty of Medicine, University of Tokyo, 7-3-1
Hongo, Bunkyo-ku, Tokyo 113-8655, Japan

**S. Kortequee, P. D. Karkos, H. Atkinson, D. C. Sylvester
and S. Sood**
Department of Otolaryngology, Bradford Royal Infirmary,
Bradford BD9 6RJ, UK

R. S. Harar and N. Sethi
Department of Otolaryngology, Pinderfields Hospital,
Wakefield WF1 4DG, UK

W. J. Issing
Department of Otolaryngology, The Freeman Hospital,
Newcastle upon Tyne NE7 7DN, UK

Daniel de SousaMichels and Márcio Nakanishi
Department of Otorhinolaryngology and Head and Neck
Surgery, Brasília University Hospital, HUB, SGAN 605,
Avenida L2Norte, 70830-200 Brasília, DF, Brazil

Amanda da Mota Silveira Rodrigues
Universidade de Brasília (UnB), Campus Universitário
Darcy Ribeiro, 70910-900 Brasília, DF, Brazil

**André Luiz Lopes Sampaio and Alessandra Ramos
Venosa**
Department of Otorhinolaryngology and Head and Neck
Surgery, Brasília University Hospital, HUB, SGAN 605,
Avenida L2Norte, 70830-200 Brasília, DF, Brazil
Universidade de Brasília (UnB), Campus Universitário
Darcy Ribeiro, 70910-900 Brasília, DF, Brazil

Larysa Sokolova
Faculty of Neurology, Bohomolets National Medical
University, Shevchenko Avenue, 13, Kiev 01601, Ukraine

Robert Hoerr
Clinical ResearchDepartment, Dr.Willmar Schwabe
GmbH&Co. KG, Willmar-Schwabe-Straße 4, 76227
Karlsruhe, Germany

Tamara Mishchenko
Institute of Neurology, Psychiatry and Narcology of the
NAMS of Ukraine SI, 46, Akademika Pavlova Street,
Kharkiv 61068, Ukraine

**Carolina Mensi, Dario Consonni, Claudia Sieno and
Luciano Riboldi**
Department of Preventive Medicine, Fondazione IRCCS
Ca' Granda—Ospedale Maggiore Policlinico, Via San
Barnaba 8, 20122Milan, Italy

Sara De Matteis
National Heart & Lung Institute, Department of
Occupational & Environmental Medicine, Imperial
College London, London SW3 6LR, UK
Department of Clinical Science and Community Health,
Universit`a Degli Studi di Milano, Via San Barnaba 8,
20122Milan, Italy

Pier Alberto Bertazzi
Department of Preventive Medicine, Fondazione IRCCS
Cá Granda—Ospedale Maggiore Policlinico, Via San
Barnaba 8, 20122Milan, Italy
Department of Clinical Science and Community Health,
Universitá Degli Studi di Milano, Via San Barnaba 8,
20122Milan, Italy

Vinaya K. C. Manchaiah
Centre for Long Term and Chronic Conditions, College
of Human and Health Sciences, Swansea University,
Swansea SA2 8PP, UK
Linnaeus Centre HEAD, Swedish Institute for Disability
Research, Department of Behavioural Sciences and
Learning, Linköping University, 58183 Linköping, Sweden

Dafydd Stephens
Department of Psychological Medicine & Neurology,
School of Medicine, Cardiff University, Cardiff CF14
4XN, UK

Thomas Lunner
Linnaeus Centre HEAD, Swedish Institute for Disability
Research, Department of Behavioural Sciences and
Learning, Linköping University, 58183 Linköping, Sweden
Eriksholm Research Centre, Oticon A/S, 20 Rørtangvej,
3070 Snekkersten, Denmark

**Ryuji Yasumatsu, Torahiko Nakashima, RinaMiyazaki,
Yuichi Segawa and Shizuo Komune**
Department of Otorhinolaryngology, Graduate School
of Medical Sciences, Kyushu University, 3-1-1 Maidashi,
Higashi-ku, Fukuoka 812-8582, Japan

**Kohichi Yamauchi, Yasunao Kogashiwa, YorihisaMoro
and Naoyuki Kohno**
Department of Otolaryngology, Head and Neck Surgery,
Kyorin University School of Medicine, 6-20-2 Shinkawa,
Mitaka, Tokyo 181-8611, Japan